Dentoalveolar Surgery

Editor

SOMSAK SITTITAVORNWONG

ORAL AND MAXILLOFACIAL SURGERY CLINICS OF NORTH AMERICA

www.oralmaxsurgery.theclinics.com

Consulting Editor
RUI P. FERNANDES

November 2020 • Volume 32 • Number 4

ELSEVIER

1600 John F. Kennedy Boulevard • Suite 1800 • Philadelphia, Pennsylvania, 19103-2899

http://www.oralmaxsurgery.theclinics.com

ORAL AND MAXILLOFACIAL SURGERY CLINICS OF NORTH AMERICA Volume 32, Number 4
November 2020 ISSN 1042-3699, ISBN-13: 978-0-323-75529-0

Editor: John Vassallo; j.vassallo@elsevier.com
Developmental Editor: Laura Fisher

Oral and Maxillofacial Surgery Clinics of North America (ISSN 1042-3699) is published quarterly by Elsevier Inc., 360 Park Avenue South, New York, NY 10010-1710. Months of issue are February, May, August, and November. Business and Editorial Offices: 1600 John F. Kennedy Blvd., Suite 1800, Philadelphia, PA 19103-2899. Periodicals postage paid at New York, NY and additional mailing offices. Subscription prices are $401.00 per year for US individuals, $756.00 per year for US institutions, $100.00 per year for US students/residents, $474.00 per year for Canadian individuals, $906.00 per year for Canadian institutions, $100.00 per year for Canadian students/residents, $525.00 per year for international individuals, $906.00 per year for international institutions and $235.00 per year for international students/residents. To receive student/resident rate, orders must be accompanied by name or affiliated institution, date of term, and the *signature* of program/residency coordinator on institution letterhead. Orders will be billed at individual rate until proof of status is received. Foreign air speed delivery is included in all *Clinics* subscription prices. All prices are subject to change without notice. **POSTMASTER:** Send address changes to *Oral and Maxillofacial Surgery Clinics of North America,* Elsevier Periodicals **Customer Service, 11830 Westline Industrial Drive, St. Louis, MO 63146. Tel: 1-800-654-2452 (U.S. and Canada); 314-447-8871 (outside U.S. and Canada). Fax: 314-447-8029. E-mail: journalscustomerservice-usa@elsevier.com (for print support); journalsonlinesupport-usa@elsevier. com (for online support)**.

Reprints. For copies of 100 or more, of articles in this publication, please contact the Commercial Reprints Department, Elsevier Inc., 360 Park Avenue South, New York, NY 10010-1710. Tel.: 212-633-3874; Fax: 212-633-3820; Email: reprints@elsevier.com.

Oral and Maxillofacial Surgery Clinics of North America is covered in *MEDLINE/PubMed (Index Medicus)*, *Science Citation Index Expanded (SciSearch®)*, *Journal Citation Reports/Science Edition*, and *Current Contents®/Clinical Medicine.*

Contributors

CONSULTING EDITOR

RUI P. FERNANDES, MD, DMD, FACS, FRCS(Ed)
Clinical Professor and Chief, Division of Head and Neck Surgery, Program Director, Head and Neck Oncologic Surgery and Microvascular Reconstruction Fellowship, Departments of Oral and Maxillofacial Surgery, Neurosurgery, and Orthopaedic Surgery and Rehabilitation, University of Florida Health Science Center, University of Florida College of Medicine, Jacksonville, Florida, USA

EDITOR

SOMSAK SITTITAVORNWONG, DDS, DMD, MS
Professor, Department of Oral and Maxillofacial Surgery, The University of Alabama at Birmingham, Birmingham Alabama, USA

AUTHORS

DAVID R. ADAMS, DDS
Associate Professor, Clinic Chief, Oral and Maxillofacial Surgery, University of Utah School of Dentistry, Salt Lake City, Utah, USA

PAMELA L. ALBERTO, DMD
Clinical Associate Professor, Department of Oral and Maxillofacial Surgery, Rutgers School of Dental Medicine, Newark, New Jersey, USA

PAUL AMAILUK, BDS, MBBS (Hons), FRACDS (OMS)
Department of Oral and Maxillofacial Surgery, Gold Coast University Hospital, Queensland, Australia

DO-YEON CHO, MD
Department of Otolaryngology–Head and Neck Surgery, Gregory Fleming James Cystic Fibrosis Research Center, The University of Alabama at Birmingham, Division of Otolaryngology, Department of Surgery, Veteran Affairs Medical Center, Birmingham, Alabama, USA

GEORGE R. DEEB, DDS, MD
Professor, Department of Oral and Maxillofacial Surgery, School of Dentistry, Virginia Commonwealth University, Richmond, Virginia, USA

JANINA GOLOB DEEB, DMD, MS
Associate Professor, Department of Periodontics, School of Dentistry, Virginia Commonwealth University, Richmond, Virginia, USA

JESSICA W. GRAYSON, MD
Department of Otolaryngology–Head and Neck Surgery, The University of Alabama at Birmingham, Birmingham, Alabama, USA

LESLIE R. HALPERN, DDS, MD, PHD, FACS, FICD
Professor, Section Head, Oral and Maxillofacial Surgery, University of Utah School of Dentistry, Salt Lake City, Utah, USA

HISHAM HATOUM, DMD, MD
Assistant Professor, Division of Oral and Maxillofacial Surgery, Department of Surgery, University of Miami, Miami, Florida, USA

MELANIE D. HICKS, MD
Department of Otolaryngology–Head and Neck Surgery, The University of Alabama at Birmingham, Birmingham, Alabama, USA

LEWIS C. JONES, DMD, MD
Private Practice, Oral and Maxillofacial Surgery, Elizabethtown, Clinical Assistant Professor, Oral and Maxillofacial Surgery, University of Louisville, Louisville, Kentucky, USA

ARSHAD KALEEM, DMD, MD
Assistant Professor, Division of Oral and Maxillofacial Surgery, Department of Surgery, University of Miami, Miami, Florida, USA

DEEPAK KRISHNAN, DDS, FACS
Chief, Oral and Maxillofacial Surgery, University of Cincinnati Medical Center, Cincinnati, Ohio, USA

STUART E. LIEBLICH, DMD
Clinical Professor, Oral and Maxillofacial Surgery, University of Connecticut Health Center, Private Practice, Avon Oral, Facial and Dental Implant Surgery, Avon, Connecticut, USA

PATRICK J. LOUIS, DDS, MD
Professor, Interim Chair, Department of Oral and Maxillofacial Surgery, The University of Alabama at Birmingham, Birmingham, Alabama, USA

JUSTIN P. McCORMICK, MD
Department of Otolaryngology–Head and Neck Surgery, The University of Alabama at Birmingham, Birmingham, Alabama, USA

WILLIAM STUART McKENZIE, DMD, MD
Private Practice, Mid-State Oral Surgery and Implant Center, Nashville, Tennessee, USA

WALLACE S. McLAURIN, DMD
Instructor of Clinical Surgery, Oral and Maxillofacial Surgery, University of Cincinnati Medical Center, Cincinnati, Ohio, USA

CHRISTOPHER C. NIQUETTE Jr. DDS
Implant and Reconstructive Surgery Fellow, Brunswick Oral and Maxillofacial Surgery, Private Practice, Third Coast Oral and Maxillofacial Surgery, Grand Rapids, Michigan, USA

DANIEL B. SPAGNOLI, DDS, MS, PhD
Private Practice, Brunswick Oral and Maxillofacial Surgery, Supply, North Carolina, USA

KYLE STEIN, DDS, FACS
Clinical Associate Professor, Department of Oral and Maxillofacial Surgery, The University of Iowa, College of Dentistry, Iowa City, Iowa, USA

WILLIAM SYNAN, DDS
Clinical Professor, Department of Oral and Maxillofacial Surgery, The University of Iowa, College of Dentistry, Iowa City, Iowa, USA

RAMZEY TURSUN, DDS, FACS
Associate Professor, Director of Oral, Head and Neck Oncology, Microvascular Reconstructive Fellowship, Division of Oral and Maxillofacial Surgery, Department of Surgery, University of Miami, Miami, Florida, USA

BRADFORD A. WOODWORTH, MD
Department of Otolaryngology–Head and Neck Surgery, Gregory Fleming James Cystic Fibrosis Research Center, The University of Alabama at Birmingham, Birmingham, Alabama, USA

Contents

Dentoalveolar surgery comprises more than 50% of the practice of oral and maxillo-facial surgeons worldwide and is the most commonly performed category of surgical procedure. Optimal strategies for management of many medical problems, however, remain unclear. Remaining current on medical and surgical perioperative strategies is a standard for best practice. This article provides contemporary approaches for the perioperative management of patients presenting for dentoalveolar surgery. Attention will be directed to the perioperative management of cardiovascular disease, diabetes, and obesity. These diseases are chosen owing to controversies with respect to good scientific evidence that supports a standard of perioperative care.

Exodontia services comprise the largest portion of clinical practice for most oral and maxillofacial surgeons in the United States. This article is an overview of the princi-ples of exodontia including the physics principles underlying the appropriate use of dental elevators and forceps. Failure to understand the instrumentation and the physics principles being used can cause prolonged operative time, iatrogenic injury to the patient, and unnecessary fatigue and/or injury to the provider. Advances in materials, technology, and innovative design have produced interesting new instru-ments for exodontia. New instruments including periotomes, piezosurgery, physics forceps, and vertical extraction systems are introduced and reviewed.

Impacted third molars occur in a significant number of patients and often require treatment because of presence of symptoms and/or disease. Management of these teeth typically involves referral to oral and maxillofacial surgeons for diagnosis, treat-ment planning, and ultimate removal if indicated. Proper diagnosis and treatment planning helps optimize surgical results at each stage of the procedure, and ulti-mately patient outcomes. Adherence to proper surgical techniques helps minimize risks and complications associated with the procedure. Multiple alternative surgical techniques also exist for uncommon, but potentially complicated, situations that arise with some impacted third molars.

Impacted incisors, canines, premolars, and second molar are problems encoun-tered frequently by general dentists, orthodontists, and oral and maxillofacial surgeons. The etiology of impacted teeth is multifactorial. Traditional radiographs can be used for location of the impacted tooth but 3-D CBCT is superior in evaluating the tooth's position. Successful management requires an interdisciplinary approach with an orthodontist responsible for the overall success of the treatment plan. Surgical exposure of these impacted teeth is accomplished using an open or closed surgical procedure. Choosing the appropriate surgical procedure and orthodontic treatment plan will result in a stable, predictable, and aesthetic result.

Although conventional endodontic procedures are very successful, failure of the initial treatment can occur. Consideration for surgical treatment versus endodontic retreatment needs to be part of the decision along with thoughts of extraction with implant replacement. Apical surgery can preserve many teeth that remain symptomatic after conventional endodontic treatment especially because endodontic failure can occur after 1 year, usually after a definitive restoration is placed. This article reviews current indications for periapical surgery and discusses factors that can predict successful outcomes.

Preprosthetic surgery remains a work horse of dentoalveolar surgery. Advances in rehabilitation of the edentulous mouth with the use of endosseous osseointegrating dental implants and dermal matrix substitutes have changed the narrative of traditional preprosthetic surgery while maintaining some fundamental principles. An outline of the basic techniques in preprosthetic dentoalveolar surgery is discussed in the setting of these technological and tissue engineering advances.

Extensive reviews have concluded that grafting of the socket reduces bone loss regardless of product or method. However, nothing has been shown to reliably and completely maintain alveolar dimensions. We advocate a biologically driven and anatomically based approach for reconstruction of the socket. There are various socket manipulations that we have found to predictably prepare a site for dental implant. The combination of graft construct design and socket management maximizes graft success for any practitioner. Each socket should be treated individually, and products or methods used that are coincident with the complexity of the defect in question.

The presence of healthy soft tissue at the tooth and implant interface correlates to long-term success and stability in function and esthetics. Grafting procedures utilizing various techniques can be performed during any stage of the implant or restorative therapy. Materials of autogenous, allogeneic, and xenogeneic sources are available for oral soft tissue grafting. This article describes the classifications of soft tissue defects, treatment modalities, and materials used to enhance soft tissue quality and quantity and to achieve optimal esthetics and function around teeth and implants.

Dental Trauma

Lewis C. Jones

Dental trauma and injuries to the dentition are difficult to treat because the treatment goals serve to restore esthetics and function. The oral and maxillofacial surgeon is often called on to coordinate the efforts of rehabilitation after a dentoalveolar injury. A comprehensive understanding of the ideal treatments and use of endodontic, orthodontic, periodontal, and pediatric dental colleagues leads to the best possible results with regards to a restoration of form and function. This article provides a succinct review of the oral and maxillofacial surgeon's treatment in dentoalveolar trauma. Epidemiology, treatment, and preventative measures are discussed in this article.

Endoscopic Management of Maxillary Sinus Diseases of Dentoalveolar Origin

Justin P. McCormick, Melanie D. Hicks, Jessica W. Grayson, Bradford A. Woodworth, and Do-Yeon Cho

Endoscopic surgery on the maxillary sinus has experienced significant advances in technique and approaches since the maxillary antrostomy was introduced in the 1980s. Disease processes that previously required open surgical approaches to the maxillary sinus can now be treated endoscopically while preserving form and function of the sinus and without injuring the maxillary sinus mucosa or disrupting normal mucociliary clearance. Understanding the techniques described in this article will allow surgeons to appropriately plan treatment strategies for patients with a variety of maxillary sinus diseases from dentoalveolar origin.

Complications of Dentoalveolar Surgery

Patrick J. Louis

This article explores how to prevent and manage complications of dentoalveolar surgery. Many complications are avoidable. Surgical skills and knowledge of anatomy play an important role in prevention of complications. Prevention starts with detailed history and physical examination of the patient. Key to perioperative management of patients is risk assessment. Without a proper history and physical examination, the clinician is unable to assess the risk of performing surgery and anesthesia for each patient. Some illnesses and medications increase the risk of complications. The following complications are discussed: alveolar osteitis, displacement, fracture, hemorrhage, infection, nonhealing wound, oroantral communication, swelling, and trismus.

The Trigeminal Nerve Injury

Arshad Kaleem, Paul Amailuk, Hisham Hatoum, and Ramzey Tursun

Trigeminal nerve branches are never far from the operating field of the oral and maxillofacial surgeon. Increasingly the surgeon is required to provide accurate diagnosis and grading of trigeminal nerve injury, and surgical management by oral and maxillofacial surgeons will become common. Although trauma and ablative procedures for head and neck pathology can cause injuries, dentoalveolar surgical procedures remain an important cause of injury to the fifth cranial nerve, with the third division being the main branch affected. Oral and maxillofacial surgeons should be aware of strategies of avoiding iatrogenic injury, and know when referral and surgical management are appropriate.

ORAL AND MAXILLOFACIAL SURGERY CLINICS OF NORTH AMERICA

FORTHCOMING ISSUES

February 2021
Modern Rhinoplasty and the Management of its Complications
Shahrokh C. Bagheri, Husain Ali Khan, and Behnam Bohluli, *Editors*

May 2021
Advanced Intraoral Surgery
Orrett E. Ogle, *Editor*

August 2021
Management of Soft Tissue Trauma
Donita Dyalram, *Editor*

RECENT ISSUES

August 2020
Global Oral and Maxillofacial Surgery
Shahid R. Aziz, Jose M. Marchena, and Steven M. Roser, *Editors*

May 2020
Orthodontics for the Craniofacial Surgery Patient
Michael R. Markiewicz, Veerasathpurush Allareddy, and Michael Miloro, *Editors*

February 2020
Orthodontics for the Oral and Maxillofacial Surgery Patient
Michael R. Markiewicz, Veerasathpurush Allareddy, and Michael Miloro, *Editors*

SERIES OF RELATED INTEREST

Atlas of the Oral and Maxillofacial Surgery Clinics
www.oralmaxsurgeryatlas.theclinics.com

Dental Clinics
www.dental.theclinics.com

THE CLINICS ARE NOW AVAILABLE ONLINE!
Access your subscription at:
www.theclinics.com

Preface
Dentoalveolar Surgery

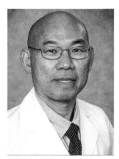

Somsak Sittitavornwong, DDS, DMD, MS
Editor

Clearly, the area of dentoalveolar surgery is undeniably the responsibility of oral and maxillofacial surgeons and dentists. Dentoalveolar surgery is one of the most common operations of the specialty of Oral and Maxillofacial Surgery. Like many other oral and maxillofacial procedures, dentoalveolar surgeries have undergone a perceptible change. The principles of any surgeries are always the same; however, the updated knowledge and techniques of dentoalveolar procedures have evolved and affected clinicians in achieving their goal. The purpose of this issue is to outline the updated principles and concepts of dentoalveolar surgery in recent years.

To address the goal of this issue of *Oral and Maxillofacial Surgery Clinics of North America*, each contributor was selected from experts who were consulted to compose articles in their skillful fields. I thoroughly discussed with each author and attempted to focus on the details of each article. In summary, dentoalveolar care and attention to its principles should be made expediently to as many fellow clinicians as possible which is the goal of this issue.

I tremendously appreciate the contributions of each one of our authors, including Dr Rui Fernandes, who is the Consulting Editor of *Oral and Maxillofacial Surgery Clinics of North America*, for asking me to edit this issue. I also would like to acknowledge the publishing staff of Elsevier for facilitating this task. Last, I must thank my wife, Suneerat, for encouraging me to accomplish this prestigious project.

Somsak Sittitavornwong, DDS, DMD, MS
Department of Oral and Maxillofacial Surgery
University of Alabama at Birmingham
419 School of Dentistry Building
1919 7th Avenue South
Birmingham, AL 35294-0007, USA

E-mail address:
sjade@uab.edu

Oral Maxillofacial Surg Clin N Am 32 (2020) ix
https://doi.org/10.1016/j.coms.2020.07.012

The Dentoalveolar Surgical Patient
Perioperative Principles Based on Contemporary Controversies

Leslie R. Halpern, DDS, MD, PHD, FICD*, David R. Adams, DDS

KEYWORDS

- Perioperative management • Preoperative lab testing • Cardiovascular disease • Diabetes
- Obesity • Controversies in dentoalveolar patient surgical workup

KEY POINTS

- As the population ages, dentoalveolar surgical outcomes become more and more reliant on perioperative medical management skills.
- New guidelines exist regarding patients presenting with hypertension in the perioperative period.
- Although there is no consensus statement in oral health, the treatment of patients on anticoagulant and/or antiplatelet therapy require an awareness of evidence-based standards that have been applied in other specialties.
- The perioperative management of diabetes and obesity in surgical patients is complex and controversial owing to a paucity of high-level evidence and expert opinion.
- The perioperative management of cardiovascular disease, diabetes, and obesity continues to be based on high level evidence trials to support a standard of care.

INTRODUCTION

Dentoalveolar surgery comprises more than 50% of the practice of oral and maxillofacial surgeons (OMFS) worldwide.[1] Procedures most commonly performed range from simple tooth extractions, implants with or without bony augmentation, preprosthetic surgical removal of tori and exostoses, exposure of impacted teeth for orthodontic treatment, and extraction of impacted third molars. More of the Baby Boomer generation are seeing the OMFS for dentoalveolar surgical intervention. Although many people aged 65 or older remain healthy and visit medical/dental providers either infrequently or for health maintenance care, their cohorts experience increased rates of age-related physiologic changes in the oral cavity, changes owing to the comorbidities of chronic illnesses and changes resulting from medications used to manage diseases.

The optimal strategies for management of many medical problems remain unclear owing to a paucity of high-level evidence and as such, the perioperative management of surgical patients remain in a dynamic state.[2,3] A quote of the late poet Emily Dickinson put it best when she said, "If you take care of the small things, the big things take care of themselves." An appropriate preoperative patient assessment is a critical component of surgical success.[2,3]

Remaining current on medical and surgical perioperative strategies form a continuum for best practice. This article provides contemporary approaches for the perioperative management of patients presenting for dentoalveolar surgery in the OMFS practice. Attention will be directed to the

Oral and Maxillofacial Surgery, University of Utah School of Dentistry, 530 South Wakara Way, Salt Lake City, UT 84108, USA
* Corresponding author.
E-mail address: Leslie.halpern@hsc.utah.edu

Oral Maxillofacial Surg Clin N Am 32 (2020) 495–510
https://doi.org/10.1016/j.coms.2020.07.004

perioperative management of cardiovascular disease, diabetes mellitus, and obesity. These systemic conditions are chosen owing to controversies in the perioperative management strategies with respect to good scientific evidence that supports a standard of care.

PREOPERATIVE SURGICAL EVALUATION

Preoperative evaluation by the OMFS is either performed the day of surgery or several days before. Each surgical patient presents with her or his own unique set of risk factors and comorbidities, and as such, there is no "standard" approach that fits all patients of all ages.[2–5] A thorough history and physical examination is always required with pertinent findings applicable to the diagnosis, as well as comorbidities that may affect surgical risk. Risk stratification that assesses the fitness of a patient is standard in practice and well characterized by the American Society of Anesthesiologists (ASA; **Box 1**). Preoperative assessment also includes a determination of how well a patient withstands the stress of surgery (as discussed elsewhere in this article; **Box 2**) and heals without any compromise.

Preoperative laboratory testing can assess risk for perioperative adverse events. Unnecessary testing, however, can lead to possible harm and undue costs.[6,7] Evidence-based meta-analyses and systematic reviews have demonstrated a lack of reliable evidence and, as such, the latest guidelines come largely from expert opinion.[6–9] In 2016 the National Guideline Center/National institute for Health and Care Excellence updated a set of guidelines based on ASA classification for routine preoperative laboratory tests in patients undergoing elective surgery.[7,9] A complete blood count is recommended in all patients undergoing high-risk procedures and in ASA class III and IV patients with cardiovascular or renal disease/symptoms. Renal function testing is recommended for ASA class III and IV patients, as well as ASA class II patients with risk for acute kidney injury. Routine coagulation with an international normalized ratio (INR) or platelet count testing should be left to the patient's cardiologist/primary care provider's discretion. Coagulation testing is recommended for ASA class III and IV patients undergoing intermediate- or high-risk procedures who also have a history of anticoagulant use and/or liver disease.[6–8] The guidelines for pregnancy testing includes qualitative beta-HCG for women of reproductive age (for further information, the reader is referred to the references). During the perioperative and postoperative period issues of malnutrition increases the risk of

---

Box 1
ASA patient classification

ASA Class 1: Normal Healthy Patient

No organic, psychiatric, or physiologic disturbance; healthy with good exercise tolerance

ASA Class 2: Mild Systemic Disease

No functional limitations; has well-controlled disease of 1 body system; that is, hypertension

And no systemic manifestations; cigarette smoking, pregnancy, mild obesity

ASA Class 3: Severe Systemic Disease

Some functional limitations with controlled disease of 1 or more body organ system or 1 major system with no immediate danger of death; that is, congestive heart failure, stable angina, hypertension that is poorly controlled, morbidly obese and chronic renal failure

ASA Class 4: Severe Systemic Disease as a Constant Threat to Life

Has at least 1 severe disease that is poorly controlled or end-stage disease with a risk of death; that is, unstable angina, symptomatic congestive heart failure, chronic obstructive lung disease, hepatic or renal disease

ASA Class 5: Moribund; not expected to live/survive without an operation

Not expected to survive more than 24 hours without surgery; imminent risk of death; multiorgan failure, sepsis with hemodynamic instability, coagulopathy that is poorly controlled

ASA Class 6: Declared Brain Dead; Possible Organ Donor

"E": If an E is added to a previously defined ASA that signifies the need for a surgical procedure to be performed emergently

Reprinted with permission of the American Society of Anesthesiologists, 1061 American Lane, Schaumburg, Illinois 60173-4973.

---

complications and wound healing in the elderly, patients with cancer, and those with immunocompromised disease states. A postoperative catabolic state and subsequent compromise in wound healing will exacerbate underlying systemic diseases. Preoperative laboratory tests for albumin and transferrin can serve as risk predictors for nutritional homeostasis during the perioperative period.[2]

The prospect of surgery provides the OMFS an opportunity to discuss smoking cessation. The

Box 2
Surgical classification system

Category 1

Minimal risk to patients independent of anesthesia; minimally invasive procedure with little or no blood loss and the operation is done in the office.

Category 2

Minimal to moderately invasive procedures; blood loss of less than 500 mL; mild risk to patients independent of anesthesia.

Category 3:

Moderately to significantly invasive procedure; blood loss of 500 to 1000 mL with a moderate risk to patients independent of anesthesia.

Category 4:

Highly invasive procedure with blood loss of greater than 1500 mL with major risk to patients independent of anesthesia.

From Fattahi T. Perioperative laboratory and diagnostic testing—what is needed and when? Oral Maxillofacial Surg Clin North Am. 2006;18(1):3; with permission.

issue of smoking and more recently vaping cessation have been under scrutiny in the surgical arena. Tobacco-related disease is the leading cause of preventable death and contributes to $200 billion annually in medical expenses and lost health productivity.[2,5] The evidence of a timeline for benefits of smoking cessation can be from 4 to 8 weeks before surgery and evidence supports a decrease in lung hyperactivity, mucociliary clearance, and improved wound healing during this time period.[5,10] Other interventions of smoking cessation well tolerated by patients can include first-line medications (varencline, bupropion, and nicotine replacement therapy) unless medically contraindicated.[11] The Affordable Care Act and 2010 Patient Protection Act has expanded the coverage for evidence-based smoking cessation.[2,5,10,11]

Perioperative management skills are significant in patients who abuse alcohol, cocaine, and other opioids before the perioperative period. According to the 2016 National Survey of Drug Use and Health, 1.8 million people had prescription pain medication use disorder, and 626,000 had a heroin use disorder.[12] In the midst of an epidemic of opioid abuse and overdose-related morbidity and mortality, the use of opioids remains the most common means of providing analgesia in the perioperative period.[12] A thorough history of abuse withdrawal and toxicity

screening can lead to cancellation of the procedure even if the drug use did not occur in the acute phase. The preoperative evaluation should identify those with opioid abuse potential to determine whether a further workup is necessary. Screening for high-risk comorbid conditions can help to guide perioperative pain management. Under special circumstances, where emergent surgical intervention is needed, the surgeon will determine whether risk assessment warrants further evaluation; that is, a preoperative urine toxicology screening for methadone, buprenorphine, and fentanyl may be done.[12] Online databases for drug monitoring should also be reviewed for abuse of controlled substance prescribing.[12] (see[8] for further interest and protocols).

Current controversies in the perioperative management of cardiovascular disease, diabetes, and obesity in the dentoalveolar patient are discussed elsewhere in this article.

PERIOPERATIVE MANAGEMENT STRATEGIES
Cardiovascular Disease

The oral and maxillofacial surgeon treats a significant number of patients with a history of cardiovascular disease in everyday practice. Cardiac issues remain a significant risk predictor of perioperative morbidity and mortality, and as such may require advanced monitoring throughout the surgical period. The perioperative management focuses on issues of coronary artery disease (CAD), hypertension, congestive heart failure, disturbances of heart rhythm (arrhythmias), and valvular heart disease. In patients with existing or potentially significant cardiovascular problems a physical examination would include an electrocardiogram, blood pressure monitoring in both arms, and auscultation for bruits, thrills, murmurs, and jugular venous distention. Further physical examination requires abdominal percussion and palpation for hepatosplenomegaly and ascites, followed by a peripheral examination of extremities for evidence of pedal edema and clubbing of the fingers. The Goldman Cardiac Risk Index has been the gold standard to assess cardiovascular risk in the noncardiac surgical patient.[13] The index is based on a series of points that, when tallied, can go from 0 signifying a 1.0% cardiac risk to more than 26 points, coinciding with a 63% risk for cardiac death. Additional cardiac risk is stratified according to the American College of Cardiology/American Heart Association 2007 guidelines on perioperative cardiovascular evaluation for noncardiac surgery (**Box 3**).[14] The Revised Cardiac Risk Index issued to estimates a patient's risk of perioperative cardiac complications by looking for an association between preoperative

Box 3
Revised Cardiac Risk Index

1. History of ischemic heart disease
2. History of congestive heart failure
3. History of cerebrovascular disease (stroke or transient ischemic attack)
4. History of diabetes requiring preoperative insulin use
5. Chronic kidney disease (creatinine >2 mg/dL [176.8 μmol/L])
6. Undergoing suprainguinal vascular, intraperitoneal, or intrathoracic surgery

Risk for cardiac death, nonfatal myocardial infarction, and nonfatal cardiac arrest:
0 predictors = 0.4%, 1 predictor = 0.9%, 2 predictors = 6.6%, ≥3 predictors = >11%

Risk Factor	Points
History of ischemic heart disease	1
History of congestive heart failure	1
History of cerebrovascular disease (stroke or transient ischemic attack)	1
History of diabetes requiring preoperative insulin use	1
Chronic kidney disease [creatinine >2 mg/dL (176.8 μmol/L)]	1
Undergoing suprainguinal vascular, intraperitoneal, or intrathoracic surgery	1

Total points:

Risk of Major Cardiac Event

Total Points	Risk (%)
0	0.4%
1	0.9%
2	6.6%
≥3	>11%

Data from Fleisher LA, Backman HA, Brown KA, et al. ACC/AHA 2007 guidelines on perioperative cardiovascular evaluation and care for noncardiac surgery: executive summary. J Amer Coll Cardiol. 2007;50(17):1707–32.

variables (eg, patient's age, type of surgery, co-morbid diagnoses, or laboratory data) and the risk for cardiac complications in a cohort of surgical patients (the derivation cohort).[14] Another risk predictor is based on the assessment of a patient's functional capacity to estimate perioperative risk of cardiovascular complication, and is determined by asking about their physical activity to estimate the metabolic equivalents they can perform without sign of myocardial ischemia.[14,15] One metabolic equivalent is the basal oxygen consumption of a 40-year-old, 70-kg man. The physical activity of a patient is quantified by a number of metabolic equivalents and when determined a patient with a MET score of greater than 4 is considered to have good functional capacity and therefore at low risk for a myocardial ischemic event (**Box 4**). Less than 4 metabolic equivalents require further cardiac risk assessment and may not be a good candidate for ambulatory center surgery.[14,15]

The following cardiovascular disease stressors in the dentoalveolar surgical patient are of consideration to the OMFS,

1. *CAD:* Patients at risk for CAD pose significant challenges for perioperative management during surgery, because 5% of patients with CAD who have noncardiac surgery can develop cardiac complications.[16] Perioperative acute events can vary from myocardial ischemia to myocardial injury to myocardial infarction. Undiagnosed heart failure, stroke, diabetes mellitus or renal insufficiency, male sex, and increasing age can all contribute as risk predictors. The administration of sedation can be challenging owing to anesthetic agents masking signs and symptoms of underlying cardiovascular disease. The diagnosis is only confirmed after preoperative laboratory testing is undertaken to determine surgical stressors (discussed elsewhere in this article). Anesthetic management must be tailored toward preventing, monitoring, and detecting any myocardial ischemia, as well as changes in hemodynamic status. Anesthetic medications should be chosen based on a favorable hemodynamic profile.[14] Hemodynamic goals include maintaining a normal heart rate, normal to high blood pressures, and avoiding fluid overload that can increase myocardial demand and decrease oxygen perfusion. If patients do complain about symptoms, all nonemergency surgical procedures are postponed and the patient is transported to the hospital emergency room for a cardiac workup.[15,16]

Box 4
Functional capacity of daily activities based on metabolic equivalents

Category of MET Activity

1	Getting dressed, eating, bathroom use
2–3	Ability to walk on level ground up to 1–2 blocks at <2 miles per hour
4–7	Ability to walk >2 blocks at a normal pace of >2–4 mph, light housework, cycling
7–10	Competitive sports, running short distances, doing heavy housework

Adapted from Weinstein AS, Sigurdsson MI, Bader AM. Comparison of preoperative assessment of patient's metabolic equivalents (METS) estimated from history versus measured by exercise cardiac stress testing. Anesthesiol Res Pract. 2018;5912726:2.

---

2. Hypertension: Hypertension is commonly seen in at least one-third of noncardiac patients scheduled for elective surgery.[16] The 2017 guidelines for hypertensive patients suggest that 50% of the population may be considered hypertensive and that early treatment can avoid morbidity and possible mortality from CVD.[16–18] The staging has the following category, systolic and diastolic numbers: <120/<80; normal; 120 to 129/<80; prehypertensive; 130 to 139/80 to 89; Stage 1 and >or = 140/> or = 90, Stage 2. The stage II hypertensive patient with a diastolic BP <110, for instance, may qualify as a candidate for elective surgery if he/she has no other comorbid conditions. Perioperatively, severe hypertension; that is, >210/110 mm, however, can have a severe hypotensive response under anesthesia and as such, office surgery should be deferred pending further medical work up. A BP of > 180/110 mm with other comorbidities should also be evaluated to prevent adverse cardiac events.[19,20] Preoperative administration of anti-hypertensive medication can be continued during the perioperative period, however, Renin-Angiotensin (ACE) inhibitors can cause intraoperative hypotension and may be held before surgery based upon the patient's need.[19–21] There is, however, controversy and evidence-based data is still under scrutiny for the perioperative use of ACE inhibitors.[19–21] Patients on Beta-blockers are advised to continue them perioperatively to avoid withdrawal

symptoms.[16,17,20] The relative risks and benefits of antihypertensive use during surgery can be decided on a case to case basis with a reasonable goal to maintain a patient's blood pressure within 20% of their respective baseline.[16,17,19,20]

3. *Heart failure:* Heart failure is a syndrome of impaired cardiac function often associated with either systolic failure or diastolic failure based on diminished ejection fractions during cardiac output. This condition can result in perioperative adverse events in up to 10% of patients during the perioperative period of noncardiac surgery.[16] Heart failure can be right sided or left sided. Left-sided symptoms include orthopnea, pedal edema, tachypnea, and crackles on auscultation of lung fields. Right sided heart failure symptomatology includes pedal edema, nausea, vomiting, and hepatic congestion. Left-sided heart failure is often the most common cause of right-sided heart failure.[16] Perioperative management begins with a thorough workup that consists of an electrocardiogram, chest radiograph, and biomarker analysis using brain natriuretic peptide, which has a high specificity for ruling in heart failure.[16] Additional testing include electrolytes, renal and liver function tests, and an echocardiogram to determine new or chronic wall motion irregularities of the heart.[21,22] Pharmacologic therapy can include angiotensin-converting enzyme inhibitor and beta blocker therapy as per American College of Cardiology/American Heart Association guidelines (see[21,22] for further interest).

4. *Symptomatic arrhythmias:* Many of the patients who present to the OMFS practice are being treated with anticoagulant or antiplatelet therapy as a result of arrhythmias associated with atrial fibrillation; that is, the lack of coordinated electrical contraction of the atria. The OMFS must monitor the patient during surgical intervention because a multitude of factors can precipitate atrial fibrillation; that is, fluid shifts, electrolyte imbalances, and catecholamine release either by the stress of surgery or administration of local anesthetics.[23] Perioperatively, these hemodynamic consequences of atrial fibrillation are of particular concern with respect to decrease in cardiac output, ventricular filling, and the formation of clots in the left atrium that predisposes the risk of a stroke.

Treatments for cardiovascular diseases such as heart valve replacement, atrial fibrillation, and venous thromboembolism have become more common and millions of patients receive anticoagulant and antiplatelet therapies to decrease thrombosis and life-threatening sequela; that is, ischemic events in the heart, lungs, and brain.[18,24,25] The medical and dental communities have sought to craft a wide variety of strategies during the perioperative period to modify anticoagulant and antiplatelet therapy and prevent an acquired bleeding dyscrasia during and after dental surgery (discussed elsewhere in this article). Other common antiarrhythmic drugs administered during the perioperative period are calcium channel blockers, beta-blockers, and digoxin (for further treatment of atrial fibrillation arrhythmias, the reader is referred to[23]).

a. *Perioperative management of acquired bleeding dyscrasias:* Perioperative medical therapy can address a significant number of patients who receive either oral anticoagulants or antiplatelet therapies as the most effective prophylactic medications to reduce thrombotic sequelae. These therapies, however, can predispose them to acquired bleeding disorders that can be life threatening. The general algorithm for managing patients on either direct or indirect anticoagulants or antiplatelet medications is to first characterize the potential for severity of bleeding based on the procedure that is planned and whether or not it will pose a significant risk. Routine dental procedures such as localized periodontal scaling or single tooth extraction may be considered low risk and as such do not require a change in anticoagulating doses. As the complexity of the procedure increases and surgical time increases, so does the potential for hemorrhage. For elective surgery, one might consider staging procedures to decrease risk for a hemorrhagic event (ie, limiting the number of extractions per visit, conservative flap design, etc).

   i. *Anticoagulants:* Several studies have suggested that often anticoagulation can continue without interruption. High-risk procedures, however, lack a consensus statement with respect to continuation of therapy. Van Diermen and colleagues[26] recommend discussion with the patient's physician if the INR is greater than 3.5 and complicated oral surgery is planned. Other studies did not confirm the association of increased risk of bleeding and a high INR.[26] Bajkin and colleagues[27] studied 54 patients with INR values between 3.5 and 4.2 who had up to 3 teeth extracted and recorded postoperative bleeding at 3.7% (2/54).

Scully and Wolff[28] found that uncomplicated extraction of 3 teeth was safe if the INR is less than 3.5, whereas Chugani[29] suggested that periodontal flaps, implant placement, and apicoectomy were not recommended in patients with INR ranges of 3.0 to 4.0. Several studies mentioned that, along with INR values and surgical trauma, an important risk predictor that is associated with a greater chance of significant bleeding is inflammation of the dental tissue environment.[29,30] Ward and Smith[18] reviewed the literature in comparison with current practice by OMFS who perform dentoalveolar procedures for the anticoagulated patient. They concluded that for moderate- to high-risk procedures warfarin discontinuation is recommended to minimal therapeutic levels as determined by the INR (as discussed elsewhere in this article).[18,25] Future prospective trials are required, however, for stronger management guidelines in this population of patients.

Newer oral anticoagulants have been developed as alternatives to warfarin. Among these are Xa inhibitors, rivaroxaban (Xarelto) and apixaban (Eliquis), as well as dabigatran (Pradaxa), a direct thrombin inhibitor. Because there are no specific tests to monitor the effects of these medications, good patient compliance is essential. For patients taking these medications, there are increased risks of life-threatening bleeding in severe trauma or nonelective major surgery because there are currently no antidotes available except for dabigatran (Praxbind: Idarucizvmab). The decision to preoperatively discontinue these medications should be based the risks of bleeding associated with the proposed procedure and in consultation with the patient's physician. In simple surgical procedures such as a single tooth extraction using local hemostatic measures, there is usually no need to discontinue these newer mediations preoperatively. In general, the risk of thromboembolism increases transiently as anticoagulants are discontinued, so careful planning of elective procedures will benefit the patient. In more complex procedures such as multiple dental extractions or more major maxillofacial surgery, anticoagulant or antiplatelet medications may need to be stopped for several days in coordination with the patient's physician.

  ii. *Antiplatelet drugs:* Surgeons are faced with the same dilemma of whether or not to discontinue antiplatelet therapy during perioperative dental and oral and maxillofacial surgical intervention because this period is associated with an increased risk of a thrombotic and/or hemorrhagic event. The latter is predicated on the timing of pharmacologic therapy; that is, when the angioplasty or stenting took place. Rebound platelet activity has the potential for a severe thrombotic event.[31,32] Patients who are on combination medicine regimens require special consideration. The most common combinations consist of anti-platelet agents and nonsteroidal anti-inflammatory drugs, as well as herbal supplements such as garlic, ginseng, fish oil, and Ginkgo. Aspirin and nonsteroidal anti-inflammatory drugs may be discontinued at the discretion of the practitioner. For most outpatient procedures, the continuation of the antiplatelet therapy outweighs risk of discontinuation. It is prudent, however, to consult with the patient's cardiologist and cardiac surgeon, because their expertise is as rigorous as ours with respect to Level A evidence (see **Table 1** for full list of anticoagulants and antiplatelet medications, as well as references for further interest).

5. *Valvular heart disease:* Surgery and anesthesia can pose significant perioperative challenges in the patient presenting with a history of valvular heart disease, aortic stenosis, aortic regurgitation, mitral valve stenosis, and mitral valve regurgitation. The OMFS should have a good understanding of the type and severity of valve heart disease because it can precipitate or exacerbate perioperative complications. Aortic stenosis is the most common form and major predictor of morbidity in patients undergoing noncardiac surgery.[16,33] There is an incidence of 3% to 8% seen in the population ages greater than 70 years and can be an incidental finding on physical examination. Calcification of the vertebral arteries can contribute to decreased cardiac reserve and its response to stressors during surgery. The latter can lead to ischemia, left ventricular failure, and cardiac arrest.[16,33] Perioperative management of valvular disease usually begins with a workup by the cardiologist consisting of a transesophageal echocardiogram, which is required if symptomatology is unknown or recurring. Invasive hemodynamic monitoring may be recommended to avoid hypovolemia, tachycardia and hypotension. Systemic vascular resistance should be maintained for physiologic coronary artery perfusion. Pharmacologic therapy may include phenylephrine and norepinephrine as per recommendations by a cardiologist. This is mostly applicable for the inpatient setting. (For further interest the reader is referred to references[16,33] in this article.)

  a. *Antibiotic prophylaxis in valvular heart disease:* The most recent literature from the American Dental Association and the American Heart Association concludes that: "there are currently relatively few patient subpopulations for whom antibiotic prophylaxis may be indicated before certain dental procedures."[34,35] This recommendation is based on a review of the scientific evidence, which showed that the risk of adverse reactions to antibiotics generally outweigh the benefits of prophylaxis for many patients who would have been considered eligible for prophylaxis in previous versions of the guidelines. Concern about the development of drug-resistant bacteria also was a factor. Infective endocarditis prophylaxis for dental procedures should be recommended only for patients with underlying cardiac conditions associated with the highest risk of adverse outcome from infective endocarditis.[34] For patients with these underlying cardiac conditions, prophylaxis is recommended for all "dental procedures that involve manipulation of gingival tissue or the periapical region of teeth or perforation of the oral mucosa".[34] The procedures and events that do not need prophylaxis are routine anesthetic injections through noninfected tissue, taking dental radiographs, placement of removable prosthodontic or orthodontic appliances, adjustment of orthodontic appliances, placement of orthodontic brackets, shedding of deciduous teeth, and bleeding from trauma to the lips or oral mucosa.

Wilson and colleagues[35] discussed a recommendation for patients who forget to premedicate before their appointments. The recommendation is that, for patients with an indication for antibiotic prophylaxis, the antibiotic be administered before the procedure for the antibiotic to reach adequate blood levels. However, the guidelines to prevent infective endocarditis state, "If the dosage of antibiotic is inadvertently not administered before the

Table 1
Antiplatelet and anticoagulant drugs

Anticoagulants (DOAC)

Generic	Proprietary	Mechanism of Action	Renal Function (Cr/Cl/min)	Discontinue (D/C) or Not (N)
Warfarin Half-life: 20–60 h	Coumadin	Antagonist of vitamin K, and affecting factors II, VII, IX, and X	>80 mL/min: Hold 48 h; 50–80 mL/min: Hold 72 h	D/C based on INR (if >4 no surgery)
Dabigatran Half-life: 12–17 h	Pradaxa	Inhibitor of free thrombin; Thrombin bound to fibrin; inhibits activity of IIa (INR not required)	≥80 mL/min	N based on number of teeth to be removed (>2 discuss with physician)
Rivaroxaban Half-life: 9–13 h	Xarelto	Selective Factor Xa inhibitors (INR not required)	≥50 mL/min	N based on the number of teeth; that is, >2–3
Apixaban Half-life: 9–14 h	Eliquis	Selective factor Xa inhibitors (INR not required)	≥50 mL/min	N based on the number of teeth; that is, >2–3
Heparin (LMWH) Enoxaparin Half-life: 4.5 h Dalteparin Half-life: 2.2 h	Lovenox Fragmin	Inhibit activity of Xa and IIa		Used for bridging to avoid undue thromboembolic events

Antiplatelet Medication (NOAP/Others)

Generic	Proprietary	Mechanism of Action	Renal Function (CR/Cl/min)	Discontinue (D/C) or Not (N)
Acetyl salicylic acid Half-life: 15–20 min	Aspirin, BioPak, Adira	Inhibits TXA_2 and platelet aggregation		D/C depends on dosing: 325 mg vs 81 mg

Dipyridamole	Persantine	Blocks adenosine transport in platelets, erythrocytes and endothelial cells. Acts on platelet A2-receptors increasing cAMP and blocks platelet aggregation	Works with ASA and not usually used alone. Short half-life D/C based on dual effects with other antiplatelet drugs
Clopidogrel bisulfate Half-life: 7–9 h	Plavix, Iscover	Inhibit platelet aggregation by blocking ADP binding to platelet receptors (P_2Y_{12}) and activation of GPIIb-IIIa complex	Do not D/C up to 1 y. After 1 y check with physician before D/C based on complexity of procedure
Ticlopidine hydrochloride	Ticlid, Ticlodone	Inhibits platelet binding to ADP-fibrinogen as well as platelet aggregation	D/C 10–14 d before elective surgery
Cilostazol	Pletal	Prevents platelet aggregation and indices vasodilatory effects	Must D/C 10–14 d before elective surgery
Prasugrel Half-life: 7 h	Effient	A thienopyridine that binds irreversibly to P_2Y_{12} platelet receptors	N: do not D/C for elective surgery
Ticagrelor Half-life: 7–9 h	Brilique	A thienopyridine that binds irreversibly to P_2Y_{12} platelet receptors	N: do not D/C for elective surgery

Abbreviations: ADP, adenosine diphosphate; cAMP, cyclic adenosine monophosphate; NOAP, novel oral antiplatelet; TXA_2, thromboxane A2.

procedure, the dosage may be administered up to 2 hours after the procedure."[33] If a patient with an indication for prophylaxis who appropriately received antibiotic premedication 1 day before a dental procedure and who is then scheduled the following day for a dental procedure also warranting premedication (eg, dental prophylaxis), the antibiotic prophylaxis regimen should be repeated before the second appointment. Another concern that dentists have expressed involves patients who require prophylaxis but are already taking antibiotics for another condition. In these cases, the guidelines for infective endocarditis recommend that the dentist select an antibiotic from a different class than the one the patient is already taking. For example, if the patient is taking amoxicillin, the dentist should select clindamycin, azithromycin, or clarithromycin for prophylaxis.[35]

Diabetes Mellitus

Hyperglycemia (blood glucose >140 mg/dL) is a frequent occurrence with a prevalence of 20% to 40% in the general surgery and 80% to 90% in the cardiac surgery populations.[36–38] During the perioperative period, hyperglycemia is an independent marker of poor surgical outcomes.[36–38] Patients with diabetes mellitus, whether type 1 or 2, are at an increased risk of intraoperative and postoperative morbidity, a 2-fold higher risk of infection and other complications such as wound healing owing to endothelial dysfunction, platelet activation, and synthesis of proinflammatory cytokines that contribute to a prothrombotic state. A prothrombotic state inhibits fibrinolysis and results in subsequent vessel occlusion with myocardial impairment. Chronic hyperglycemia, a potential consequence of surgical stress, can result in significant microvascular and macrovascular disease; that is, diabetic neuropathy, diabetic retinopathy, cerebrovascular disease, and peripheral vascular disease. All contribute to heart disease as a cause of death in 80% of diabetic patients.[39] The main objectives of the perioperative management of type 1 or type 2 diabetes mellitus is to prevent the consequences of hyperglycemia and hypoglycemia. The following provides an approach to the perioperative management to achieve good glucose control during the perioperative period.

1. *Preoperative assessment*: The OMFS must take a detailed history of the type of Diabetes and whether or not there have been exacerbation of disease and concomitant complications (as discussed elsewhere in this article). This also involves whether the patient is susceptible to bouts of hypoglycemia or hyperglycemia based on the present medicine regimen (as discussed elsewhere in this article). A decision must also be made as to whether the surgery will be done in the inpatient setting or in the office during the early part of the day.

2. *Perioperative blood glucose targeting*: Although there are no prospective randomized trials in relation to blood glucose control during the perioperative period several laboratory risk predictors can help in perioperative care. Glycosylated hemoglobin (HbA_{1c}) is tested to monitor the long-term control of diabetes mellitus. The level of HbA_{1c} is increased in the red blood cells of persons with poorly controlled diabetes mellitus and can aid in determining the overall blood glucose over a 2- to 3-month period. The preoperative determination of the HbA_{1c} is associated with a lower incidence of complications, and decreased mortality, whereas an elevated preoperative HbA_{1c} can result in adverse outcomes after surgery regardless of a previous diagnosis of diabetes mellitus.[40] There is no consensus, however, regarding whether to determine the HbA_{1c} in all patients who will undergo surgery. Several studies support routine measure of HbA_{1c} in nondiabetics, as well as measurement in diabetic patients who have not had their values determined in the past 3 months.[41] A systematic review by Bock and colleagues[41] concluded that HbA_{1c} is not required in the nondiabetic undergoing elective, vascular and orthopedic surgery unless there are clinical symptoms indicative of diabetes mellitus. In 2018, the American Diabetes Association guidelines were updated to reflect limitations in HbA_{1c} measurements owing to hemoglobin variants, ethnicity, age and altered red blood cell turnover. They have recommended the use of a new term, estimated average glucose that expresses the HbA_{1c} in the same units (mg/dL or mmol/L) as the average glucose levels self-monitored by the patient.[42] This strategy provides a better comparison to improve the discussion of glucose control with patients. Although there are no well-validated cutoff HbA_{1c} values, elective surgery should be postponed if the HbA_{1c} is greater than 10% (see **Box 5** for correlation of Blood glucose, HbA_{1c} and estimated average glucose).

Monitoring of blood glucose levels during the perioperative period is controversial owing to the lack of high quality evidence (see above references). The World Health Organization (WHO) surgical safety target is blood glucose maintained between 108 to 180 mg/dl with a range

Box 5
The relationship among Hba1c, blood glucose, and estimated average glucose

Hb_{a1c} %	Blood Glucose (mg/dL)	Estimated Average Glucose (mmol/L)
6.0	126	7.0
6.5	140	7.8
7.0	154	8.6
7.5	169	9.4
8.0	183	10.1
8.5	197	10.9
9.0	212	11.8
9.5	226	12.6
10.0	240	13.4

Reprinted with permission from The American Diabetes Association. Copyright 2020 by the American Diabetes Association.

between 76 to 216 mg/dl.[42] This is in accordance with the position statement of the American Diabetes Association/American Association of Clinical Endocrinologists (AACE) and Endocrine society.[43] It still remains to be determined if these levels of blood glucose during surgery will decrease intraoperative and postoperative complications in diabetes mellitus patients undergoing noncardiac elective surgery. (please review the references for further data interpretation)

3. Perioperative management of oral agents and insulin

   a. *Oral agents:* The OMFS sees a large percentage of patients with diabetes mellitus type 2 who are taking oral antihyperglycemic agents. Insufficient evidence, however, exists regarding the optimal perioperative management of oral antihyperglycemic agents and, as such, controversial recommendations exist, especially for the agent metformin.[39] The latter can lead to lactic acidosis with subsequent renal dysfunction. Studies suggest to hold metformin for 24 to 48 hours before surgery and resume dosing after a postoperative meal. Sodium glucose cotransporter-2 inhibitors should be held within 24 hours before the surgical procedure and then continued when the patient is discharged.[39]

   b. *Insulin agents:* Insufficient evidence exists regarding a uniform perioperative management algorithm for insulin-treated patients undergoing surgery. Recommendations are based on safety, avoidance of

hypoglycemia, and adequate perioperative glucose control. Patients who require insulin therapy, either alone or with oral agents, should decrease the dose of long-acting insulin by 25% the evening before.[39,44] Those who take insulin in the morning should hold it before surgery. Patients who take high does or a total daily dose of 80 units should decrease the dose by 50% to 75% to minimize the risk of hypoglycemia. These recommendations are based on the avoidance of hypoglycemia and a maintenance of adequate glucose control (**Table 2**).[39,44] The intraoperative management must be carefully monitored and after recovery ambulatory patients who are stable and taking in nutrition can be discharged to home on their normal antihyperglycemic regimens.

4. *Perioperative infections*: Diabetic patients are highly susceptible to perioperative infections (as stated elsewhere in this article). Hyperglycemia can alter leukocyte function, degranulation, phagocytosis, and expression of cellular adhesion, all of which impair the ability to fight off pathogens. Studies have shown that a combination of intravenous and subcutaneous insulin can decrease the rate of infection during the postoperative period.[43,44] Controversy remains as to developing a standard for optimal glycemic control and there are many random control trials being crafted with respect to optimum control and its influence on comorbidities and surgical outcomes in the diabetic patient population.

The Obese Patient

The World Health Organization and US Centers for Disease Control and Prevention define obesity as a body mass of index greater than or equal to 30 and current figures estimate that one-third of adults in the United States are obese.[45,46] The estimated prevalence in middle-age adults varies from 20% to 25% and severe obstructive sleep apnea (OSA) can occur in 10% of the population seen.[47,48] The OMFS is becoming a center for referrals of obese patients owing to their comorbidity of OSA. Comorbidities associated and exacerbated by OSA include hypotension, arrhythmias, heart failure diabetes mellitus type 2, and mortality from cardiovascular disease.[47,49,50] A recent study involving more than 0.5 million patients suggested that even in the absence of these metabolic derangements, obese patients are more likely to develop cardiovascular disease complications.[51]

Perioperative management in obese patients becomes challenging owing to the complexity of

Table 2
Insulin regimen algorithms during the perioperative period of surgical intervention**

Insulin Therapy	24 h Before Surgery	Day of Surgery
Continuous subcutaneous Insulin infusion	No change in dose or decrease by 20%–30% of base if history of hypoglycemia	
Long-acting insulin analogue	No dose change or decrease by 20%–30% evening dose if history of nocturnal or morning hypoglycemia	No dose change or decrease by 20%–30% morning dose if history of hypoglycemia
Intermediate-acting insulin	No change of morning dose or decrease evening dose by 20%–30%	Decrease morning dose by 25%–50% No change of meal evening dose
Prefixed combination of insulins	No dose change	Decrease morning dose by 25%–50% of intermediate-acting insulin Component. Omit short-acting insulin component in morning. Omit lunchtime dose and no change in evening dose.
Short and rapid acting insulins	No dose change	Omit morning and lunchtime dose

** There is insufficient evidence regarding a consensus for perioperative management of insulin-treated diabetic patients undergoing surgery.
From Soldevila B, Lucas AM, Zavala R, et al. Perioperative management of the diabetic patient. In: Stuart-Smith K, editor. Perioperative medicine — current controversies. Cham: Springer International Publishing Switzerland; 2016. pp.165–92; with permission.

medical and surgical disease management. The primary concern will be in assessing the degree of upper airway obstruction because obesity is an independent predictor of difficult mask ventilation and laryngoscopy. Assessing the airway preoperatively is most critical and is accomplished using awake nasopharyngoscopy, lateral cephalograms, and the use of cone beam or hospital grade computed tomography scans. This imaging provides a 3-dimensional view of the airway for measuring the degree of narrowing and how this will affect airway manipulation during dentoalveolar surgery. Controversies exist throughout the literature with respect to the use of the lateral cephalogram. Yet it remains as an adjunct to other imaging tools.[48] Medical considerations are complex and grouped by what is referred to as the metabolic syndrome, whose criteria are at least 3 of the following: abdominal obesity, glucose intolerance, hypertension, hypertriglyceridemia, and/or high-density lipoprotein cholesterol of less than 40 mg/dL in men and less than 50 mg/dL in women.[50,51] Obese noncardiac surgical patients with this syndrome and airway compromise are at increased risk for mortality, stroke, wound complications, and possible sepsis postoperatively.[51]

Perioperative management is challenging with respect to nil per on (NPO) status and gastric emptying time, which will be longer than the 6- to 8-hour regimens in adults. An electrocardiogram and echocardiogram may be used to assess ventricular and valvular function and so medical clearance is advocated to optimize a patient's cardiopulmonary disease status. The STOP-BANG score (STOP; snoring, tiredness, observed apnea, high blood pressure, BANG; body mass index, age, neck circumference, and sex) has been extensively applied with high validity in obese surgical patients.[51] A value of more than 3 has a high positive predictive value for detecting OSA (85%); greater than 5 a high specificity of 70% in moderate to severe OSA and concomitant adverse events perioperatively.[52]

Pharmacologic considerations are challenging because drug dosing must be adjusted owing to an increase in adipose tissue in proportion to body weight and lean body mass. Drug pharmacokinetic profiles and the volume of distribution of lipophilic drugs will be greater than in the normal adult.[53] Lipophilic drugs, however, such as barbiturates, benzodiazepines, and volatile inhalation agents should be given with caution.[53,54] Propofol has been found to be appropriate without evidence of increased drug accumulation. Desflurane is the volatile agent of choice in obese patients, as well as sevoflurane.[53,54] For opioid coverage, remifentanil is the drug of choice because it does not accumulate in the fat.[47,54] Postoperative pain management can be challenging owing to the need to have the patient become mobile and reestablish a good pulmonary toilet. A patient-controlled analgesia pump may be a good choice if a dosage regimen is carefully titrated to avoid respiratory depression. Dosing should be based on lean body mass. Nasal continuous positive airway pressure may be recommended postoperatively, along with supplemental oxygen.[47,51,54]

Other physiologic complications during perioperative management include pulmonary mishaps, cardiovascular morbidities, postoperative cognitive decline, and wound infections.[51] Obese patients have an increased incidence of asthma precipitated by lung mechanics, inflammation, immune function, and risk of atelectasis.[47,53,54] Noninvasive positive pressure ventilation following intubation can improve oxygenation, as well as the use of positive end-expiratory pressure during the maintenance of anesthesia if the patient is intubated. Obesity in of itself is not necessarily a risk factor for cardiovascular disease, but must be evaluated along with the other risk predictors of the metabolic syndrome, discussed elsewhere in this article. Patients who are obese and have insulin resistance can have an increased risk of a perioperative myocardial infarction. A high risk for venous thromboembolic event is likely during the perioperative period and is exacerbated by increase surgical time, male sex, older age, and a previous history of deep vein thrmobosis.[51,52]

Postoperative cognitive decline has been a controversy of debate because it is associated with increased morbidity and mortality in obese surgical patients.[52] Investigation has focused on a role for neuroinflammatory mechanisms based on proinflammatory cytokines and their ability to potentiate a correlation between learning and retaining ones memory.[55] Obesity is associated with both a low-grade inflammatory state and an insulin-resistant state. The latter is responsible for elevated levels of proinflammatory mediators that correlate with learning and memory, as well as increasing the risk of dementia by 64%.[56] The OMFS may decide to apply "care bundles," which modify and decrease precipitating factors for postoperative delirium (refer to reference[52] for interest).[52] The pathophysiology of wound infections in this patient group can also be attributed to mechanisms of adipose tissue breakdown and production of excessive cytokines (tumor necrosis factor-alpha and IL-1, -6, -8, and -10) impairing mononuclear cell function with decreased lymphocyte activity, both of which disrupt the immune response. Diabetes, depression, and anxiety can also contribute to impaired wound healing.[57,58] Strategies that can be applied to avoid this event include weight-adjusted antibiotic dosing, careful layered closure of wounds, and minimally invasive alternatives to surgical intervention.

Considerable controversy still exists in the perioperative management of obese surgical patients owing to the complexity of issues and the OMFS will continue to require an integrative multidisciplinary team to meet the challenges for safe practice in this patient population. Multiple outcome metrics will include optimal airway management, biomarkers for risk predictors of surgical success and a closer examination of "obesity type" to differentiate between a healthy obese patient and one with a hazardous risk during the perioperative period.

SUMMARY AND FUTURE DIRECTIONS

The perioperative management whether hospital-based, or within the private practice setting, is a process of "clinical assessment that precedes the delivery of anesthetic and surgical care. It includes a review of past medical records, recent lab analyses and a comprehensive physical examination of the pulmonary, cardiovascular, airway and systemic homeostasis."[2,3] As the surgical population ages their dentoalveolar surgical needs become more dependent on perioperative management skills that must meet the dynamics of total body wellbeing. Management strategies should be tailored according to both the characteristics of the surgical procedure, as well as the patient's treatment schedule.

Evidence-based guidelines on perioperative management continue to be monitored owing to insurance company criteria for reimbursement and issues of reimbursement to decrease the rate of hospital readmission. As such, there remains the need for high quality evidence-based studies to further define the ideal preoperative algorithm specific to the patient, which will also be cost effective. The risk assessments discussed in patients with cardiovascular disease, diabetes, and/or obesity must be carefully weighed against the surgical stress even in situations of in-office procedures. Future trials should involve an interdisciplinary approach that will reflect the current state of scientific evidence based on randomized, controlled studies coupled with expert opinion. The strongest predictors of perioperative risk of complications will continue to be predicated on preexisting illnesses, as revealed by a thorough history and the nature of the surgery to be performed. The preoperative evaluation by the OMFS can offer patients an opportunity to optimize their health status before surgical intervention. This is the first step in developing a therapeutic alliance so that shared decision making can improve surgical outcomes.

DISCLOSURE

The authors have nothing to disclose.

REFERENCES

1. Bagheri SC. Clinical review of oral and maxillofacial surgery. 2nd edition. Elsevier; 2014.
2. O'Donnell FT. Preoperative evaluation of the surgical patient. Sci Med 2016;113(3):196–201.
3. Miloro M, Yang B, Halpern LR. Patient assessment: In: Parameters of Care. J Oral Maxillofac Surg 2017;75(Suppl 1):e12–33.
4. Niederman R, Richards D. What is evidence-based dentistry and do oral infections increase systemic morbidity or mortality? Oral Maxillofac Surg Clin North Am 2011;23(4):491–6.
5. Krishnan DG. Controversies in dentoalveolar and pre-prosthetic surgery. Oral Maxillofac Surg Clin North Am 2017;29:383–90.
6. Fattahi T. Perioperative laboratory and diagnostic testing: what is needed and when? Oral Maxillofac Surg Clin North Am 2006;18(1):3–7.
7. Martin SK, Cifu AS. Routine preoperative laboratory tests for elective surgery. JAMA 2017;318:567–8.
8. Routine perioperative tests for elective surgery. London: National Institute for Health and Excellence; 2016. NICE guideline 45.
9. Bock M, Fritsch G, Hepner DL. Preoperative laboratory testing. Anesthesiol Clin 2016;34(1):43–58.
10. King BA, Dube SR, Tynan MA. Current tobacco use among adults in the United States: findings from the national adult tobacco survey. Am J Public Health 2012;102(11):e93–100.
11. Wong J, Lam DP, Abrishami A, et al. Short-term preoperative smoking cessation and postoperative complications: a systematic review and meta-analysis. Can J Anaesth 2012;59:268–79.
12. Alexander JC, Patel Biral, Girish P, et al. Perioperative use of opioids: current controversies and concerns. Best Pract Res Clin Anaesthesiol 2019; 33(3):341–51.
13. Goldman L, Caldera DL, Nussbaum SR, et al. Multifactorial index of cardiac risk in noncardiac surgical procedures. N Engl J Med 1977;297:26.
14. Fleischer LA, Beckman JA, Brown LA, et al. American college of Cardiology/American Heart Association (ACC/AHA) 2007 guidelines on perioperative cardiovascular evaluation and care for noncardiac surgery: a report of the American College of cardiology/American Heart Association Task force on Practice Guidelines). Circulation 2007;116:418–99.
15. Weinstein AS, Sigurdsson MI, Bader AM. Comparison of preoperative assessment of patient's metabolic equivalents (METS) estimated from history versus measured by exercise cardiac stress testing. Anesthesiol Res Pract 2018. Available at: https://doi.org/10.1155/2018/5912726. Accessed December 31 2019.
16. Shear T, Katz J, Greenberg SB, et al. Perioperative approach to the high-risk cardiac patient. In: Kaplan JA, Cronin B, Maus TM, editors. Kaplan's essentials of cardiac anesthesia for noncardiac surgery. Philadelphia: Elsevier; 2019. p. 16–32.
17. Whelton PK, Carey RM, Wilbert S, et al. 2017ACC/AHA/AAPA/ABC/ACPM/AGS/APhA/ASH/ASPC/NMA/PCNA Guideline for the Prevention, Detection, Evaluation, and Management of High Blood Pressure in Adults. A Report of the American College of Cardiology/American Heart Association Task Force on clinical practice guidelines. J Am Coll Cardiol 2018;71(19). https://doi.org/10.1016/j.jacc.2017.11.006.
18. Ward BB, Smith MH. Dentoalveolar procedures for the anticoagulated patients: literature recommendations versus current practice. J Oral Maxillofac Surg 2007;65(8):1454–60.
19. Matei V, Sami Haddadin A. Systemic and pulmonary arterial hypertension. In: Hines RL, Marschall KE, editors. Stoelting's anesthesia and co-existing disease. 6th edition. Philadelphia: Elsevier Saunders; 2012. p. 104–19.
20. Abramowicz S, Roser SM. Medical management of patients undergoing dentoalveolar surgery. Oral Maxillofac Surg Clin North Am 2015;27:345–52.
21. Roshanov PS, Rochwerg B, Patel A, et al. Withholding versus continuing angiotensin-converting enzyme inhibitors or angiotensin II receptor blockers before noncardiac surgery: an analysis of the vascular events in noncardiac surgery patients. Anesthesiology 2017;126:16.
22. Yancy CW, Jessup M, Bozkurt B, et al. 2017 ACC/AHA focused update of the 2013 guideline for the management of heart failure. J Am Coll Cardiol 2017;70(6):776–97.
23. January CT, Wann LS, Alpert JS, et al. ACC/AHA Task force Members. 2014 AHA/ACC/HRS guideline for the management of patients with atrial fibrillation: a report of the American College of Cardiology/American Heart Association Task force on practice guidelines and the Heart Rhythm Society. Circulation 2014;130:e199–267.
24. Steed MB, Swanson MT. Warfarin and newer agents: what the oral surgeon needs to know. Oral Maxillofac Surg Clin North Am 2016;28:151–521.
25. Bruno EK, Bennett JD. Platelet abnormalities in the oral and maxillofacial surgery patient. Oral Maxillofac Surg Clin North Am 2016;28:473–80.

26. Van Diermen DE, van der Waal I, Hoogstraten J. Management recommendations for invasive dental treatment in patients using oral antithrombotic medication, including novel oral anticoagulants. Oral Surg Oral Med Oral Pathol Oral Radiol 2013; 116(6):709–16.

27. Bajkin BV, Vujkov SB, Milekic BR, et al. Risk factors for bleeding after oral surgery in patients who continued using oral anticoagulant therapy. J Am Dent Assoc 2015;146(6):375–81.

28. Scully C, Wolff A. Oral surgery in patients on anticoagulant therapy. Oral Surg Oral Med Oral Pathol Oral Radiol Endod 2002;94(1):57–84.

29. Chugani V. Management of dental patients on warfarin therapy in a primary care setting. Dent Update 2004;31(7):279–382.

30. Yan S, Shi Q, Liu J, et al. Should oral anticoagulant therapy be continued during dental extraction? A meta-analysis. BMC Oral Health 2016;16:1–9.

31. Ghantous AE, Ferneini EM. Aspirin, Plavix, and other antiplatelet medications: what the oral and maxillofacial surgeon needs to know. Oral Maxillofac Surg Clin North Am 2016;28:497–506.

32. Mauer P, Conrad-Hengerer I, Hollstein S, et al. Orbital hemorrhage associated with orbital fractures in geriatric patients on antiplatelet or anticoagulant therapy. Int J Oral Maxillofac Surg 2013;42(12): 1510–4.

33. Nishimura RA, Otto CM, Bonow RO, et al. ACC/AHA Task force Members. 2014 AHA/ACC guidelines for the management of patients with valvular heart disease: a report of the American college of Cardiology/American Heart association Task force on Practice Guidelines. Circulation 2014;129: pe521–643.

34. American Dental Association. Oral health topics. Chicago: Center for Scientific Information, ADA Science Institute; 2017. Available at: www.ada.org/en/member-center/oral-health-topics/antibiotic-prophylaxis.

35. Wilson W, Taubert KA, Gewitz M, et al. Antibiotic prophylaxis prior to dental procedures. Oral Health Topics. 2017. Available at: http://www.ada.org/en/member-center/. Accessed March 31, 2019.

36. Kotagal M, Symons RG, Hirsch IB, et al, SCOAP-CERTAIN Collaborative. Perioperative hyperglycemia and risk of adverse events among patients with and without diabetes. Ann Surg 2015;261(1): 97–103.

37. Frisch A, Chandra P, Smiley D, et al. Prevalence and clinical outcome of hyperglycemia in the perioperative period in noncardiac surgery. Diabetes Care 2010;33(8):1783–8.

38. Dogra P, Jialal I. Diabetic perioperative management. Available at: https://www.ncbi.nlm.nih.gov/books/NBK540965/?report=reader. Accessed January 1 2020.

39. Soldevila B, Lucas AM, Zavala R, et al. Perioperative management of the diabetic patient. In: Stuart-Smith K, editor. Perioperative medicine-current controversies. Zurich: Springer International Publishing; 2016. p. 165–92.

40. Underwood P, Askari R, Hurwitz S, et al. Preoperative A_{1c} and clinical outcomes in patients with diabetes undergoing major noncardiac surgical procedures. Diabetes Care 2014;37(3): 611–6.

41. Bock M, Johansson T, Fritsch G, et al. The impact of preoperative testing for blood glucose concentration and Hemoglobin A_{1c} on mortality, changes in management and complications in noncardiac elective surgery: a systematic review. Eur J Anaesthesiol 2015;32:152–9.

42. American Diabetes Association. Pharmacologic approaches to glycemic treatment: standards of medical care in diabetes-2018. Diabetes Care 2018; 41(Suppl 1):S73–85.

43. Dhatariya K, Levy N, Kilvert A, et al. Joint British Diabetes Societies NHS diabetes guideline for the perioperative management of the adult patient with diabetes. Diabet Med 2012;29:420–33.

44. Vann MA. Management of diabetes medications for patients undergoing ambulatory surgery. Anesthesiol Clin 2014;32:329–39.

45. Flegal KM, Carroll MD, Kit BK, et al. Prevalence of obesity and trends in the distribution of body mass index among US adults. 1999-2010. JAMA 2012; 307:491–7.

46. Obesity: preventing and managing the global epidemic. Report of a WHO consultation. World Health Organ Tech Rep Ser 2000;894(i-xii): 1–253.

47. Leonard KL, Davies SW, Waibel BH. Perioperative management of obese patients. Surg Clin North Am 2015;95:379–90.

48. Dicus-Brookes CC, Boyd SB. Controversies in obstructive sleep apnea surgery. Oral Maxillofac Surg Clin North Am 2017;29:503–13.

49. Marin JM, Carrizo SJ, Vicente E, et al. Long-term cardiovascular outcomes in men with obstructive sleep apnea-hypopnea with or without treatment with continuous positive airway pressure: an observational study. Lancet 2005;365:1046.

50. Wang X, Bi Y, Zhang Q, et al. Obstructive sleep apnoea and the risk of type 2 diabetes: a meta-analysis of prospective cohort studies. Respirology 2013;18:140.

51. Lang LH, Parekh K, Tsui YK, et al. Perioperative management of the obese surgical patient. Br Med Bull 2017;124:135–55.

52. Chung F, Yang Y, Liao P. Predictive performance of the STOP-BANG score for identifying obstructive sleep apnea in obese patients. Obes Surg 2013; 23:2050–7.

53. Cullen A, Ferguson A. Perioperative management of the severely obese patient: a selective pathophysiological review. Can J Anaesth 2012;59: 974–96.

54. Servin F. Ambulatory anesthesia for the obese patient. Curr Opin Anaesthesiol 2006;19:597–9.

55. Terrando N, Eriksson LI, Ryu JK, et al. Resolving postoperative neuroinflammation and cognitive decline. Ann Neurol 2011;70:986–95.

56. Anstey KJ, Cherbuin N, Budge M, et al. Body mass index in midlife and late-life as a risk factor for dementia: a meta-analysis of prospective studies. Obes Rev 2011;12:e426–37.

57. Guo S, Dipietro LA. Factors affecting wound healing. J Dent Res 2010;89:219–29.

58. Wilson JA, Clark JJ. Obesity: impediment to postsurgical wound healing. Adv Skin Wound Care 2004;17: 426–35.

Principles of Exodontia

William Stuart McKenzie, DMD, MD

KEYWORDS

- Exodontia • Elevators • Dental forceps • Dental extractions

KEY POINTS

- Exodontia services comprise the largest portion of clinical practice for most oral and maxillofacial surgeons in the United States.
- This article is an overview of the principles of exodontia including the physics principles underlying the appropriate use of dental elevators and forceps.
- New instruments including periotomes, piezosurgery, Physics Forceps, and vertical extraction systems are also introduced and reviewed.

The most common procedure performed by most oral and maxillofacial surgeons is extraction of decayed or impacted teeth. According to the National Institute of Dental and Craniofacial Research, 92% of US citizens age 20 to 64 have had dental caries in their permanent dentition, with 26% of adults in this age range with current untreated caries.[1] Many patients require one or more extractions throughout their lifetime because of impaction, caries, periodontal disease, fracture of teeth from mastication or previous dental procedures, and failed root canal therapy. The ideal principles of exodontia should allow the efficient, effective, and safe removal of teeth with a primary focus on minimizing complications and maximizing comfort for the patient and provider. Failure to understand the instrumentation and the physics principles being used can cause prolonged operative time, iatrogenic injury to the patient, and unnecessary fatigue and/or injury to the provider. This article reviews the principles, techniques, and instrumentation of exodontia, and presents new instruments being currently marketed for exodontia.

PREOPERATIVE ASSESSMENT

Before any surgical procedure, a thorough history and physical examination must be completed. Although most patients can safely undergo basic exodontia procedures, medical history and current medications can allow the surgeon to anticipate and avoid intraoperative and postoperative complications including bleeding issues, bone and/or soft tissue healing issues, and the best pain management strategy for the individual patient. This assessment also includes forecasting the specific instrumentation that may be needed for the procedure. Communication of the need for special instrumentation or hemostatic agents to the surgical team maximizes procedural efficiency. The examination process also includes diagnostic radiographs of the teeth requiring removal to confirm necessity of removal and to assess for possible complications. The radiograph also allows the patient to visualize the teeth that are to be removed, and to participate in the informed consent process by seeing the structures that may be at risk, such as the maxillary sinus cavity, the inferior alveolar nerve canal, or adjacent restorations.

The use of cone beam computed tomography (CBCT) scan by oral and maxillofacial surgeons has become increasingly popular in the United States. Although most patients having routine exodontia do not require CBCT, CBCT may be indicated when impacted mandibular wisdom teeth are in close proximity to the inferior alveolar canal. Matzen and Wenzel[2] performed a comprehensive and well-designed review of the efficacy of CBCT before mandibular wisdom tooth extraction. They found a paucity of randomized controlled trials in their review of more than 300 articles, and ultimately concluded that periapical

Mid-State Oral Surgery and Implant Center, 445 Henslee Drive, Dickson, TN 37055, USA
E-mail address: mckenzieomfs@gmail.com

Oral Maxillofacial Surg Clin N Am 32 (2020) 511–517
https://doi.org/10.1016/j.coms.2020.06.001
1042-3699/20/© 2020 Elsevier Inc. All rights reserved.

and panoramic imaging is sufficient for most patients undergoing wisdom tooth removal. However, they did find that CBCT may be indicated if traditional imaging suggested high risk of inferior alveolar nerve proximity, and that the CBCT would change clinical decision making, such as performing coronectomy instead of extraction.[2]

INSTRUMENTATION/STAFFING

The instrumentation necessary for successful dental extractions includes optimal lighting, suction, and proper retraction of the soft tissue. A well-trained assistant is a critical component to any successful procedure by providing suction, irrigation, and anticipating instrument needs as the procedure progresses. The assistant can also serve as a last line of defense for verification of correct patient, procedure, allergy profile, consent completion, and preprocedural sedation requirements (eg, NPO status, adult driver). The value of a formal "time-out" checklist and strict adherence of the surgical team to the checklist cannot be understated.

Patient positioning is important for visualization of the surgical field by the entire surgical team and for the appropriate posture of the surgeon. Patient positions that cause unnecessary bending or twisting of the neck or back can cause significant disability for the surgeon over time.

Dental elevators come in a wide array of designs to facilitate luxation of the tooth. However, the forces applied to the tooth are encompassed by three principles of physics: (1) a lever, (2) a wedge, and (3) a wheel. It behooves the oral and maxillofacial surgeon to understand these principles to maximize the effectiveness of the elevators, while minimizing excessive or ill-directed force. The goal of the dental elevators is to luxate the tooth in a manner that disrupts the periodontal ligament, thus allowing removal of the tooth with a forceps.

The elevator is used as a wedge when the thin sharp edge of the instrument is directed parallel to root surface with apical force. This transects the periodontal ligament, but also expands the periradicular bone laterally, and displaces the tooth coronally.

The elevator is used as a class I lever (fulcrum located between the source of effort and the source of resistance) when the tip of the instrument is placed between the bone and the root surface using the crest of the alveolar bone as a fulcrum (**Fig. 1**). The longer the lever arm, the greater the force that is generated by the working end of the elevator. A stable purchase point on the tooth is necessary to allow the force to be adequately applied to the tooth. If the tooth has

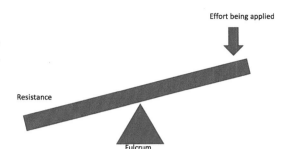

Fig. 1. Class I lever.

significant caries, a trough or sectioning of the tooth may need to be completed to achieve a purchase on stable tooth structure. Another technique is to create a purchase point on the tooth with a drill to allow the use of a Crane pick to be used as a lever.

Finally, the elevator (particularly the Cryer-type elevators) is used as a wheel and axle. With a Cryer elevator, the handle acts as an axle, and the working end of the elevator acts as a wheel to generate increased force and arc of rotation to elevate a root. This is primarily used in the mandibular molar region.

Often, a combination of all three physics principles are used simultaneously to wedge the elevator as apical as possible for optimum purchase/fulcrum, then apply lever and rotational forces to the tooth to quickly and efficiently extract the tooth. The development of a feel for the correct application of these forces is critical and must be carefully and continually reassessed as surgeon skill develops. With time, one can quickly assess by feel whether the tooth can be successfully elevated, or whether the use of a drill would be most effective.

Dental forceps also have a multitude of designs to adapt to the specific teeth that they are being used on. The fundamental principle of the forceps is as a lever; however, some designs also create a wedge effect (eg, #23 forceps or forceps with thin beaks). As with the elevators, prudent use of force is key to avoiding complications. The lever that is created by the conventional forceps is that of two type I levers connected by a hinge.[3] In this configuration, the hinge is acting as the fulcrum with the handle being the long lever and the beaks being the short lever.

Perhaps the greatest advance in modern exodontia is the drill. The modern surgical drill is a sophisticated instrument that creates high-speed, high-torque rotation of the bur that can function in the presence of water and blood and withstand repeated sterilization cycles. The drill allows for efficient removal of cortical bone and sectioning of teeth. The liberal use of irrigation to minimize overheating and subsequent necrosis of surrounding bone is critical. Adequate lighting, retraction, and suctioning is important to avoid iatrogenic injury to adjacent tissues. The impact of the surgical drill on the efficiency of office-based exodontia cannot be understated and is an invaluable surgical tool. The use of the drill allows significant mechanical advantage by allowing apical position of the elevators, increased purchase, and dividing of multirooted teeth.

NOVEL INSTRUMENTATION/EXTRACTION TECHNIQUES

Advances in materials, technology, and innovative design have produced interesting new instruments for exodontia. Here we review some of the new products that have been marketed.

Physics Forceps

The Physics Forceps (GoldenDent, Roseville, MI) uses a class I lever by placing a bumper in the buccal vestibule and a thin beak on the lingual aspect of the tooth. Constant pressure is then applied for several minutes to the tooth, which elevates the root from the socket 1 to 3 mm. Per the manufacturer, the combination of the lever arm combined with release of hyaluronidase within the periodontal ligament space causes release of the periodontal ligament. The tooth can then be removed with rongeur or other tooth forceps. The manufacturer claims that the forceps provides atraumatic extractions that minimize root or alveolar bone fractures and preserves surrounding bone. **Fig. 2** shows the instrument design, and **Fig. 3** shows how the forceps is positioned to create a class I lever. El-Kenawy and Ahmed[3] compared the Physics Forceps with conventional forceps with regard to incidence of root, crown, and buccal plate fracture. The authors found a significant reduction in incidence of crown and root fracture with the Physics Forceps.[3] The design of the Physics Forceps replaces the buccal beak on a traditional forceps with a rubber bumper that seats against the soft tissue deep in the vestibule. This creates a significant mechanical advantage with the class I lever analogous to using the claw of a hammer to remove a nail from a board. The manufacturer intends for the forceps to be used with gentle constant pressure applied over several minutes in contrast to traditional forceps, where squeezing and rotation are often used. Patel and colleagues[4] used a split-mouth prospective methodology to compare the Physics Forceps with conventional forceps for orthodontic extractions. The study found a significant reduction in

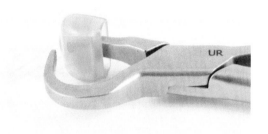

Fig. 2. Physics Forceps instrument. (*Courtesy of* GoldenDent/Directa Inc, Roseville, MI.)

operative time and immediate postoperative marginal bone and soft tissue loss with the Physics Forceps. Hariharan and coworkers[5] found advantages with the Physics Forceps over conventional forceps with regards to pain scores.

Periotomes

Advances in material physical properties have allowed for the creation of extremely thin and sharp instruments, such as the Luxator (Directa Inc, Newtown, CT) style periotome (**Fig. 4**). The extremely thin edge can be inserted between the root surface and the alveolar bone directly transecting the periodontal ligament while simultaneously acting as a wedge (**Fig. 5**). Even though less force is used than a traditional elevator, the resistance to instrument fatigue and fracture is an achievement in material science. The periotome is most effective on single-rooted teeth

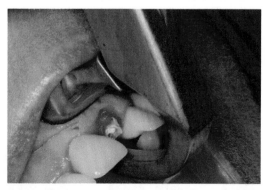

Fig. 3. Physics Forceps being used for extraction. (*Courtesy of* GoldenDent/Directa Inc, Roseville, MI.)

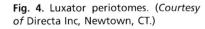
Fig. 4. Luxator periotomes. (*Courtesy of* Directa Inc, Newtown, CT.)

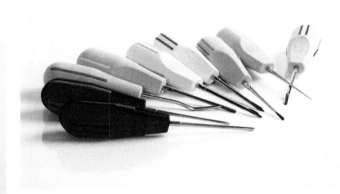

where the working tip of the instrument is used to transect the gingival fibers and crestal periodontal ligament fibers.[6] The instrument is then inclined mesial and distal and advanced apically. This sweeping motion transects the periodontal ligament while simultaneously expanding the bone. The instrument is advanced approximately two-thirds of the distance to the apex. The procedure is repeated on the lingual side of the tooth. The periotome is then removed and forceps is used to complete the extractions. Sharma and co-workers[6] completed a randomized, double blinded trial of periotome/forceps versus periosteal/forceps extraction of single-rooted teeth. The study found a significant reduction in operative time, pain scores, and gingival laceration with the use of a periotome.[6] In the age of implant dentistry, the periotome may certainly have a role in preserving bone and gingival architecture. The concept of directly transecting the fibers as opposed to tearing the fibers through luxation and bone expansion is intellectually valid if the aim is maximizing bone and soft tissue preservation. A motorized version of the handheld periotome is available that uses a reciprocating motion. This can theoretically reduce buccal plate fractures by reducing the amount of torque force that may be inadvertently applied when using the hand periotomes.[7]

Piezosurgery

Piezosurgery refers to the use of an ultrasonic transducer using piezoelectric crystal to convert oscillating electrical fields applied to the crystal into mechanical vibration. **Fig. 6** shows an example of a piezoelectric surgical unit. The mechanical vibrations produced are in the ultrasonic frequency (>20 kHz). These vibrations can cause fragmentation of solid structures and cavitation of liquid structures to which they are applied. The frequency of the ultrasonic waves used by the surgical units is specific for hard tissue, which allows minimal impact on surrounding soft tissue.[8] The ability to avoid mechanical injury of adjacent soft tissue with this technology is a significant advantage over rotary instruments, particularly in close proximity to neurovascular structures or sinus membranes. Advantages also include precise bone cutting to the depth of 20 to 200 μm depending on the tip in use and less force required when performing osteotomies compared with rotary instruments. Piezoelectric surgery has two unique

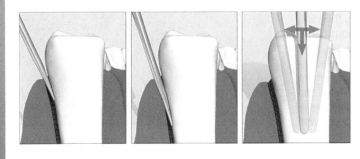

Fig. 5. Luxator periotomes being used for extraction. (*Courtesy of* Directa Inc, Newtown, CT.)

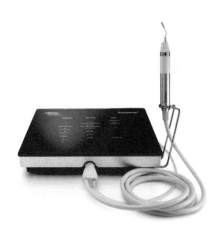

Fig. 6. Piezoelectric surgery unit. (*Courtesy of* mectron s.p.a., Italy.)

properties because of how the energy is transferred to the bone. The first is minimal bleeding while operating, which is caused by microcoagulation of the vessels caused by the shockwaves from implosion of bubbles (cavitation effect).[9] This leads to increased visibility while operating. The second unique property of piezosurgery is release of oxygen molecules while cutting, which is antiseptic and promotes healing of the area.[9] This not only reduces discomfort but improves healing and preserves bone if implant placement is indicated. The piezosurgery blades also allow for precise osteotomies, which can improve bone preservation (**Fig. 7**). The limitation of piezosurgery is increased time to complete osteotomies compared with rotary drills. In a review of the literature, Al-Moraissi and coworkers[10] found statistically significant reduction in swelling, pain, and trismus, but a significant increase in the operative time compared with rotary drills.

Vertical Extraction System

There have been several studies on a vertical tooth extraction system (Benex, Lucerne, Switzerland).[11,12] **Fig. 8** shows the Benex device. The earliest was by Muska and colleagues[11] who

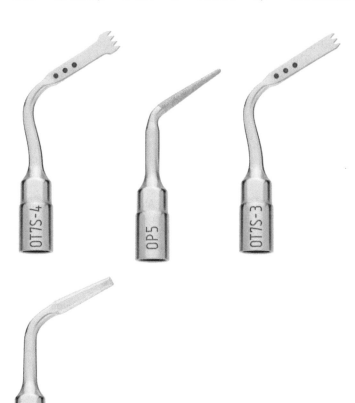

Fig. 7. Piezoelectric inserts/blades in a variety of configurations for clinical use. (*Courtesy* of mectron s.p.a., Italy.)

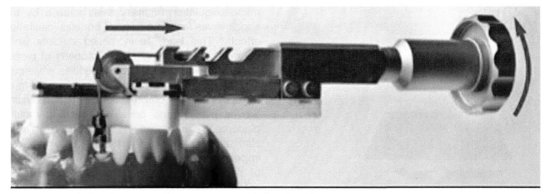

Fig. 8. Benex device. (*Courtesy of* Benex, Lucerne, Switzerland.)

demonstrated the principle of this system, which includes placement of a pin into the canal of the tooth followed by placement of the extractor apparatus (occasionally requiring silicone impression material on adjacent dentition for stabilization). A traction wire is attached from the pin to the extraction apparatus so that vertical traction is applied to the tooth. The traction is increased until extraction is completed successfully. The system is most successful in single-rooted teeth and in non–root canal treated teeth.[11,12] The advantage of the system when used successfully allows for extraction of severely decayed teeth without having to elevate a flap or remove buccal/interproximal bone. This is advantageous in highly esthetic areas where implant restorations are planned. Although likely not a first-line option, the technology certainly has a role in maximal preservation of gingival and alveolar architecture.

SUMMARY

Exodontia is the cornerstone of most oral and maxillofacial surgery practices. Although each surgeon has their routine instruments and techniques, it is important to occasionally re-evaluate how and why your "routine" method was established. By taking the time to reconsider the patient evaluation, instrumentation/staffing, and techniques surrounding exodontia, we can often find subtle ways to improve the efficiency, comfort, and safety for ourselves and our patients. We must also always stay current on new techniques and technologies that enter the field. The apt surgeon has a thorough understanding of how, why, and when a certain instrument would be the most effective. It is hoped this article allows reflection on and introduction to the most current techniques of exodontia.

DISCLOSURE

The author has nothing to disclose.

REFERENCES

1. Dental caries (tooth decay) in adults (age 20 to 64). In: National Institute of Dental and Craniofacial Research. 2018. Available at: https://www.nidcr.nih.gov/research/data-statistics/dental-caries/adults. Accessed February 29, 2020.
2. Matzen LH, Wenzel A. Efficacy of CBCT for assessment of impacted mandibular third molars: a review-based on a hierarchical model of evidence. Dentomaxillofac Radiol 2015;44(1): 20140189.
3. El-Kenawy M, Ahmed W. Comparison between physics and conventional forceps in simple dental extraction. J Maxillofac Oral Surg 2015;14(4): 949–55.
4. Patel HS, Managutti AM, Menat S, et al. Comparative evaluation of efficacy of Physics Forceps versus conventional forceps in orthodontic extractions: a prospective randomized split mouth study. J Clin Diagn Res 2016;10(7):ZC41–5.
5. Hariharan S, Narayanan V, Soh CL. Split-mouth comparison of Physics Forceps and extraction forceps in orthodontic extraction of upper premolars. Br J Oral Maxillofac Surg 2014;52(10): e137–40.
6. Sharma S, Vidya B, Alexander M, et al. Periotome as an aid to atraumatic extraction: a comparative double blind randomized controlled trial. J Maxillofac Oral Surg 2015;14(3):611–5.
7. Jain S, Oswal R, Purohit B, et al. Technological advances in extraction techniques and outpatient oral surgery. Int J Prev Clin Dental Res 2017;4(4):295–9.
8. Rahnama M, Czupkałło L, Czajkowski L, et al. The use of piezosurgery as an alternative method of minimally invasive surgery in the authors'

experience. Wideochir Inne Tech Maloinwazyjne 2013;8(4):321–6.

9. Schlee M, Steigmann M, Bratu E, et al. Piezosurgery: basics and possibilities. Implant Dent 2006; 15(4):334–40.

10. Al-Moraissi EA, Elmansi YA, Al-Sharaee YA, et al. Does the piezoelectric surgical technique produce fewer postoperative sequelae after lower third molar surgery than conventional rotary instruments? A systematic review and meta analysis. Int J Oral Maxillofac Surg 2016;45(3):383–91.

11. Muska E, Walter C, Knight A, et al. Atraumatic vertical tooth extraction: a proof of principle clinical study of a novel system. Oral Surg Oral Med Oral Path Oral Rad 2013;116(5):e303–10.

12. Hong B, Bulsara Y, Gorecki P, et al. Minimally invasive vertical versus conventional tooth extraction. J Am Dent Assoc 2018;149(8):688–95.

Management of Impacted Third Molars

William Synan, DDS*, Kyle Stein, DDS

KEYWORDS

- Impacted third molars • Assessment and treatment planning • Surgical management
- Radiographic evaluation

KEY POINTS

- Management of impacted third molars constitutes a major portion of contemporary oral and maxillofacial surgery practice.
- Diagnosis and treatment planning involves obtaining a comprehensive history and obtaining detailed clinical and radiographic examinations, which may include cone beam computed tomography imaging.
- Surgical considerations include localized tooth and site anatomy, flap design, bone removal, tooth sectioning, closure, and alternative techniques for special cases.

INTRODUCTION

Management of impacted third molars constitutes a major portion of contemporary oral and maxillofacial surgery practice. It is a complex topic and controversial, particularly with regard to surgical techniques used and the management of systemic and disease-free teeth. Proper management of impacted third molars involves appropriate diagnosis using detailed clinical and radiographic examinations, treatment planning with emphasis on modifying risk factors that may be present, and appropriate surgical techniques to minimize the risks of complications and ensure an efficient procedure and optimal patient outcomes.

CLASSIFICATION OF IMPACTED TEETH

There are a variety of classification systems available to categorize impacted teeth. Most of these systems rely on radiological assessment and clinical examination.

Classification of impacted third molars has often been used as a predictor regarding degree of surgical difficulty. However, this is not universally reliable. Other factors that can influence the surgical difficulty in removal of third molars may include dental-related factors and patient-related factors.

Dental-related factors may include:

1. Morphology of roots
2. Number of roots
3. Diameter of periodontal ligament
4. Presence or absence of a dental follicle
5. Proximity to adjacent teeth
6. Proximity to vital structures (ie, inferior alveolar nerve, lingual nerve, maxillary sinus)

Patient-related factors may include:

1. Bone density
2. Advanced age
3. Tongue size
4. Maximum interincisal opening
5. Size of oral aperture
6. Exaggerated gag reflex
7. Body mass index
8. Level of anxiety
9. Obstreperous behavior
10. Anesthetic management

The more common classification systems of impacted third molars analyze either the

Department of Oral and Maxillofacial Surgery, The University of Iowa, College of Dentistry, 451 Dental Science S, 801 Newton Road, Iowa City, IA 52242-1001, USA
* Corresponding author.
E-mail address: william-synan@uiowa.edu

Oral Maxillofacial Surg Clin N Am 32 (2020) 519–559
https://doi.org/10.1016/j.coms.2020.07.002
1042-3699/20/© 2020 Elsevier Inc. All rights reserved.

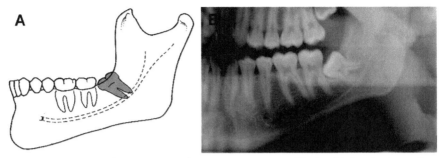

Fig. 1. (*A*) Mesioangular mandibular impaction, the most common mandibular third molar impaction and usually the least difficult to remove. (*B*) Radiograph of a mesioangular impacted mandibular third molar. (*From* [*A*] Hupp JR. Principles of management of impacted teeth. In: Hupp JR, Ellis E III, Tucker MR, editors. Contemporary oral and maxillofacial surgery. 6th edition. Philadelphia: Elsevier; 2013. p. 151; with permission; and [*B*] Rafetto LR, Synan W. Surgical management of third molars. Atlas Oral Maxillofacial Surg Clin N Am. 2012;20(2):198; with permission.)

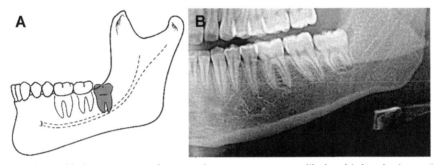

Fig. 2. (*A*) Vertical mandibular impaction, the second most common mandibular third molar impaction. Its long axis runs parallel to the long axis of the second molar. (*B*) Radiograph of vertical impacted mandibular third molar. (*From* [*A*] Hupp JR. Principles of management of impacted teeth. In: Hupp JR, Ellis E III, Tucker MR, editors. Contemporary oral and maxillofacial surgery. 6th edition. Philadelphia: Elsevier; 2013. p. 151; with permission; and [*B*] Rafetto LR, Synan W. Surgical management of third molars. Atlas Oral Maxillofacial Surg Clin N Am. 2012;20(2):198; with permission.)

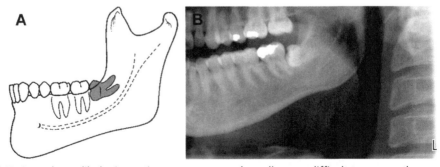

Fig. 3. (*A*) Horizontal mandibular impaction; uncommon and usually more difficult to remove than a mesioangular impaction. (*B*) Radiograph of horizontal impacted third molar. (*From* [*A*] Hupp JR. Principles of management of impacted teeth. In: Hupp JR, Ellis E III, Tucker MR, editors. Contemporary oral and maxillofacial surgery. 6th edition. Philadelphia: Elsevier; 2013. p. 151–2; with permission; and [*B*] Rafetto LR, Synan W. Surgical management of third molars. Atlas Oral Maxillofacial Surg Clin N Am. 2012;20(2):199; with permission.)

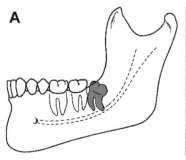
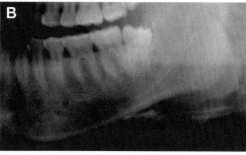

Fig. 4. (*A*) Distoangular mandibular impaction; uncommon and usually the most difficult to remove of the 4 types of mandibular third molar impactions. This difficulty is caused by the path of withdrawal into the ramus and often the close proximity of the mesial root to the distal root of the second molar. (*B*) Radiograph of distoangular mandibular third molar. (*From* [A] Hupp JR. Principles of management of impacted teeth. In: Hupp JR, Ellis E III, Tucker MR, editors. Contemporary oral and maxillofacial surgery. 6th edition. Philadelphia: Elsevier; 2013. p. 152; with permission; and [*B*] Rafetto LR, Synan W. Surgical management of third molars. Atlas Oral Maxillofacial Surg Clin N Am. 2012;20(2):199; with permission.)

angulation of the long axis of the third molar or its degree of depth of impaction. These systems may provide a preliminary analysis of the potential surgical difficulty that may be encountered during removal of third molars. However, astute clinicians will also pay close attention to the other aforementioned factors.

Winter Classification of Impacted Third Molars

This system classifies impacted third molars according to angulation of the long axis of the impacted third molar with respect to the long axis of the second molar (**Figs. 1–6**).

Pell and Gregory Classification of Impacted Mandibular Third Molar

This system is based on the relationship of the anterior border of the ramus to the impacted tooth. Surgical removal usually becomes more difficult as more of the third molar is embedded in the ramus (**Fig. 7**).

Pell and Gregory Classification of Maxillary and Mandibular Third Molars

This system is based on the relationship of the impacted tooth to the occlusal surface of the adjacent second molar. Typically, the deeper the impaction, the more difficult it is to remove (**Fig. 8**).

Classification System Based on Dental Procedure Codes (ie, American Dental Association Current Dental Terminology Codes)

These codes focus on the degree of impaction based on clinical and radiographic interpretation of the type of tissue overlying the impacted tooth (**Figs. 9–12**).

CLINICAL EVALUATION

A clinical examination should start by obtaining the patient's medical history. This evaluation usually begins by determining the patient's chief complaint and then eliciting the history

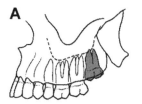
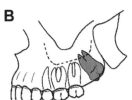
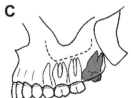
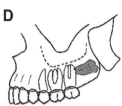

Fig. 5. (*A*) Vertical impaction of maxillary third molar, the most common maxillary third molar impaction. (*B*) Distoangular impaction of maxillary third molar. (*C*) Mesioangular impaction of maxillary third molar. (*D*) Horizontal impaction of maxillary third molar, the least common maxillary third molar impaction. (*Modified from* Hupp JR. Principles of management of impacted teeth. In: Hupp JR, Ellis E III, Tucker MR, editors. Contemporary oral and maxillofacial surgery. 6th edition. St. Louis: Mosby; 2013. p. 158; with permission.)

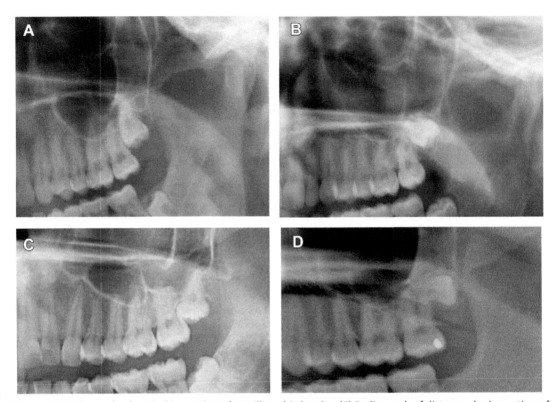

Fig. 6. (*A*) Radiograph of vertical impaction of maxillary third molar. (*B*) Radiograph of distoangular impaction of maxillary third molar. (*C*) Radiograph of mesioangular impaction of maxillary third molar. (*D*) Radiograph of horizontal impaction of maxillary third molar. (*Modified from* Rafetto LR, Synan W. Surgical management of third molars. Atlas Oral Maxillofacial Surg Clin N Am. 2012;20(2):200; with permission.)

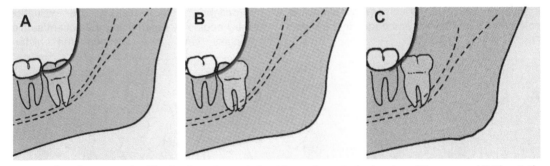

Fig. 7. Pell and Gregory classification based on relationship to the anterior border of the ramus. (*A*) Class I: the mandibular third molar has sufficient space anterior to the anterior border of the ramus to erupt. The whole crown of the third molar is anterior to the anterior border. (*B*) Class II: the distal portion of the third molar crown is covered by bone from the ascending ramus. (*C*) Class III: the third molar crown is completely embedded in bone posterior to the anterior border of the ramus. (*From* Hupp JR. Principles of management of impacted teeth. In: Hupp JR, Ellis E III, Tucker MR, editors. Contemporary oral and maxillofacial surgery. 6th edition. Philadelphia: Elsevier; 2019. p. 152–3; with permission.)

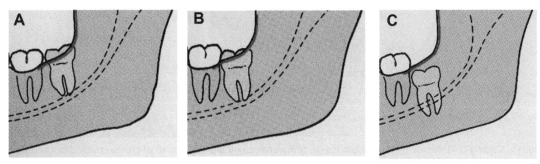

Fig. 8. Depth classification of maxillary and mandibular third molars. Surgery usually becomes more difficult as the depth of impaction increases. (*A*) Class A: occlusal plane of the third molar is at or above the occlusal plane of the second molar. (*B*) Class B: occlusal plane of the third molar is between the occlusal plane and cervical line of the second molar. (*C*) Class C: occlusal plane of the third molar is beneath the cervical line of the second molar. (*From* Hupp JR. Principles of management of impacted teeth. In: Hupp JR, Ellis E III, Tucker MR, editors. Contemporary oral and maxillofacial surgery. 6th edition. Philadelphia: Elsevier; 2013. p. 152–3; with permission.)

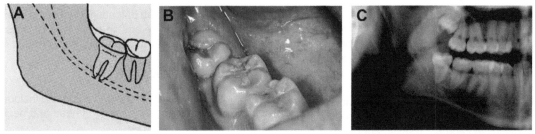

Fig. 9. Code D7220: removal of impacted tooth, soft tissue. (*A*) Occlusal surface of tooth is covered by soft tissue. Surgery requires reflection of a mucoperiosteal flap. (*B*) Soft tissue impacted mandibular third molar. (*C*) Radiograph of soft tissue impacted mandibular third molar. (*From* [*A*] Hupp JR. Principles of management of impacted teeth. In: Hupp JR, Ellis E III, Tucker MR, editors. Contemporary oral and maxillofacial surgery. 6th edition. Philadelphia: Elsevier; 2013. p. 157; with permission; and [*B, C*] Rafetto LR, Synan W. Surgical management of third molars. Atlas Oral Maxillofacial Surg Clin N Am. 2012;20(2):201; with permission.)

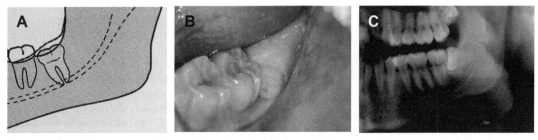

Fig. 10. Code D7230: removal of impacted tooth, partially bony. (*A*) Part of crown covered by bone. Surgery requires reflection of mucoperiosteal flap and removal of bone. (*B*) Partial bone impacted mandibular third molar. (*C*) Radiograph of partial bone impacted mandibular third molar. (*From* [*A*] Hupp JR. Principles of management of impacted teeth. In: Hupp JR, Ellis E III, Tucker MR, editors. Contemporary oral and maxillofacial surgery. 6th edition. Philadelphia: Elsevier; 2013. p. 157; with permission; and [*B, C*] Rafetto LR, Synan W. Surgical management of third molars. Atlas Oral Maxillofacial Surg Clin N Am. 2012;20(2):202; with permission.)

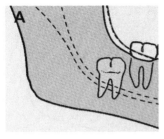
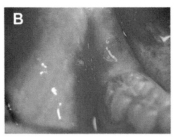
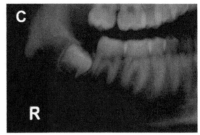

Fig. 11. Code D7240: removal of impacted tooth, completely bony. (*A*) Most or all of crown covered by bone. Surgery requires reflection of a mucoperiosteal flap and removal of bone. (*B*) Complete bone impacted mandibular third molar. (*C*) Radiograph of complete bone impacted mandibular third molar. (*From* [*A*] Hupp JR. Principles of management of impacted teeth. In: Hupp JR, Ellis E III, Tucker MR, editors. Contemporary oral and maxillofacial surgery. 6th edition. Philadelphia: Elsevier; 2013. p. 157; with permission; and [*B, C*] Rafetto LR, Synan W. Surgical management of third molars. Atlas Oral Maxillofacial Surg Clin N Am. 2012;20(2):203; with permission.)

regarding the chief complaint or present illness. This information can give insight as to whether or not the patient is in pain or discomfort and is seeking urgent care versus being asymptomatic and seeking consultation regarding elective care.

The medical history should include a review of any existing systemic disorders, previous surgeries and hospitalizations, medications, allergies, and social history. Patients should be assessed for undergoing certain therapies such as radiation therapy or bisphosphonate therapy, which may have a detrimental effect on bone and soft tissue healing. Any previous anesthesia exposure should be discussed and an assessment of the patient's level of anxiety should be performed.

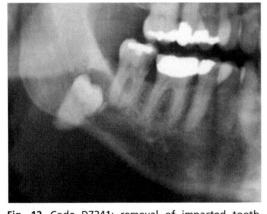

Fig. 12. Code D7241: removal of impacted tooth, completely bony with unusual surgical complications. Radiograph of deep full bone impacted mandibular third molar. Most or all of the crown is covered by bone and unusually difficult or complicated because of factors such as nerve dissection required, separate closure of maxillary sinus required, or aberrant tooth position.

Increasing age and systemic comorbidities have the potential of increasing the degree of difficulty associated with surgery. Therefore, a thorough medical history helps the surgeon determine the patient's American Society of Anesthesiologists status and whether or not the patient is a candidate for surgery either as an outpatient or hospital inpatient. It also helps determine what type of anesthesia may be required for patient management.

PHYSICAL EXAMINATION

Physical examination of the patient should include a thorough extraoral and intraoral head and neck examination.

EXTRAORAL EXAMINATION

This examination should note any abnormal size or asymmetry about the head and neck. Any suspicious masses or enlargements should be noted along with any changes in color, such as redness, paleness, or purpura. Extraoral palpation should be performed to detect any enlargement or tenderness of salivary glands, lymph nodes, or anatomic spaces. The presence of painful facial swelling or enlarged tender lymph nodes could indicate the presence of an active infection.

A temporomandibular joint (TMJ) examination should be included. The patient should be asked to open as wide as possible and close. The range of motion and maximum opening should be measured to determine normalcy or whether any trismus or deviation is present. At the same time, the size of the oral aperture can be appraised along with the laxity of the soft tissue of the lips and cheeks. As the patient opens and closes, the joints can be palpated to detect tenderness and observed for the presence of joint noises such as clicking, popping, or crepitus. This examination can help determine the existence of any preexisting TMJ disorders and may influence the surgical management of the patient.

INTRAORAL EXAMINATION

This examination should include soft and hard tissue evaluation. The soft tissue of the labial and buccal mucosa, soft and hard palate, gingiva, floor of mouth, tongue, and oropharynx should be inspected for any color changes, swelling, elevated or depressed lesions, masses, or ulcerations. These soft tissues should also be palpated to elucidate any tenderness, firmness, or fluctuance.

The hard tissues, such as teeth, alveolar bone, mandible, and maxilla, should be examined. The overall condition of the teeth should be assessed. Any missing, malposed, or supernumerary teeth should be noted. The alveolar bone, mandible, and maxilla should be evaluated for any asymmetry or enlargement. In addition, a more focused examination of the third molar area is performed.

THIRD MOLAR FOCUSED EXAMINATION

Examination of the third molars should determine the following:

- Eruption status: erupted, partially erupted, completely unerupted
- Position in the arch: any buccal, palatal, or lingual displacement
- Functional status: in occlusion
- Any presence of local infection or inflammation of soft tissue adjacent to third molar (pericoronitis)
- Periodontal status of third molar and adjacent second molar, including probing depths, bleeding on probing, or the ability to detect the third molar with probing
- Presence of caries, restorations, or resorption of third molar or adjacent second molar
- Third molar impingement on second molar
- Available access for surgery and oral hygiene maintenance
- Any limited opening caused by TMJ disorder, small aperture, submucosal fibrosis, scarring
- Thickness of overlying bone
- Any orthodontic considerations
- Any restorative considerations
- Any prosthetic considerations
- Any presurgical considerations

On completion of the clinical examination, any positive findings should be noted and considered during the decision-making process regarding removal or retention of the third molar. This process takes place following an adequate radiographic evaluation.

RADIOGRAPHIC EVALUATION

In addition to a thorough clinical examination, a radiographic evaluation is required to confirm whether disease is associated with the third molar and to assist in the formulation of an appropriate treatment plan. The radiographic images should provide information pertaining to the third molar, the adjacent teeth, the surrounding bone, and adjacent anatomic structures.

Oral surgeons have traditionally used conventional two-dimensional radiographic images such as bitewing, periapical, occlusal, cephalometric, and panoramic radiographs to diagnose and treat patients.

An advantage of an intraoral radiograph (ie, bitewing, periapical) is the sharpness of the image. It is higher than that of a panoramic image, and the magnification factor when using a paralleling technique is around 1.05 with minimal image distortion.[1]

An intraoral periapical radiograph may be sufficient for the assessment of a third molar before surgical removal. The image should show the whole third molar, the size of the follicle, the adjacent second molar, the surrounding bone, and the relation to the inferior alveolar canal (IAC). If there appears to be overlap between the roots of the molar and the IAC, a modification of the tube shift method along the vertical plane can be implemented. This technique was described by Richards.[2] The SLOB (same side lingual, opposite side buccal) rule can be applied.

An advantage of an intraoral occlusal radiograph is the capability to determine whether an impacted third molar is in buccal version or lingual version. This image may also identify the presence of additional roots.

However, there are potential disadvantages of intraoral radiographs. Positioning of the intraoral receptor may be difficult because of the size of the film or digital receptor. The film or receptor can be deflected by the soft tissue in the floor of the mouth. This deflection can cause gagging or discomfort for the patient. Another potential disadvantage is the inability to fully visualize a deeply impacted third molar. In about 25% to 36% of patients, the whole third molar and adjacent anatomic structures are not imaged by the intraoral imaging method.[3,4]

Thus, periapical radiographs tend to be used as a supplement to panoramic radiographs if indicated. They can provide more detailed imaging of caries, root contour, and alveolar bone height adjacent to the second molar.

Orthopantomography (OPG) is still the most common imaging technique for evaluating impacted third molars. It is readily available, inexpensive, and provides visualization of both the upper and lower jaw with minimal discomfort and at a low radiation dose.

OPG can provide information regarding angulation of teeth, number of roots, morphology of roots, and associated hard tissue disorder. It can detect the presence (or absence) of third molars and supernumerary third molars. It can also show the relationship of upper third molars to the maxillary sinus and the proximity of the lower third molar to the IAC, albeit in a two-dimensional view. This evaluation is essential because the anatomic relationship between the mandibular third molar and the IAC may be the most predictable risk factor for inferior alveolar nerve (IAN) injury.[5–8]

Rood and Shehab[9] found 3 radiological diagnostic signs to be significantly related to IAN injury:

1. Darkening of the roots, which has been attributed to impingement of the canal on the tooth root causing a loss of density of the root (**Fig. 13**A). Darkening of the roots has also been attributed to thinning or perforation of the lingual cortex by the roots when evaluated by cone beam computed tomography (CBCT) imaging.[10]
2. Diversion of the IAC. If the IAC changes its direction as it crosses the mandibular third molar, then it is considered to be divergent (**Fig. 13**C).
3. Interruption of the white lines of the IAC (**Fig. 13**D). Interruption of the cortical roof and floor of the IAC may indicate either deep grooving of the root if it appears alone or perforation of the root if the interruption is seen in conjunction with narrowing of the inferior alveolar canal.

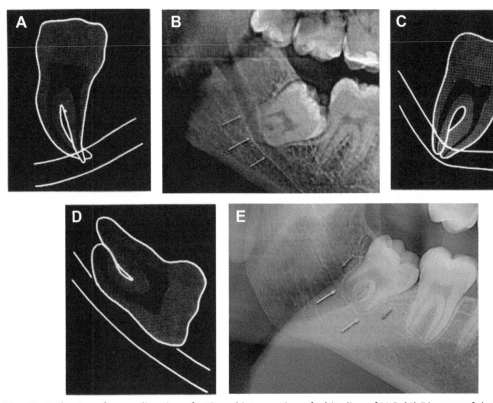

Fig. 13. Darkening of roots, diversion of IAC, and interruption of white line of IAC. (*A*) Diagram of darkening of roots. (*B*) Section of a pantomograph of a lower right third molar with 2 roots showing overlap of the IAC, darkening of roots, and diversion of the canal. Green arrows show diversion of canal. Yellow arrow shows darkening of roots. (*C*) Inferior alveolar canal diversion. (*D*) Interruption of white line of IAC. (*E*) Section of a pantomograph of a lower right third molar showing interruption of the superior white line of the IAC. Yellow arrows show inferior border of IAC. Superior border of IAC appears absent in between the orange arrows. ([*A, C, D*] *From* Rood JP, Shehab BA. The radiographic prediction of inferior alveolar nerve injury in third molar surgery. Br J Oral Maxillofac Surg. 1990;28(1):22; with permission.)

Additional studies seem to confirm that darkening of the roots and interruption of the white lines are the most frequently observed signs of risk of injury to the IAN and most strongly associated with contact between the tooth and the canal.[11–14]

These high-risk signs identified by OPG images are significantly associated with the absence of cortication between the mandibular third molar and the IAC.[15] However, the absence of these signs does not guarantee a lack of close contact.[16]

Another panoramic radiographic marker viewed by clinicians as an indicator of a close relationship between the third molar and the IAC is the vertical relationship between the IAC and the roots of the third molar (**Fig. 14**). The risk of IAN injury is increased significantly in a class I vertical relationship where the superimposition of the third molar roots extend beyond the inferior border of the IAC[17] or when the canal is superimposed over more than one-half of the root.[18,19] It is suspected that the risk of injury increases because of the increased surface area of contact between the third molar and the IAC.

Therefore, when a traditional two-dimensional image reveals 1 or more of these high-risk signs, it may be beneficial to assess the relationship via a three-dimensional evaluation using CBCT, especially if the apices appear to be touching or crossing the inferior border of the canal or floor of the maxillary sinus. CBCT can provide information in the axial, coronal, and sagittal planes and has been shown to be more accurate than panoramic images in identifying direct contact where there is no bony separation between the third molar and the IAC.[5,20–22] It can also identify absence of cortication between maxillary roots and the maxillary sinus.

Several studies have indicated that contact between the IAC and the mandibular third molar seems to occur more frequently when the IAC is positioned on the lingual side of the impacted tooth.[8,22–24] The degree of this proximity or contact between the IAC and the mandibular third molar also seems to be related to the shape of the IAC as seen on a CBCT image.[17,25]

Canal shapes can be described as round, oval, teardrop, or dumbbell. The dumbbell shape has been referred to as invagination, narrowing, or flattening of the canal, presumably caused by intimate contact with the mandibular molar. These dumbbell-shaped canals are seen more frequently on the lingual side of the lower third molar roots and are at high risk of IAN injury.[17,23]

Overall, there seems to be a significant association between the lingual position of the IAC and an increased risk of IAN injury following third molar removal.[8,17,18,23,26] There is also a significant correlation between narrowing/flattening of the IAC at the contact area of the third molar and an increased risk of IAN injury following third molar removal.[17,25,26]

In summation, CBCT images that are associated with higher risk of IAN injury show:

1. Direct contact between the IAC and the roots
2. Absence of IAC cortication
3. Lingual position of the IAC relative to the roots (**Fig. 15**A)
4. Dumbbell shape/narrowing of the IAC (see **Fig. 15**A)
5. Interradicular position of the IAC (**Fig. 15**B)

Additional advantages of CBCT imaging compared with OPG include:

1. More reliability in detecting multiple roots of mandibular third molars (**Fig. 16**B, C) and detecting supernumerary third molars (**Fig. 17**B, C)[24,27,28]
2. Better assessment of the relationship between the maxillary sinus and molar root apices (**Fig. 18**B, C)[29–31]
3. Confirmation of pathosis either at the distal surface of the second molar or in association with the third molar (ie, internal or external resorption, marginal bone loss, cyst formation) (**Figs. 19**B and **20A**)[32]

OPG images may be sufficient in most cases before removal of impacted third molars.

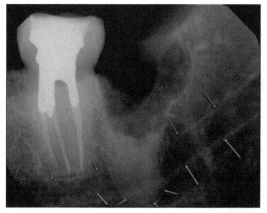

Fig. 14. Section of a pantomograph of a lower left third molar postcoronectomy. There is a class 1 vertical relationship between the IAC and the roots of the third molar. The complete canal is superimposed by the third molar roots; the apex lies beneath the inferior border of the IAC. Orange arrows indicate superior border of IAC. Yellow arrows indicate inferior border of IAC. Green arrows indicate apex of root structure of third molar.

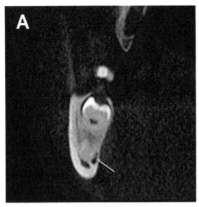
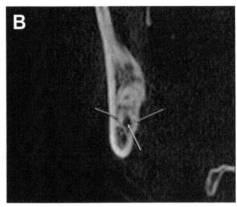

Fig. 15. Coronal views of CBCT showing shape and anatomic position of IAC. (*A*) Lingual dumbbell-shaped IAC. Coronal CBCT image. Yellow arrow indicates a lingual dumbbell-shaped IAC between third molar roots and lingual cortex of mandible. (*B*) Interradicular IAC. Coronal CBCT shows an impacted mandibular right third molar with an interradicular position of the IAC. Yellow arrow indicates inferior alveolar canal is between the mesiobuccal and mesiolingual roots (*orange arrows*) of a 3-rooted impacted mandibular right third molar. Orange arrows indicate mesiobuccal and mesiolingual roots.

However, preoperative assessment using CBCT images may be justified in high-risk cases where a more accurate assessment of the anatomic relationship between the third molar and vital structures is warranted. If this additional information can influence the surgeon's decision-making process and ultimately change the treatment or the treatment outcome for the patient, then it may be deemed beneficial.

Until recently, the use of CBCT did not seem to reduce the number of neurosensory disturbances after surgical removal of mandibular third molars.[17,28,33] In addition, the cost associated with this imaging was estimated to be 3 to 4 times the cost of panoramic imaging.[34,35] The CBCT radiation exposure of the mandible was also estimated to be 4 to 5 times higher than OPG imaging.[36,37] If CBCT imaging were to become routine before surgical removal of mandibular third molars, it has been projected that the annual cancer risk would increase 0.46-fold.[34] Therefore, CBCT should be used only when necessary. The potential benefits need to be weighed against the potential risks of exposure to additional ionizing radiation.

Several recent studies have shown evidence that the use of CBCT can alter the treatment or surgical approach before surgical intervention of mandibular third molars.[15,21,22,32]

However, as yet, there are no standard eligibility criteria that necessitate the use of CBCT examination before removal of third molars. Ultimately,

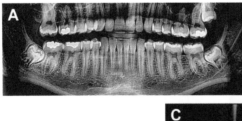
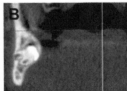
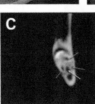

Fig. 16. Impacted mandibular right and left multirooted third molars. (*A*) Cropped panoramic image showing impacted mandibular right and left third molars. (*B*) Coronal CBCT image showing lingual version and multiple roots of the mandibular right and left third molars. (*C*) Coronal CBCT image of the mandibular left third molar showing 3 roots with the IAC positioned interradicularly between a mesiobuccal and mesiolingual root. Yellow arrow points to IAC. Orange arrows show 3 separate roots. Superior orange arrow points to distal root.

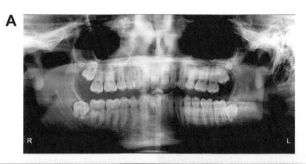

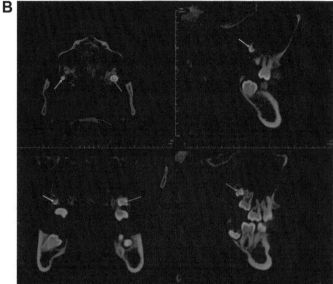

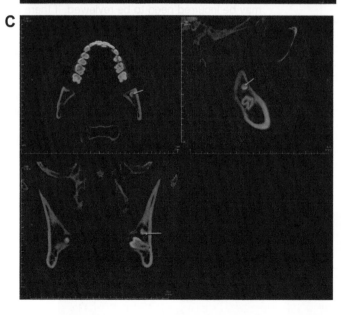

Fig. 17. Impacted maxillary right and left supernumerary third molars and supernumerary mandibular left third molar. (*A*) Pantomograph showing evidence of maxillary right, left, and possibly mandibular left supernumerary third molars. (*B*) Multiplanar reconstruction (MPR) of CBCT. Yellow arrows indicate maxillary right supernumerary third molar. Orange arrows indicate maxillary left supernumerary third molar. (*C*) MPR of CBCT. Green arrows indicate supernumerary mandibular left third molar.

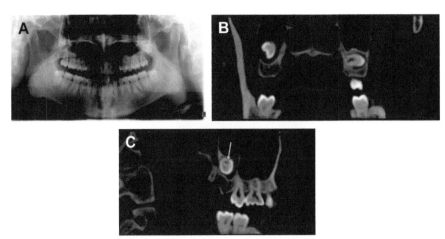

Fig. 18. High impacted maxillary right and left third molars. (*A*) Pantomograph showing high impacted maxillary right and left third molars. Upper right third molar is superimposed by the maxillary sinus. Upper left third molar is horizontally inclined. (*B*) Coronal CBCT image of maxillary right third molar appears to indicate the tooth is alongside the posterior wall of the sinus. (*C*) Sagittal CBCT view confirms the maxillary right third molar is alongside the posterior wall of the maxillary sinus (*arrow*).

further studies and randomized clinical trials will be needed to determine whether CBCT imaging decreases the incidence of complications following the removal of impacted third molars compared with two-dimensional imaging.

TREATMENT PLANNING

On completion of the history, clinical, and radiographic examinations, the clinician should determine whether the patient is symptomatic. If symptomatic, are the symptoms related to the third molars? Is there a presence or absence of disease related to the third molars?

Whether the patient is symptomatic or not, if a disease or aberrant condition is noted, the clinician should strive to make an evidence-based decision regarding what treatment option is most appropriate for management of the third molar

or molars in question. The treatment option should be reasonably effective and the patient should be informed of the potential risks and complications associated with treatment versus no treatment.

In addition, any potential effects on health-related quality-of-life issues and any costs that may be incurred need to be reviewed. If there are any reasonable alternative treatment options, then those too should be discussed.

In most cases, the management of third molars is predicated on the presence or absence of symptoms and disease (**Boxes 1** and **2**).

In an effort to facilitate the clinical decision-making process, Dodson[38] developed an intuitive and useful classification system (**Table 1**).

Via this system, a patient's symptoms are designated as either present (S+) or absent (S−).

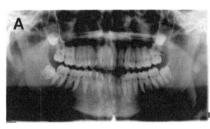
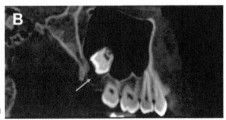

Fig. 19. Imaging of high impacted maxillary right and left third molars. (*A*) Pantomograph showing high impacted maxillary right and left third molars. Uncertainty regarding possible presence of cyst associated with upper left third molar or whether the third molar is in the maxillary sinus. (*B*) Sagittal CBCT image of maxillary left third molar. Orange arrow identifies associated cyst with impacted third molar. Extremely thin sinus floor separates third molar from the sinus cavity.

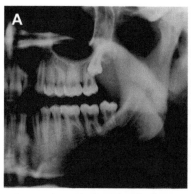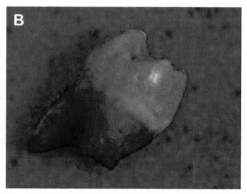

Fig. 20. Imaging and surgical removal of a maxillary second molar with buccal root resorption caused by impacted third molar. (*A*) Section of a panoramic image showing superimposition of roots of the maxillary second molar by the mesioangular impacted third molar. The image does not clearly depict any resorption of the second molar. (*B*) Extracted second molar with obvious buccal root resorption.

Likewise, clinical or radiographic evidence of disease is designated either present (D+) or absent (D−).

It is recommended that the probing status of the third molar be evaluated during the clinical examination. This evaluation is done to assess the periodontal health status of the third molar and adjacent second molar because clinical evidence of periodontal disease may be subtle at times, especially if the third molar is not visible. If it is not visible, but can be detected on probing, this may indicate that the tooth is chronically contaminated with oral flora and prone to developing inflammatory disease. A probing depth (PD) greater than or equal to 4 mm in the third molar region is an indicator of chronic oral inflammation and incipient periodontal disease.

MANAGEMENT OF GROUP A PATIENTS: SYMPTOMS PRESENT (S+) AND DISEASE PRESENT (D+)

Management of these patients is fairly straightforward. The associated disease is determined by clinical, radiographic, and laboratory data. The cause may be one of the more common disorders, such as pericoronitis, caries, or periodontal disease. Less frequent disease entities may be related to root resorption of the adjacent second molar, the presence of an odontogenic cyst or tumor, or traumatic ulceration of buccal mucosa caused by a buccally malpositioned third molar. Treatment depends on the diagnosis, eruption status, and anatomic location of the third molar, associated risk factors, cost, and patient preference. Treatment may range from oral hygiene care to restorative treatment, periodontal therapy, coronectomy, or extraction.

MANAGEMENT OF GROUP B PATIENTS: SYMPTOMS PRESENT (S+) AND DISEASE ABSENT (D−)

Patients presenting with symptoms purportedly related to third molars but showing no evidence of related disease are seen less frequently than patients in groups A, C, and D.[39] Management of these patients can be perplexing.

Box 1
Commonly reported symptoms

- Pain
- Pressure
- Swelling
- Limited opening
- Foul odor or taste
- Shifting or crowding of teeth

Box 2
Disease or pathologic changes associated with third molars

- Inflammation (pericoronitis)
- Caries/resorption of third molar
- Caries/resorption of second molar
- Marginal bone loss, periodontal disease of third molar/second molar
- Infection (cellulitis, abscess)
- Development of cysts or tumors
- Adjacent soft tissue trauma/sequela (ie,. ulcerations, irritative fibroma)

Table 1
Classification of third molars based on symptom and disease status

Symptoms Attributable to Third Molars	Clinical or Radiographic Evidence of Disease	
	Yes (D+)	No (D−)
Yes (S+)	A	B
No (S−)	C	C

A, symptoms present (S+) and disease present (D+) or S+/D+.

B, symptoms present (S+) and disease absent (D−) or S+/D−.

C, no symptoms present (S−) and disease present (D+) or S−/D+.

D, no symptoms present (S−) and disease absent (D−) or S−/D−.

From Dodson TB. The management of the asymptomatic, disease-free wisdom tooth: removal versus retention. Atlas Oral Maxillofacial Surg. Clin. N Am. 2012;20(2):170; with permission.

Sometimes patients in group B report vague pain associated with an erupting third molar. Occasionally, mild inflammation is seen. Typically, there is no evidence of disease radiographically and there appears to be enough dental arch space to accommodate eruption of the tooth into a normal occlusion. In this situation, the discomfort may be attributed to a teethinglike pain. Management may include reassurance, analgesics, perhaps an antimicrobial mouth rinse, and observation.

Other clinical disorders that may be associated with symptomatic, disease-free patients are TMJ disorders, myalgia, and atypical facial pain. Another scenario involves pain referred from an adjacent carious or periodontally compromised tooth.

Ideally, a proper diagnosis is established and then the appropriate treatment can be rendered. If the clinician is unable to identify the source of the symptoms, then observation may be warranted to see whether the source eventually presents itself. Otherwise, the clinician needs to thoroughly review the possible benefits and alternatives to third molar removal and inform the patient of the possibility that the symptoms may not resolve if the third molar is removed.

MANAGEMENT OF GROUP C PATIENTS: SYMPTOMS ABSENT (S−) AND DISEASE PRESENT (D+)

Management of the patients in group C is similar to the management of patients in group A, mainly because the existence of disease associated with the third molar has been established. Therefore, the goal is to treat the disease. Periodically, the use of the term asymptomatic has been ambiguous in the literature. Asymptomatic does not necessarily mean disease free. A patient can be asymptomatic but still have evidence of third molar–associated disorder.

For example, periodontal disorder can be associated with asymptomatic third molars.

Twenty-five percent (82 of 329) of enrolled asymptomatic healthy patients in a 30-month longitudinal study had at least 1 PD equal to or greater than 5 mm on the distal aspect of a second molar or around a third molar. The mean age of the patients was 25 years. PD equal to or greater than 5 mm was also associated with periodontal attachment loss of at least 1 mm in every patient and 2 mm in 80 of 82 patients.[40]

White and colleagues[41] examined the microbial complexes in subgingival plaque taken from the distal surfaces of all second molars in 295 young, periodontally healthy patients with asymptomatic third molars. Periodontal pathogenic orange and red complex microorganisms were detected at levels of at least 10^5 more often if the patients had a PD of at least 5 mm with periodontal attachment loss at the distal of second molars or around third molars at baseline.

These clinical findings of increased periodontal PDs and periodontal attachment loss, coupled with colonization of periodontal pathogens, support the concept that clinical and microbial changes associated with the initiation of periodontitis may manifest first in the third molar region of young adults.[41]

Caries can also be associated with asymptomatic third molars. Prospective studies of occlusal caries in patients with asymptomatic third molars have reported an increasing frequency of caries with age and erupted third molars. At baseline, 28% of 303 asymptomatic patients had at least 1 third molar with occlusal caries (39% in patients ≥25 years old). Lower third molars were affected more often than upper third molars. Less than 2% of third molars had occlusal caries if first molars and second molars were without caries.[42]

Another study that examined the progression of third molar occlusal caries in 211 patients with asymptomatic third molars found that 33% had third molar caries compared with 29% at baseline. This finding was at a median 2.9-year follow-up. The increase in caries occurred primarily in the mandible. Only 1% of the third molars had occlusal caries if the first molars and second molars were caries free.[43]

The incidence of cysts or tumors related to an impacted third molar is low (2.77%–3.1%).[44,45] However, it is common for these patients to be asymptomatic and learn of presence of a pathologic entity during a routine radiographic examination. This situation is another example of being symptom free but disease present.

MANAGEMENT OF GROUP D PATIENTS: SYMPTOMS ABSENT (S−) AND DISEASE ABSENT (D−)

Management of patients in group D remains controversial. Patients in group D typically report no symptoms and there is no clinical or radiographic evidence of disease present. Clinical examination may reveal that the third molar is completely erupted, functional, in occlusion, and has PDs less than 4 mm.

Examination could also reveal that the third molar is impacted, cannot be seen, cannot be probed, and PDs are less than 4 mm.

Erupting, disease-free third molars with potentially adequate space to accommodate a functional tooth can also be included in this group (**Box 3**).

To remove or not remove, that is the question. Is there justification for removal of an asymptomatic, disease-free third molar? The clinician needs to make a decision whether or not the removal of a symptom-free and disease-free impacted third molar is more beneficial than its retention. There needs to be an evaluation of the risk factors involved and a comparison of the potential outcomes. However, clinical expertise alone cannot be relied on because of an inherent risk of bias. Therefore, randomized controlled trials with minimal risk of bias should be used to help guide the decision-making process and assist in the resolution of this controversial topic. Without scientifically valid external evidence, there will always be some ambiguity regarding the management of these patients.

In 2000, the National Institute for Health and Care Excellence (NICE) published guidelines advising that the routine practice of prophylactic removal of disorder-free impacted third molars should be discontinued. NICE's clinical indications for removal of third molar teeth were limited to patients with evidence of disease, including patients who had more than 1 episode of pericoronitis.[46]

Twelve years later, in 2012, McArdle and Renton[47] investigated the effects of the NICE guidelines. Before the implementation of the guidelines, 80% of the National Health Service (NHS) codes for oral surgery procedures were related to the removal of third molars. The average age was 25 years. Ten percent of removal reasons were caries related. Shortly after the implementation of the guidelines, the number of NHS codes for third molar removal decreased 50%. Ten percent of removal reasons were caries. However, 10 years later there was a significant increase in third molar removals: 97% of NHS code numbers for oral surgery were third molar removals. Average age was 32 years and 30% were caries related.

Given the evolution of these statistics, McArdle and Renton[47] concluded that the guidelines did not reduce the number of third molar removals but instead shifted the moment of removal to an older age with a higher incidence of caries. Some retained third molars that are initially asymptomatic and disease free can and do become symptomatic and diseased later in life. The ensuing dilemma is whether a clinician will be able to predict which asymptomatic third molar will become symptomatic and diseased later in life.

There have been numerous studies published regarding indications for removal or retention of asymptomatic third molars. The conflicting results of these studies have made the decision-making process difficult for clinicians. Many studies have been considered inadequate because of flaws pertaining to study design, sample size, or insufficient follow-up time.

Since 2005 the Cochrane group has conducted several systematic reviews[48–50] examining this controversial topic. The conclusion of each review was that there was insufficient evidence to support or refute the routine prophylactic removal of asymptomatic third molars. Evidence may be lacking because it is extremely difficult to conduct randomized controlled trials with follow-up beyond 30 years.

Eventually it may be determined which patients are at high risk of developing disease associated with third molars. This goal may be achievable if the prevalence of disease and associated risk factors are determined in the general population. The

---

Box 3
Characteristics of asymptomatic, disease-free third molars

Patient history:

  No symptoms or vague, nonspecific complaints

Clinical examination:

1. Impacted third molar cannot be seen, cannot be probed, and PDs are less than 4 mm

2. Erupting third molar with adequate space to accommodate a functional tooth

3. Erupted third molar has reached the occlusal plane; is functional and hygienic; with PDs less than 4 mm; with no caries, restorable caries, or restored caries; all 5 surfaces can be examined clinically; as well as attached tissue along the distal surface of the tooth

Radiographic examination:

  No evidence of radiographic disease is present

From Dodson TB. The management of the asymptomatic, disease-free wisdom tooth: removal versus retention. Atlas Oral Maxillofacial Surg. Clin. N Am. 2012;20(2):172; with permission.

prevalence of complications associated with removal of third molars and their risk factors also needs to be determined. If these data can be obtained, then the probability of developing disease and experiencing a complication may become predictable. To date, the evidence from studies investigating these issues indicates the following conclusions:

- The prevalence of caries and periodontal attachment loss greater than 4 mm associated with asymptomatic third molars is high in the older population, whereas the prevalence of cysts and tumors associated with asymptomatic third molars is low in the older population.[51,52]
- The prevalence of periodontal disorders of the distal of second molars adjacent to soft tissue/partial bone impactions is significantly greater than for second molars adjacent to an absent third molar, erupted third molar, or a bony impacted third molar.[53]
- Progression of periodontal disease is often found in the third molar region of asymptomatic patients who have at least PD greater than or equal to 4 mm.[54]
- Almost all resorption and marginal bone loss along the distal aspect of second molars is observed in relation to mesioangular and horizontally positioned third molars.[55]
- The presence of a partially erupted horizontal or mesioangular mandibular third molar is a significant factor for caries on the distal surface of the mandibular second molar.[56–58]
- The periodontal health of a second molar can improve significantly after surgical removal of the adjacent impacted mandibular third molar.[59]

These findings may support the prophylactic removal of asymptomatic third molars in young patients who present with:

- Soft tissue/partially impacted third molars, or
- Bone impacted third molars that are mesioangulated or horizontally positioned and have associated PD greater than 4 mm

Prophylactic removal would not be recommended for fully erupted, functional, third molars with good oral hygiene or to prevent cyst or tumors.

There are other clinical indications that may necessitate the removal of symptom-free, disease-free third molars.

Systemic Health-Related Indications

To date, most studies do not seem to establish a clear cause-effect relationship between oral health and systemic health. In most instances, studies seem to indicate more of an association type of relationship. Therefore, current evidence does not necessarily support the assumption that treatment of oral disease prevents systemic morbidity and mortality.

However, there are systemic physiologic conditions that may adversely affect a patient's health if a third molar is removed. This situation can occur in medical conditions requiring treatment with radiation therapy or bisphosphonates, which can result in osteonecrosis of the jaw.

Radiation Therapy for Head and Neck Malignancies

Radiation therapy is a common modality for treating malignancies of the head and neck. The radiotherapy selectively destroys neoplastic cells. However, normal tissues with rapid turnover rates, such as epithelial cells, endothelial cells, and hematopoietic cells, can also be adversely affected, which can subsequently lead to adverse radiation effects on oral mucosa, salivary glands, mandibular mobility, and bone. Oral mucosa can become erythematous and progress to mucositis. Eventually, the epithelium can become thin and less keratinized, making the mucosa less pliable and prone to ulcerations, which are difficult to heal.

Radiation can induce inflammation of muscle and connective tissue, which can progress to muscle fibrosis and can decrease the patients' ability to open their mouths. Food intake and oral hygiene maintenance can become compromised.

Salivary glands sustain significant damage stemming from the destruction of fine vasculature by the radiation. Patients may develop severe xerostomia, which can lead to a multitude of disorders, including increased susceptibility to mucosal injury and rampant caries.

The radiation effects on bone can also be severe and problematic. The radiation can devitalize bone because of elimination of the fine vasculature within bone. This condition can progress to osteoradionecrosis, where bone becomes nonvital and remaining viable bone may be unable to remodel and repair itself. This condition is more prevalent in the mandible because of its limited vascularity.

The risks of xerostomia and osteoradionecrosis increase dramatically as the dose of radiation increases beyond 50 Gy (5000 rad). Therefore, it may be prudent to remove a partially erupted S−/D− mandibular third molar to prevent the risk of infection and the subsequent debilitating effects of osteoradionecrosis. If possible, this should be performed at least several weeks before initiation of radiotherapy to allow sufficient healing to take place. It may be more prudent to retain a complete bone impacted disease-free third molar and monitor its condition.

Bisphosphonate Therapy for Osteoporosis and Malignant Bone Metastases

Bisphosphonates are drugs that inhibit bone resorption by suppressing the recruitment and activity of osteoclasts. Bisphosphonates can also help control bone loss from metastatic skeletal lesions in patients with cancer. These drugs can remain in the body for years depending on the duration of treatment and type of bisphosphonate used.

Bone deposition and remodeling are significantly compromised in patients receiving bisphosphonates. A potential adverse effect of bisphosphonate therapy is the development of devitalized areas of bone in the jaws, which has been referred to as medication-related osteonecrosis of the jaws (MRONJ). Other medications can also lead to MRONJ, including receptor activator of nuclear factor kappa-B (RANK) ligand inhibitors (denosumab) used for similar indications as bisphosphonates as well as numerous antiangiogenic agents used for cancer treatment.

This condition typically presents with areas of chronically exposed necrotic bone, which are usually painful and difficult to manage. Often, they do not respond to conventional treatment such as debridement and antibiotics or hyperbaric oxygen therapy. Patients receiving intravenous bisphosphonates for management of metastatic skeletal lesions are more susceptible to MRONJ than those who are taking oral bisphosphates for osteoporosis.

Prevention of MRONJ is critical to the management of patients who are taking this medication, especially for cancer-related management. Any questionable third molars should be removed before the institution of bisphosphonate therapy for management of cancer-related metastatic bone disease.

Prosthodontic Indications

If there is an impacted third molar in an area where a removable prosthesis will be seated, it should be considered for removal. The third molar is at risk of irritation by the overlying prosthesis if it is exposed to the oral cavity, covered by soft tissue, or beneath a thin layer or cortical bone. This chronic irritation can lead to inflammation, swelling, and ulceration of the soft tissue. The patient may experience chronic pain and the condition may eventually progress toward a frank infection.

Restorative Indications

A partially impacted third molar may be considered for removal if it is in intimate contact with the distocervical portion of an adjacent second molar that is planned for either a full crown or distal restoration. This situation may simplify the restorative procedure for the clinician and improve the patient's access for oral hygiene maintenance.

Orthodontic Indications

There is justification for the removal of a symptom-free, disease-free (S−/D−) third molar if it is preventing the eruption of a second molar or if additional arch space is required for the distalization of molars.

However, evidence-based research seems to refute the need for prophylactic removal of S−/D− third molars as a means of preventing lower anterior arch crowding or postorthodontic relapse.[60,61] Controversy still exists regarding this subject. Other studies have indicated that insufficient arch space for eruption of third molars can aggravate dental crowding,[62] and patients who have third molars with a Pell and Gregory class III B position at the beginning of root formation, undergo orthodontic treatment, and finish without the use of a retainer have a greater chance of developing crowding of anterior teeth.[63]

Presurgical Indications

Many clinicians consider early removal of impacted mandibular third molars before performing sagittal split ramus osteotomies. This procedure is done with the intention of minimizing the risk of unfavorable fractures, nerve injuries, and postoperative neurosensory disturbances. It is also done to maintain ample bone for rigid fixation.

Some clinicians may advocate the opposite and recommend removal of third molars concomitantly with the sagittal split osteotomy, citing limitations of risk and cost-efficiency.[64,65]

Another presurgical indication for removal of an S−/D− third molar can occur when an impacted third molar is in the line of a mandibular angle fracture and prevents the reduction of the fracture. In this situation, the third molar should be removed because mandibular angle fractures pose a high risk for postoperative complications such as infection and malunion.

Advocating for the removal of asymptomatic, disease-free third molars to prevent jaw fractures is more controversial. The angle of the mandible is a recognized area of reduced bone strength and is more prone to fracture. The lateral and medial cortices of bone approximate each other in this region. As this occurs, the medullary space between them diminishes. This decreased volume of bone can be compounded by the presence of a space-occupying impacted third molar, which can further weaken the angle of the mandible.

However, the incidence of mandibular fractures is low in the general population (11.5 per 100,000 individuals per year).[66] Therefore, it does not seem justifiable to promote prophylactic removal of mandibular third molars based on this variable alone.

The prophylactic removal of S−/D− third molars to prevent cysts and tumors is also controversial. The overall incidence rate of these pathologic lesions is low (2.7%–3.1%), with cysts accounting for 2.14% to 2.31% and tumors 0.61% to 0.79%.[44,45] Malignant tumors are rare. These statistics lean against prophylactic removal. In contrast, 2 other separate studies have shown a statistically high incidence (23%–24%) of dentigerous cystic changes in radiographically normal–appearing follicles around impacted mandibular third molars.[67,68] These statistics could weigh in favor of prophylactic removal of impacted mandibular third molars because the treatment of odontogenic cysts and tumors can be devastating to the patients, both from cost and quality-of-life standpoints.

At present, there still seems to be insufficient evidence available to advocate for or against the routine removal of asymptomatic, disease-free impacted third molars. Therefore, clinicians need to review the risks and benefits of extractions versus retention and take into consideration the patients' own preferences. If the decision is made to retain an asymptomatic, disease-free, impacted third molar, clinical assessment at regular intervals is advised to either prevent or minimize undesirable outcomes.

SURGICAL MANAGEMENT

Once a decision has been made to proceed with surgery, a proper and detailed surgical plan should be formulated. The surgeon will require instrumentation, which will help enable performance of the surgery in a safe and efficient manner. It will also be necessary to adhere to sound surgical principals in an effort to achieve a positive outcome.

ARMAMENTARIUM

The surgeon should have an in-depth knowledge of the instrumentation available and its proper usage. The surgical equipment may include nondisposable and disposable instruments (**Figs. 21** and **22**).

Box 4 lists the most common instruments used and their purpose.

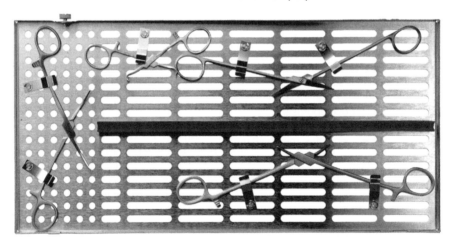

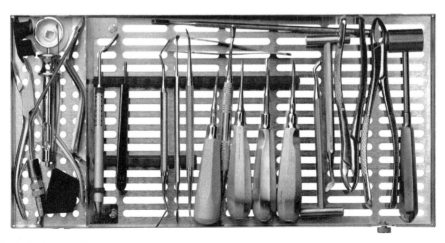

Fig. 21. Sterile instrument tray.

BASIC SURGICAL TECHNIQUE

The removal of an impacted third molar should proceed in an orderly, stepwise fashion. The first step should be to provide adequate access and visibility of the surgical site. This step is accomplished by reflection of a full-thickness mucoperiosteal flap. Various designs of soft tissue flaps have been advocated for a variety of reasons. All should follow sound principles of flap design.

SURGICAL FLAP

The surgical approach to access an impacted third molar often begins with an incision after appropriate anesthesia has been delivered. Two of the most commonly used flap designs are the envelope flap and the 3-cornered (triangular) flap. Both provide favorable access for the buccal-occlusal removal of impacted third molars.

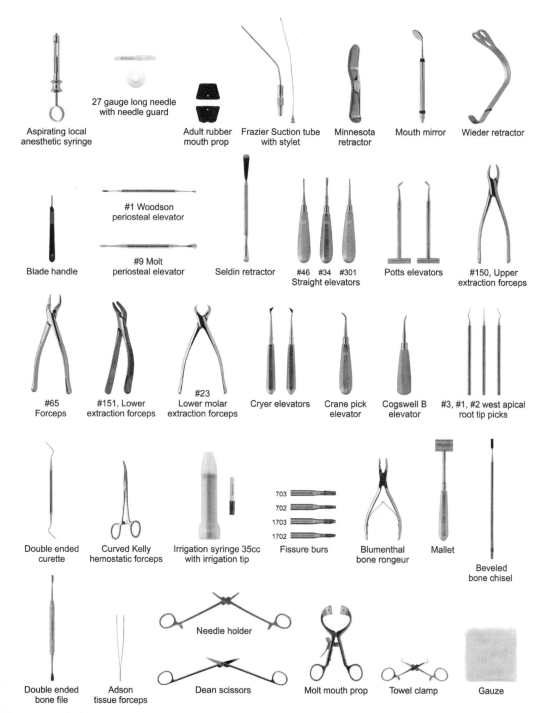

Fig. 22. Surgical instruments.

Box 4
The most common instruments used and their purpose

Instrument	Purpose
Scalpel (composed of a blade and handle, most commonly used blade is #15)	Primary instrument used to make incision
Scissors	Used to undermine or cut soft tissue, cut sutures
Eg, Metzenbaum, Dean	
Periosteal elevators	Used to reflect a mucoperiosteal flap off the bone
Eg, #1 Woodson, #9 Molt	
Soft tissue retractors	Can retract the cheek, lips, and mucoperiosteal flap
Eg, right angle retractors, Minnesota retractor, Seldin retractor	
Tongue retractor	Keeps tongue protected and away from the surgical field
Eg, mouth mirror, tongue depressor, Weider retractor	
Instruments to Grasp Soft Tissue	
Adson tissue forceps College pliers	Stabilize soft tissue when incising or suturing the tissue
Instruments to Control Hemorrhage	
Curved Kelly hemostatic forceps (curved hemostat)	Used to clamp small blood vessels and ligate with suture
Electrocautery	Used for thermal coagulation of soft tissue
Pressure packs	Gauze used to tamponade bleeding
Instruments to Remove Bone	
Rongeurs bone forceps (side cutting, end and side cutting)	Used to trim bone
Mallet and chisel	Removes bone; occasionally used to remove palatal and lingual tori and exostosis
Bur and handpiece (high speed and high torque)	Used to remove bone quickly and under copious irrigation to prevent overheating of the underlying bone. Must not exhaust air into the operative field to prevent tissue emphysema
#6, #8 round burs	Used to remove bone and section teeth
#702, #703 fissure burs	
#1701, #1703 fissure burs	
Double-ended bone file	Smooths bone via a pulling motion
Instruments to Remove Soft Tissue from Bone Cavity	
Double-ended curette	Double-ended instrument used to remove granulomas or cysts from bone cavities
Curved hemostatic forceps	Removes soft tissue debris
Rongeur forceps	Removes soft tissue debris
Instruments for Suturing	
Needle holder	Holds and directs suture needle
Suture needles (half circle or three-eighths circle in shape, cutting or tapered)	Used to approximate tissue
Suture material (classified by diameter: 3.0, 4.0)	Used to approximate tissue and hold in place
Resorbable: plain gut resorbs in 3–5 d, chromic gut resorbs in 10 d	
Nonresorbable: silk, nylon, stainless steel	
Monofilament: plain gut, chromic gut, nylon	
Polyfilament: silk, polylactic	
Instruments to Hold the Mouth Open	
Rubber molt prop	Inserted between the maxillary and mandibular teeth. Helps to support the mandible and prevent stress or torquing of the TMJ

(continued on next page)

Box 4
(continued)

Instrument	Purpose
Molt mouth prop	Operates via a ratchet-type action. Can open the mouth wider as the handle is squeezed. Can be useful in patients who have trismus
Instruments for Irrigation	
Sterile irrigation water	Cools the surgical bur and prevents overheating of bone. Also prevents clogging of the flutes of the bur
Plastic 35-mL syringe with irrigation tip Eg, smooth, blunted, 18-gauge irrigation tip	Cools the surgical bur and prevents overheating of bone. Also prevents clogging of the flutes of the bur
Instruments for Suctioning	
Frazier surgical suction tube	Provides visualization of surgical site by evacuation of pooled blood, saliva, and irrigation fluid. Small hole in the handle allows operator to control the degree of suction force supplied by the suction apparatus
Wire stylet	Cleans debris from lumen of the suction tip
Suction tubing and vacuum	Evacuates fluid and debris from mouth and transports to a vacutainer
Towel clamp	Clamps patient's drapes and can support the suction tubing
Instruments Used to Luxate and Remove Teeth	
Dental elevators	Instruments used to luxate (loosen) teeth from the alveolar bone and remove broken or sectioned roots. These tools can potentially minimize the occurrence of fractured roots, teeth, and bone
Straight elevators	301 (small), 46 (medium), and 34 (large)
Straight elevators with angled blades Eg, paired Potts elevators	Used to access and elevate posterior maxillary molars
Triangular elevators Eg, paired Cryer elevators	Used via a wheel-and-axle motion to elevate and remove a retained root adjacent to an empty socket
Pick-type elevators Eg, Crane pick, Cogswell B	A Crane pick or Cogswell B can act as a lever to elevate a root or tooth from the socket via a purchase point in the tooth. A hole is made in the tooth adjacent to the bone with a bur. The pick leverages off the buccal plate to elevate the tooth or root. This is more applicable to mandibular molars
Root tip picks 1, 2, 3	These are thin, fine instruments used to tease root tips from the socket by wedging the tip of the instrument into the periodontal ligament space between the root tip and alveolar bone
Extraction forceps Eg, maxillary universal forceps, #150 maxillary root forceps, #65 mandibular universal forceps, #151 mandibular cow-horn forceps #23	Instruments used to remove teeth from the alveolar bone

An envelope flap is initiated with a #15 blade. The incision is made intrasulcularly around the necks of the adjacent teeth. When this type of flap is used to expose an impacted mandibular third molar, it may extend posteriorly from the mesial aspect of the first molar up to the anterior ramus. A lateral (buccal) divergent incision is made at this point to minimize risk of injury to the lingual nerve.

Sometimes a 3-cornered (triangular) flap may be performed in an attempt to gain increased exposure of the operatory site with less subsequent tissue trauma. The vertical releasing incision of this design may be placed either anteriorly or just posteriorly to the second molar. It is the clinician's preference whether or not to include a papilla in the design. A papilla can provide a definitive stop while the flap is repositioned and sutured, which may reposition the flap more precisely.

On completion of the incision, the flap is reflected subperiosteally with a sweeping motion of a mucoperiosteal elevator. Reflection of the flap is carried to the edge of the external oblique ridge of the mandible. Once fully reflected, the flap can be retracted with a Minnesota retractor just lateral to the external oblique ridge (**Figs. 23–25**).

BONE REMOVAL

Once the mucoperiosteal flap has been reflected, the clinician needs to determine how much bone needs to be removed to gain access to the impacted tooth. The amount of bone is determined by (1) angulation of the tooth, (2) depth of the impaction, (3) number and morphology of the roots, and (4) size and density of the mandible.

Only enough bone should be removed to provide visibility and access to perform sectioning, if needed, and elevation of the crown and roots from the bony crypt. Usually a bur and a high-speed handpiece are used for bone removal. A mallet and a chisel are an alternative to a handpiece, but are perhaps better reserved for removal of thin, porous bone in the maxilla rather than the dense, cortical bone of the mandible. Gross bone removal can be performed with either a 703-fissure bur or a #8 round bur.

Bone reduction is typically performed over the occlusal aspect of the tooth and along the buccal bone adjacent to the crown. The extent of buccal bone removal can vary. It often extends either to or just beyond the height of contour of the crown. However, it may approach the cervical margin of the tooth if deemed appropriate.

Final bone removal may be accomplished with a narrower 702-fissure bur. This bur can create a buccal bone trough between the cortical plate of bone and the tooth. The blade of a dental elevator such as a #301 can be positioned in the trough and rotated, which can create a lever-type force to initiate elevation of the tooth from the alveolar bone (**Fig. 26**).

Rarely is bone ever removed from the lingual or palatal aspect of the impacted third molar. This precautionary measure helps avoid injury to the lingual nerve and is usually not necessary in the maxilla because of the thin buccal plate of bone and the buccally inclined path of withdrawal of maxillary third molars.

TOOTH SECTIONING

After the tooth has been adequately exposed, a decision is made whether or not sectioning of the tooth is required. This decision is usually based on angulation of the tooth and the morphology of its roots. Other determining factors may include size and density of the mandibular bone, age of the patient, presence and size of a dental follicle, and proximity to vital structures such as the IAN and maxillary sinus.

If sectioning is deemed necessary, it is typically performed either with a fissure bur or round bur. Sectioning of mandibular third molars is more common than sectioning maxillary third molars, and the extent of sectioning can vary. Sometimes only a portion of the crown needs to be sectioned and removed, whereas other situations may necessitate vertical sectioning of the tooth into mesial and distal halves. More complex impactions may require removal of the crown followed by sectioning of the roots, or perhaps multiple sectioning of the crown followed by additional sectioning of the roots.

While sectioning an impacted mandibular third molar, caution should be exercised that the cut is not carried through the entire tooth. This precaution ensures that the lingual cortex, and thus the lingual nerve, is not encroached on by the bur, otherwise there is the potential risk of injury to the lingual nerve.

Similarly, the depth of the cut should not extend past the furcation in order to minimize the risk of injury to the IAN. Avoidance of adjacent crowns and roots of other teeth also needs to be considered while sectioning third molars.

Occasionally, purchase points may be placed during the sectioning of third molars. A purchase point needs to be large enough and deep enough to accommodate the tip of a Cogswell B or Crane pick elevator. If it does not meet these requirements, then there is a high likelihood of fracture of the tooth segments during elevation. Excessive force should also be avoided while elevating. If too

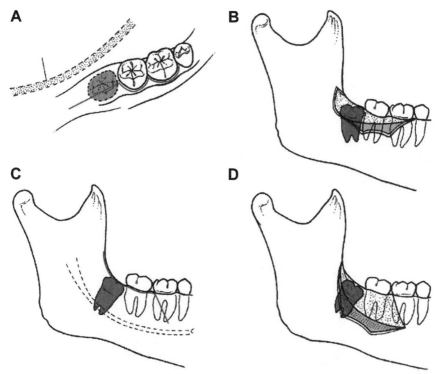

Fig. 23. (*A*) Envelope incision is commonly used to reflect soft tissue for the removal of impacted mandibular third molars. The posterior extension should diverge laterally to avoid injury to the lingual nerve. (*B*) Envelope incision. Soft tissue is reflected laterally to expose bone overlying the impacted tooth. (*C*) Three-cornered flap incision. Releasing incision is made at the mesial aspect of the second molar. (*D*) Three-cornered flap, lateral reflection of soft tissue exposing bone overlying the impacted tooth. (*From* Hupp JR. Principles of management of impacted teeth. In: Hupp JR, Ellis E III, Tucker MR, editors. Contemporary oral and maxillofacial surgery. 6th edition. Philadelphia: Elsevier; 2013. p. 172; with permission.)

much force is used, there is the possibility of bone or jaw fracture, soft tissue trauma, and displacement of roots and teeth.

Figs. 28–36 show some examples of third molar sectioning.

VERTICAL IMPACTIONS

This type of impaction may only require a disto-buccal bone trough. The tooth may be delivered with lever-type elevation via a straight elevator. Otherwise, the tooth may be divided in half along the vertical axis and each half removed separately (**Fig. 27**).

MESIOANGULAR IMPACTIONS

If it is a slight mesioangular impaction, the crown may be divided obliquely with the distal portion of the crown removed. The remainder of the tooth may be elevated and delivered (**Figs. 28** and **29**). Otherwise, the tooth may be divided in half along

the long vertical axis and each half removed separately (**Figs. 30** and **31**).

HORIZONTAL IMPACTIONS

The crown is sectioned from its roots and removed. The roots are sectioned and removed into the space occupied by the crown (**Figs. 32** and **33**).

DISTOANGULAR IMPACTIONS

The crown may be sectioned from the roots with the roots being elevated into the space vacated by the crown. Sometimes the roots themselves may need to be sectioned from each other and removed separately (**Figs. 34–36**).

REMOVAL OF IMPACTED MAXILLARY THIRD MOLARS

Sectioning is often not required. An envelope flap is usually sufficient to access a low, soft tissue–

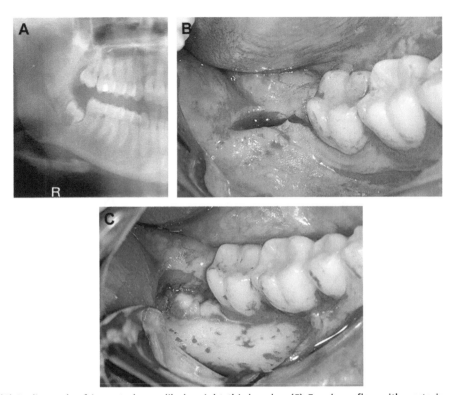

Fig. 24. (*A*) Radiograph of impacted mandibular right third molar. (*B*) Envelope flap with posterior divergent lateral incision. (*C*) Envelope flap, soft tissue reflected laterally. Flap retracted by Minnesota retractor. (*From* Rafetto LR, Synan W. Surgical management of third molars. Atlas Oral Maxillofacial Surg Clin N Am 2012;20(2):205; with permission.)

type impaction. A 3-cornered (triangular) flap may be necessary to access a high partial or full bone type of impaction (**Figs. 37–39**).

WOUND CLOSURE

After the impacted third molar has been removed, the socket should be examined for presence of a dental follicle or its remnants. This follicle can be managed with curettage by a double-ended curette and removed by grasping it with a curved hemostat or rongeurs. The bone should be inspected for any sharp or rough edges, which can be removed and smoothed with a rongeur and bone file. Thorough irrigation of the site should be performed with sterile saline. This irrigation should be done all along the exposed surgical site and along the underside and full depth of the reflected mucoperiosteal flap. Evacuation of all bone chips and debris helps reduce the risk of postoperative infection.

Lastly, the wound should be inspected for any signs of residual bleeding. Specific bleeding points, whether they are in bone or soft tissue,

should be controlled. This control can be achieved via direct pressure or ligation, application of a hemostatic agent, or electrocautery.

On completion of these final postoperative checks, the flap may be sutured. The flap should be repositioned into its original preoperative position and sutured, usually with 2 or 3 resorbable sutures. Patients seem to prefer resorbable sutures because they do not want the site manipulated within a short time frame after surgery.

ALTERNATE SURGICAL TECHNIQUES FOR MANAGING IMPACTED THIRD MOLARS

Sometimes an alternate surgical approach may be warranted to remove an impacted third molar. This option may be indicated in situations where the roots of the third molar are in intimate contact with the IAN canal or where the nerve itself may course through the roots of the molar.

Another indication for an alternate surgical approach is when surgical access is compromised via a traditional buccal/lateral approach. This

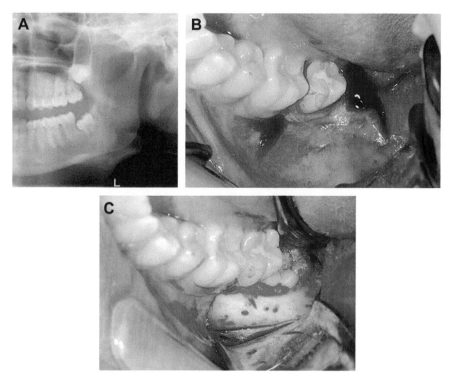

Fig. 25. (*A*) Radiograph of impacted mandibular left third molar. (*B*) Three-cornered flap with anterior vertical release and posterior divergent lateral incision. (*C*) Three-cornered flap, soft tissue reflected laterally. Flap retracted by Minnesota retractor. (*From* Rafetto LR, Synan W. Surgical management of third molars. Atlas Oral Maxillofacial Surg Clin N Am. 2012;20(2):205; with permission.)

indication can occur where there is an aberrant positioning of the impacted third molar. The molar may be deeply impacted and lie either partially or totally below the IAN canal, or it may be located in the ramus of the mandible. Because of its unusual location, an excessive amount of bone removal may be required to remove the tooth. This excessive bone removal can subsequently lead to displacement of either the tooth or a portion of the tooth into an adjacent anatomic space, such as the submandibular, sublingual, or pterygoid space. Excessive bone removal can also weaken the mandible and cause an immediate or delayed mandibular fracture.[69–71]

If the risk of these potential complications seems to be high, then other techniques should

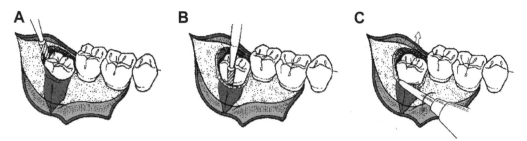

Fig. 26. Surgical removal of impacted teeth. (*A*) Soft tissue flap reflected to expose vertical impacted tooth. If bone is overlying occlusal surface, then remove bone with a fissure bur. (*B*) Bone along the buccodistal aspect of the crown of a vertically impacted tooth is removed to the cervical line with a fissure bur. (*C*) The edge of a small straight elevator is placed in the buccal groove of bone and rotated to elevate the tooth upward. (*Modified from* Hupp JR. Principles of management of impacted teeth. In: Hupp JR, Ellis E III, Tucker MR, editors. Contemporary oral and maxillofacial surgery. 6th edition. Philadelphia: Elsevier; 2013. p. 173; with permission.)

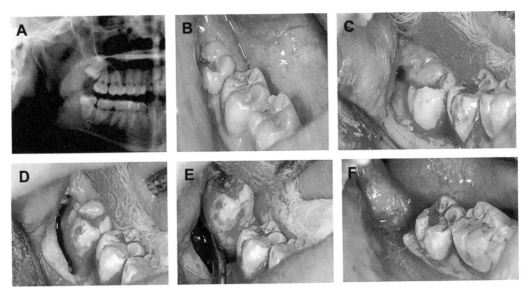

Fig. 27. (*A*) Panorex of vertical soft tissue impaction right mandibular third molar. (*B*) Vertical soft tissue impacted right mandibular third molar. (*C*) Envelope flap incision. (*D*) Distobuccal bone removed along cervical margin. (*E*) Small straight elevator placed in buccal trough of bone, rotated, tooth elevated and delivered. (*F*) Flap sutured. ([*A, B*] *From* Rafetto LR, Synan W. Surgical management of third molars. Atlas Oral Maxillofacial Surg Clin N Am. 2012;20(2):207; with permission; and [*C–F*] Rafetto LR, Synan W. Surgical management of third molars. Atlas Oral Maxillofacial Surg Clin N Am. 2012;20(2):208; with permission.)

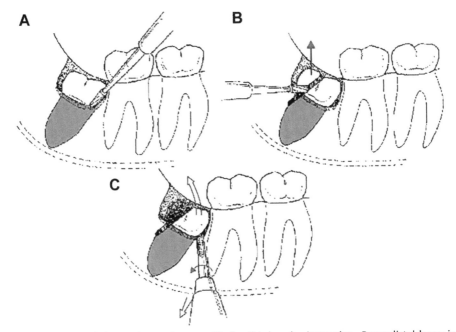

Fig. 28. (*A*) Removal of a slight mesioangular mandibular third molar impaction. Buccodistal bone is removed along the cervical line to expose the crown of the tooth. (*B*) Distal aspect of crown may be sectioned from tooth. (*C*) After distal portion of crown is removed, a small straight elevator is inserted into purchase point along the mesial aspect of the third molar. The tooth is delivered with rotational and lever motion of the elevator. (*From* Hupp JR. Principles of management of impacted teeth. In: Hupp JR, Ellis E III, Tucker MR, editors. Contemporary oral and maxillofacial surgery. 6th edition. Philadelphia: Elsevier; 2013. p. 163; with permission.)

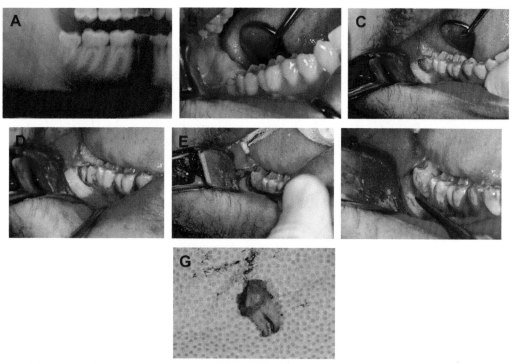

Fig. 29. (*A*) Panorex of slight mesioangular mandibular third molar impaction. (*B*) Mesioangular impacted third molar. (*C*) Envelope flap reflected and buccodistal bone trough created along cervical margin of crown. (*D*) Distal aspect of crown sectioned with fissure bur. (*E*) Distal portion of crown removed. (*F*) Remainder of tooth elevated with a straight elevator. (*G*) Tooth delivered.

be considered. These techniques may include lingual split technique/lingual corticotomy, mandibular sagittal split osteotomy (MSSO), extraoral approach, and partial odontectomy/coronectomy. Each of these techniques may have its own risks and complications.

An innovative recommendation was made by Abu-El Naaj and colleagues[72] in 2010. They presented a new third molar classification (TMC) system for the surgical management of mandibular third molars. The premise behind this new classification was to help surgeons in the decision-making process during treatment planning with the intention of limiting risks associated with extraction of impacted mandibular third molars. The mandibular third molar is classified according to its position relative to the mandibular canal using a standard panoramic radiograph. Surgical approach for removal depends upon the third molar classification type (TMC).

There are 3 major types: TMCI, TMCII, and TMCIII. TMCII is subdivided into TMCIIa and TMCIIb (**Figs. 40–42, Table 2**).

LINGUAL SPLIT TECHNIQUE

This technique promotes the delivery of a mandibular third molar from the alveolus in a distolingual direction. This delivery is accomplished via the reflection of buccal and lingual mucoperiosteal flaps and the use of 3-mm and 5-mm chisels. Potential risks and complications include displacement of the tooth, postoperative patient discomfort, bone exposure, and possible injury to the lingual nerve.

After a comprehensive review of the literature, Pichler and Beirne[73] reported that there was a 3-fold increase in the incidence of permanent lingual nerve injury involving a bur technique with a lingual flap compared with a bur technique without a lingual flap.[73] Due to concern regarding potential injury of the lingual nerve, this technique is used infrequently in the United States.

MANDIBULAR SAGITTAL SPLIT OSTEOTOMY

The MSSO is a commonly used procedure in orthognathic surgery. Some surgeons have

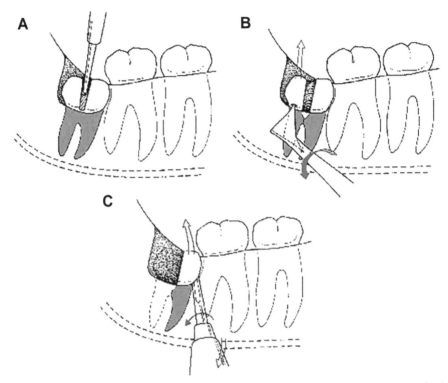

Fig. 30. (*A*) Buccodistal bone removed to expose crown of mesioangular impacted mandibular third molar. (*B*) Occasionally it is necessary to section the entire tooth into 2 halves. Distal half of tooth removed via elevator. (*C*) Elevator is inserted into a purchase point along the mesial half. The remaining mesial half is delivered with rotational and lever motion of the elevator. (*From* Hupp JR. Principles of management of impacted teeth. In: Hupp JR, Ellis E III, Tucker MR, editors. Contemporary oral and maxillofacial surgery. 6th edition. Philadelphia: Elsevier; 2013; with permission.)

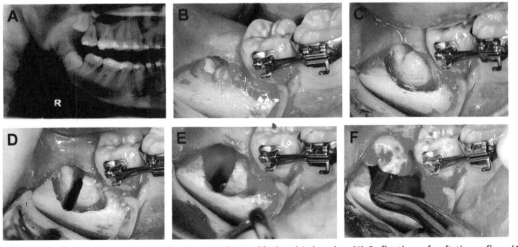

Fig. 31. (*A*) Radiograph of mesioangular impacted mandibular third molar. (*B*) Reflection of soft tissue flap. (*C*) Buccodistal bone removed to expose crown. (*D*) Mesioangular third molar sectioned in half vertically. (*E*) Distal half of crown removed. (*F*) Mesial half of crown removed with elevator. (*From* Rafetto LR, Synan W. Surgical management of third molars. Atlas Oral Maxillofacial Surg Clin N Am. 2012;20(2):210; with permission.)

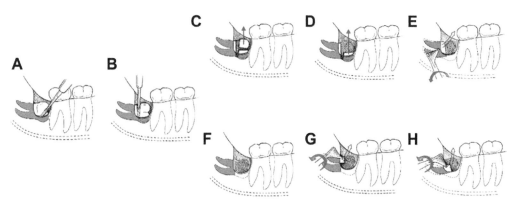

Fig. 32. (*A*) During removal of a horizontal impaction approximately two-thirds to three-fourths of the buccal and distal bone overlying the crown is removed. The inferior one-third to one-quarter of bone is often left intact. (*B*) Crown is sectioned from the roots and removed if there is enough space available. (*C*) If there is insufficient space for crown removal, a second horizontal (T) cut is made through the crown. The superior half of the crown is removed. (*D*) Next, inferior half of the crown is removed with an elevator. (*E*) Roots are removed together via a purchase point at the furca. An elevator is used to advance the roots forward of an elevator and sometimes a purchase point. (*F*) If roots cannot be removed via purchase point, they are sectioned. (*G*) Superior root removed. (*H*) Inferior root removed. (*Adapted from* Hupp JR, Ellis E III, Tucker MR, editors. Contemporary oral and maxillofacial surgery. 5th edition. St. Louis: Mosby Elsevier; 2008; with permission.)

advocated the removal of impacted third molars concomitantly with sagittal split osteotomies if mandibular orthognathic surgery is performed.[74]

A prospective study by Doucet and colleagues[75] found that the presence of third molars during sagittal split osteotomies is not associated with an increased frequency of unfavorable fractures. Performing both procedures at the same time can potentially limit risk, reduce overall cost, and minimize the postsurgical

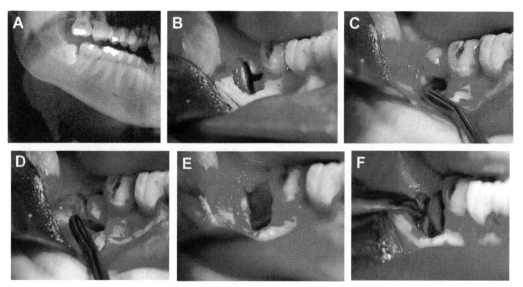

Fig. 33. (*A*) Radiograph of horizontal impacted right mandibular third molar. (*B*) Envelope flap reflected, three-quarters of buccal bone removed from overlying crown, vertical and horizontal T cut made with fissure bur through crown. (*C*) Superior half of crown is delivered with elevator. (*D*) Inferior half of crown of horizontal impaction removed with elevator. (*E*) Purchase point made in furca. (*F*) Cogswell B pick inserted into purchase point and roots advance forward into socket. (*From* Rafetto LR, Synan W. Surgical management of third molars. Atlas Oral Maxillofacial Surg Clin N Am. 2012;20(2):212; with permission.)

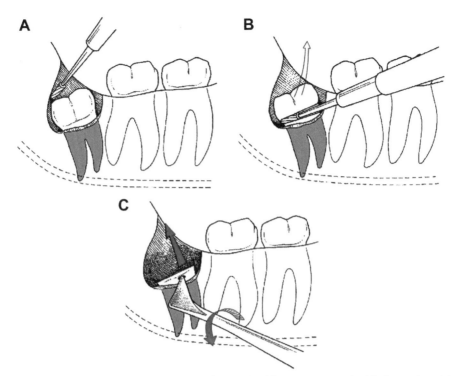

Fig. 34. (*A*) Distoangular impaction. Occlusal, buccal, and distal bone is removed with fissure bur. (*B*) Crown of distoangular impaction is sectioned off with a fissure bur and removed with straight elevator. (*C*) Purchase point is made in furca region of remaining root structure. Roots are removed with either a pick elevator or triangular elevator. If roots are divergent, they may need to be sectioned, separated, and removed separately. (*From* Hupp JR. Principles of management of impacted teeth. In: Hupp JR, Ellis E III, Tucker MR, editors. Contemporary oral and maxillofacial surgery. 6th edition. Philadelphia: Elsevier; 2013; with permission.)

sequelae. However, the application of the MSSO technique with the sole purpose of removing a deeply impacted mandibular third molar is limited.

Indications for using the MSSO approach include deeply impacted teeth associated with an intimate relationship between the IAN and the dental roots with or without an associated large lesion such as a cyst and/or tumor as shown on computed tomography or CBCT scan images.[76] Extensive bone removal via a conventional buccal/lateral approach can increase the risk of mandibular fracture.[69,77] In these situations, the MSSO approach may be an alternative option for the surgeon.

Advantages of the MSSO approach are:

1. Excellent access
2. Direct vision of the IAN
3. Bone preservation
4. Reduced risk of potential mandibular fracture[3,9]

Disadvantages of the MSSO approach are:

1. IAN neurosensory deficit
2. TMJ disorder
3. Infection
4. Nonunion
5. Malocclusion
6. Bad split
7. Cost/operating room (OR) procedure

It has been suggested that, if radiographic evidence shows bone remodeling caused by chronic inflammation, presence of large lesions such as cysts or tumors, or the mandibular canal is within the buccal cortex, then there may be an associated increased risk of potential complications associated with the MSSO procedure[76]

EXTRAORAL APPROACH

The extraoral approach is another less conservative and infrequently used procedure to remove impacted mandibular third molars. Indications for this approach are similar to those for the MSSO. It may be chosen for situations that pose a high

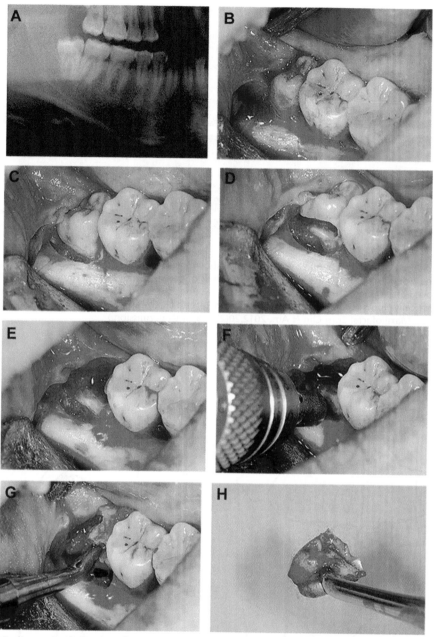

Fig. 35. (*A*) Radiograph of distoangular impacted mandibular right third molar. (*B*) Envelope flap reflection to expose distoangular impaction. (*C*) Buccodistal bone trough. (*D*) Sectioning of crown from roots. (*E*) Crown removed, root structure visualized. (*F*) Purchase point made in furca region of root structure with fissure bur. (*G*) Roots elevated and delivered with pick elevator. (*H*) Roots removed with pick elevator. (*From* Rafetto LR, Synan W. Surgical management of third molars. Atlas Oral Maxillofacial Surg Clin N Am. 2012;20(2):215; with permission.)

risk of injury to the IAN and a significant loss of alveolar bone if a traditional conservative intraoral approach is taken. The submandibular and preauricular approaches are the more commonly used extraoral approaches. These approaches are usually reserved for cases where an impacted mandibular third molar is totally below the IAC or positioned high in the ramus/subcondylar region and associated with inflammation, infection, cyst, or tumor.[78,79]

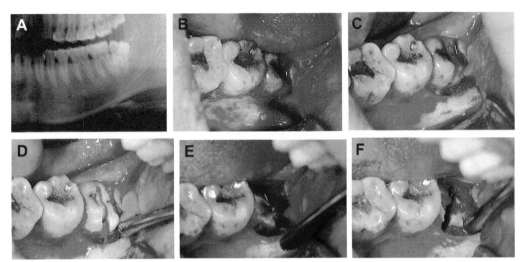

Fig. 36. (*A*) Radiograph of distoangular impacted mandibular left third molar. (*B*) Surgical flap reflected. (*C*) Buccodistal bone trough made with fissure bur. (*D*) Distal half of crown sectioned and removed. (*E*) Mesial half of crown removed after failed attempt to mobilize tooth. (*F*) Root structure of distoangular molar visualized and sectioned vertically. Roots separated and removed. (*From* Rafetto LR, Synan W. Surgical management of third molars. Atlas Oral Maxillofacial Surg Clin N Am. 2012;20(2):216; with permission.)

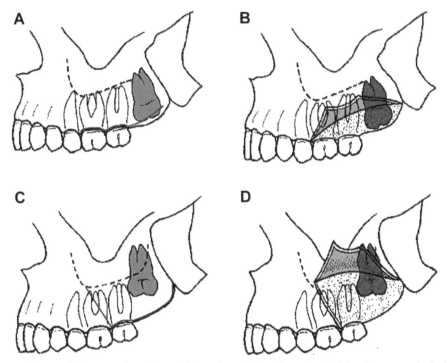

Fig. 37. Surgical access for impacted maxillary third molars. (*A*) Envelope flap incision for removal of a low maxillary impacted third molar. (*B*) Envelope flap soft tissue reflected laterally to expose bone overlying third molar. (*C*) Three-cornered flap incision used to access high impacted maxillary third molar. (*D*) Releasing incision of 3-cornered flap provides greater visibility and access to the apical portion of the surgical field. (*From* Hupp JR. Principles of management of impacted teeth. In: Hupp JR, Ellis E III, Tucker MR, editors. Contemporary oral and maxillofacial surgery. 6th edition. Philadelphia: Elsevier; 2013; with permission.)

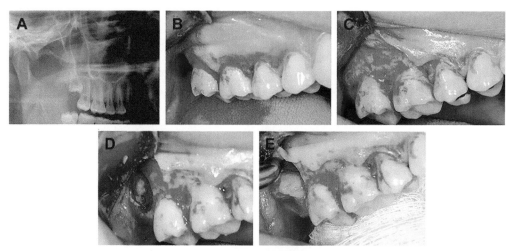

Fig. 38. (A) Radiograph of impacted maxillary right third molar. (B) Envelope flap incision. (C) Reflection of envelope flap to access impacted maxillary third molar. (D) Bone removed from overlying crown with fissure bur. (E) Impacted maxillary third molar delivered via rotation of Potts elevator. (*From* Rafetto LR, Synan W. Surgical management of third molars. Atlas Oral Maxillofacial Surg Clin N Am. 2012;20(2):219; with permission.)

Advantages of the extraoral approach are:

1. Good access and visibility
2. Bone preservation
3. Reduced risk of potential mandibular fracture

Disadvantages of extraoral approach are:

1. Technically more difficult
2. Risk of facial nerve injury
3. Skin scar
4. Cost/OR procedure

CORONECTOMY

Coronectomy is the removal of the crown of an impacted tooth with purposeful retention of the roots in a nonmobile state. This technique is most commonly indicated to reduce the risk of IAN injury with impacted third molars at moderate to high risk for neurosensory disturbance, based on evaluation of a panoramic radiograph and with confirmation of IAN position via CBCT.[80] Another common indication is for patients at high

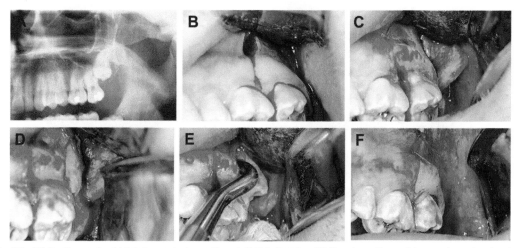

Fig. 39. (A) Radiograph of high impacted maxillary left third molar. (B) Envelope flap with anterior releasing incision. (C) Three-cornered flap reflected to expose high impacted maxillary third molar. (D) Buccal bone overlying impacted third molar is removed. (E) Potts elevator used to deliver impacted third molar from site. (F) Flap sutured. (*From* Rafetto LR, Synan W. Surgical management of third molars. Atlas Oral Maxillofacial Surg Clin N Am. 2012;20(2):220; with permission.)

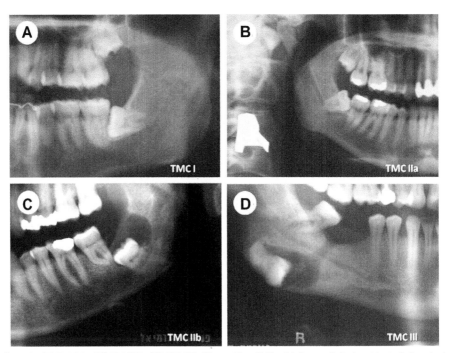

Fig. 40. (*A*) TMCI. (*B*) TMCIIa. (*C*) TMCIIB. (*D*) TMCIII. (*From* Abu-El Naaj I, Braun R, Leiser Y, et al. Surgical approach to impacted mandibular third molars—operative classification. J Oral Maxillofac Surg 2010;68(3):630; with permission.)

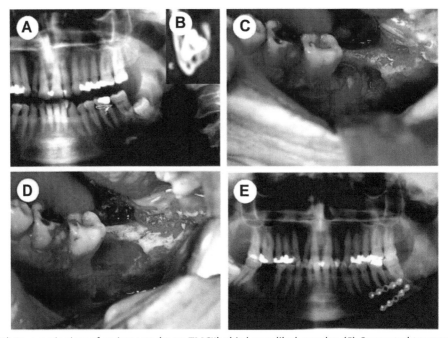

Fig. 41. (*A*) Panoramic view of an impacted type TMCIIb third mandibular molar. (*B*) Computed tomography (CT) DentaScan view of the impacted molar in coronal view. (*C*) The sagittal split osteotomy, which exposed the impacted tooth. (*D*) Surgical field after removal of the tooth and enucleation. (*E*) Panoramic view of postoperation fixation. (*From* Abu-El Naaj I, Braun R, Leiser Y, et al. Surgical approach to impacted mandibular third molars—operative classification. J Oral Maxillofac Surg 2010;68(3):631; with permission.)

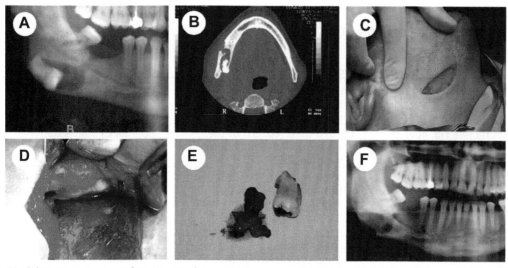

Fig. 42. (*A*) Panoramic view of an impacted type TMCIII mandibular third molar with radiolucent fistula. (*B*) CT DentaScan view of the impacted molar in axial view; note lingual and buccal bony destruction. (*C*) Surgical incision 1 cm below the mandible. (*D*) Exposure of the impacted third molar. (*E*) The tooth and the dentigerous cyst that surrounded the crown. (*F*) Postsurgical panoramic view showing the beginning of healing in the surgical area. (*From* Abu-El Naaj I, Braun R, Leiser Y, et al. Surgical approach to impacted mandibular third molars—operative classification. J Oral Maxillofac Surg 2010;68(3):631; with permission.)

risk of mandible fracture with extraction of impacted third molars, particularly when mandibular atrophy and deep impactions are present. Contraindications to coronectomy include disorder involving the roots (eg, caries, infection, cysts), mobility of the tooth/roots, the need to distalize second molars orthodontically, and impactions where the tooth lies parallel to the IAN, because the risk of crown/enamel removal is similar to or higher than with extraction.[80]

Proper coronectomy technique involves removal of the crown at or just below the cementoenamel junction and subsequent removal of all remaining traces of enamel with a bur (**Fig. 43**). The surrounding crest of alveolar bone should be 3 to 4 mm coronal to the remaining roots to allow for boney overgrowth and possible root migration (**Fig. 44**). The vital pulpal tissues should not be removed from the remaining roots and the site should be closed primarily. Although the risk of potentially mobilizing the roots is higher, the junior author advocates avoidance of sectioning completely across the crown, which risks perforating the lingual plate and damaging the lingual nerve. These injuries are poorly tolerated by patients and most agree that it is a much worse outcome than the IAN injury that the coronectomy is attempting to avoid. Elevation of a lingual flap

and placement of a retractor to help protect the lingual nerve is an option, but carries with it the inherent risk of traction injury to the lingual nerve.

Complications unique to coronectomy include root migration and mobility. Root migration has been found to average 2.82 mm over a study timespan of 4 to 8.5 years.[81] Another long-term study has shown that less than 5% of roots migrate after 24 months, with more than 90% of root migration occurring in the first 6 months after the procedure.[82] A recent systematic study has found an overall failure rate for coronectomies of 7%, mainly caused by mobility and root migration or clinical root exposure.[83] An overall IAN injury rate of 0.5% and a permanent injury rate of 0.05% for successful coronectomies, increasing to 2.6% and 1.3% respectively for failed coronectomies, has been reported.[83] Proponents of the procedure note that, should removal of the residual roots be required, they are likely to have migrated some distance away from the IAN, thereby decreasing the risk of IAN injury. Therefore, during the informed consent process, clinicians must be sure the patient understands the potential for a second surgery and that some form of clinical and radiographic follow-up is required, although, to date, no such standardized follow-up protocol has been widely accepted.

Table 2
Third molar classification system (TMC)

Type	Molar and Root Position	Recommended Surgical Approach
TMCI (see **Fig. 40**A)	Erupted or impacted molar. Roots are entirely above the mandibular canal	Intraoral buccal (or lingual) approach
TMCIIa (see **Fig. 40**B)	Up to a third (<0.333) of the molar root length is below the mandibular canal	Dental CT scan is optional. Intraoral buccal (or lingual) approach
TMCIIb (see **Fig. 40**C)	More than a third (>0.333) of the molar root length is below the mandibular canal	Dental CT scan is mandatory to localize the impacted tooth in 3 dimensions MSSO approach if indications for extraction are present
TMCIII (see **Fig. 40**D)	Mandibular third molar is completely localized below the mandibular canal	Dental CT scan is mandatory. Extraoral approach if indications for extraction are present

Abbreviation: CT, computed tomography.

POSTOPERATIVE MANAGEMENT FOR THIRD MOLAR REMOVAL

Postoperative care begins with obtaining complete hemostasis by firmly biting on gauze for approximately 60 minutes after the procedure. If bleeding continues after this time, repeating the process is indicated, although the patient should be advised that the gauze and saliva could have traces of blood for some time after surgery. The

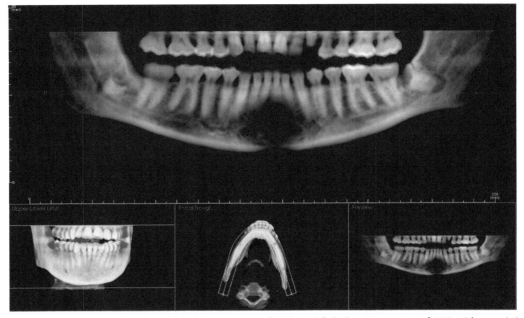

Fig. 43. Patient presenting 3 years after coronectomy of #32 and failed coronectomy of #17 with remaining enamel present, thus preventing bone overgrowth. Site #32 healed well with site #17 becoming symptomatic and requiring extraction.

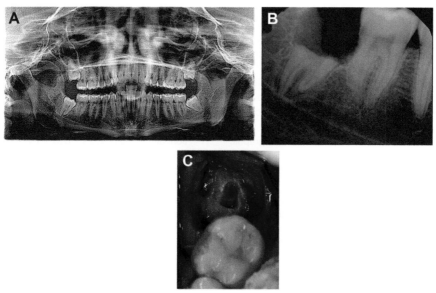

Fig. 44. (*A*) Preoperative panoramic film showing increased risk of IAN damage with extraction of #32. (*B*) Postoperative periapical view of completed coronectomy. (*C*) Intraoperative view of completed coronectomy.

patient is instructed to start with a soft diet and advance as tolerated, taking care to avoid hot foods while any numbness is still present to prevent burning. Oral hygiene should consist of a return to normal tooth brushing as soon as possible, with the surgical sites initially being treated gently or avoided. The surgical sites can be kept clean before regular brushing resumes by gently rinsing with salt water or chlorhexidine, which also helps to disinfect the areas.

Analgesia is often obtained with over-the-counter medications such as high-dose ibuprofen and acetaminophen (600–800 mg and 500–1000 mg respectively) every 6 to 8 hours. Opioid medications can be prescribed if needed, although few, if any, are typically required. Scheduled use of analgesics for 2 to 3 days after surgery, with as-needed use thereafter, is adequate for most patients. Postoperative antibiotics are a controversial topic, although many studies show that their use is not indicated for uncomplicated procedures in healthy patients. Follow-up for uncomplicated third molar surgery is not typically required, although patients should always be given verbal and written postoperative directions and contact information for the on-call surgeon to reach in case questions or concerns arise.

SUMMARY

Management of impacted third molars is a complex topic and controversial, particularly with regard to surgical techniques used and the management of asymptomatic and disease-free teeth. Continued research is necessary to better understand and predict the likelihood of which teeth will become symptomatic and/or develop disease, especially regarding the eruption and root development of these teeth. A predictive model would indicate not only which teeth to remove but also when to remove them, therefore helping minimize risks such as nerve damage and other postoperative complications for each individual patient.

REFERENCES

1. Schropp L, Stavropoulos A, Gotfredsen E, et al. Calibration of radiographs by a reference metal ball affects preoperative selection of implant size. Clin Oral Investig 2009;13(4):375–81.
2. Richards AG. Roentographic localization of the mandibular canal. J Oral Surg (Chic) 1952;10: 325–9.
3. Matzen L, Christensen J, Wenzel A. Patient discomfort and retakes in periapical examination of mandibular third molars using digital receptors and film. Oral Surg Oral Med Oral Pathol Oral Radiol Endod 2009;107(4):566–72.
4. Matzen LH, Petersen LB, Wenzel A. Radiographic methods used before removal of mandibular third molars among randomly selected general dental clinics. Dentomaxillofac Radiol 2016;45(4): 20150226.

5. Nakayama K, Nonoyama M, Takaki Y, et al. Assessment of the relationship between impacted mandibular third molars and inferior alveolar nerve with dental 3-dimensional computed tomography. J Oral Maxillofac Surg 2009;67(12):2587–91.

6. Tay AB, Go WS. Effect of exposed inferior alveolar neurovascular bundle during surgical removal of impacted lower third molars. J Oral Maxillofac Surg 2004;62(5):592–600.

7. Leung YY, Cheung LK. Correlation of radiographic signs inferior dental nerve exposure and deficit in third molar surgery. J Oral Maxillofac Surg 2011; 69(7):1873–9.

8. Xu GZ, Yang C, Fan XD, et al. Anatomic relationship between impacted third mandibular molar and the mandibular canal as the risk factor of inferior alveolar nerve injury. Br J Oral Maxillofac Surg 2013; 51(8):e215–9.

9. Rood JP, Shehab BA. The radiological prediction of inferior alveolar nerve injury during third molar surgery. Br J Oral Maxillofac Surg 1990;28(1):20–5.

10. Tantanapornkul W, Okochi K, Bhakdinaronk A, et al. Correlation of darkening of impacted mandibular third molar root on digital panoramic images with cone beam computed tomography findings. Dentomaxillofac Radiol 2009;38(1):11–6.

11. Sedaghatfar M, August MA, Dodson TB. Panoramic radiographic findings as predictors of inferior alveolar nerve exposure following third molar extraction. J Oral Maxillofac Surg 2005;63(1):3–7.

12. Sanmartí-Garcia G, Valmaseda-Castellón E, Gay-Escoda C. Does computed tomography prevent inferior alveolar nerve injuries caused by lower third molar removal? J Oral Maxillofac Surg 2012;70(1): 5–11.

13. Şekerci AE, Şişman Y. Comparison between panoramic radiography and cone-beam computed tomography findings for assessment of the relationship between impacted mandibular third molars and the mandibular canal. Oral Radiol 2014; 30(2):170–8.

14. Winstanley KL, Otway LM, Thompson L, et al. Inferior alveolar nerve injury: correlation between indicators of risk on panoramic radiographs and the incidence of tooth and mandibular canal contact on cone-beam computed tomography scans in a Western Australian population. J Investig Clin Dent 2018;9(3):e12323.

15. Umar G, Obisesan O, Bryant C, et al. Elimination of permanent injuries to the inferior alveolar nerve following surgical intervention of the "high risk" third molar. Br J Oral Maxillofac Surg 2013;51(4): 353–7.

16. Su N, van Wijk A, Berkhout E, et al. Predictive value of panoramic radiography for injury of Inferior alveolar nerve after mandibular third molar surgery. J Oral Maxillofac Surg 2017;75(4):663–79.

17. Ghaeminia H, Gerlach NL, Hoppenreijs TJ, et al. Clinical relevance of cone beam computed tomography in mandibular third molar removal: a multicentre, randomised, controlled trial. J Craniomaxillofac Surg 2015;43(10):2158–67.

18. Hasegawa T, Ri S, Shigeta T, et al. Risk factors associated with inferior alveolar nerve injury after extraction of the mandibular third molar–a comparative study of preoperative images by panoramic radiography and computed tomography. Int J Oral Maxillofac Surg 2013;42(7):843–51.

19. Hasegawa T, Ri S, Umeda M, et al. Multivariate relationships among risk factors and hypoesthesia of the lower lip after extraction of the mandibular third molar. Oral Surg Oral Med Oral Pathol Oral Radiol Endod 2011;111(6):e1–7.

20. Matzen LH, Christensen J, Hintze H, et al. Diagnostic accuracy of panoramic radiography, stereoscanography and cone beam CT for assessment of mandibular third molars before surgery. Acta Odontol Scand 2013;71(6):1391–8.

21. Matzen LH, Christensen J, Hintze H, et al. Influence of cone beam CT on treatment plan before surgical intervention of mandibular third molars and impact of radiographic factors on deciding on coronectomy vs surgical removal. Dentomaxillofac Radiol 2013; 42(1):98870341.

22. Ghaeminia H, Meijer GJ, Soehardi A, et al. The use of cone beam CT for the removal of wisdom teeth changes the surgical approach compared with panoramic radiography: a pilot study. Int J Oral Maxillofac Surg 2011;40(8):834–9.

23. Ghaeminia H, Meijer GJ, Soehardi A, et al. Position of the impacted third molar in relation to the mandibular canal. Diagnostic accuracy of cone beam computed tomography compared with panoramic radiography. Int J Oral Maxillofac Surg 2009;38(9): 964–71.

24. Peker I, Sarikir C, Alkurt MT, et al. Panoramic radiography and cone-beam computed tomography findings in preoperative examination of impacted mandibular third molars. BMC Oral Health 2014;14:71.

25. Ueda M, Nakamori K, Shiratori K, et al. Clinical significance of computed tomographic assessment and anatomic features of the inferior alveolar canal as risk factors for injury of the inferior alveolar nerve at third molar surgery. J Oral Maxillofac Surg 2012; 70(3):514–20.

26. Shiratori K, Nakamori K, Ueda M, et al. Assessment of the shape of the inferior alveolar canal as a marker for increased risk of injury to the inferior alveolar nerve at third molar surgery: a prospective study. J Oral Maxillofac Surg 2013;71(12):2012–9.

27. Soumalainen A, Ventä I, Mattila M, et al. Reliability of CBCT and other radiographic methods in preoperative evaluation of lower third molars. Oral Surg Oral Med Oral Pathol Oral Radiol Endod 2010;109(2):276–84.

28. Guerrero ME, Botetano R, Beltran J, et al. Can preoperative imaging help to predict postoperative outcome after wisdom tooth removal? A randomized controlled trial using panoramic radiography versus cone-beam CT. Clin Oral Investig 2014;18:335.

29. Shahbazian M, Vandewoude C, Wyatt J, et al. Comparative assessment of panoramic radiography and CBCT imaging for radiodiagnostics in the posterior maxilla. Clin Oral Investig 2014;18:293–300.

30. Sheran A. Correlation between maxillary sinus floor topography and related root position. Oral Surg Oral Med Oral Pathol Oral Radiol Endod 2006;102(3):375–81.

31. Lopes LJ, Gamba TO, Bertinato JVJ, et al. Comparison of panoramic radiography and CBCT to identify maxillary posterior roots invading the maxillary sinus. Dentomaxillofac Radiol 2016;45(6):20160043.

32. Matzen LH, Schropp L, Spin-Neto R, et al. Radiographic signs of pathology determining removal of an impacted mandibular third molar assessed in a panoramic image or CBCT. Dentomaxillofac Radiol 2017;46(1):20160330.

33. Petersen LB, Vaeth M, Wenzel A. Neurosensoric disturbances after surgical removal of the mandibular third molar based on either panoramic imaging or cone beam CT scanning: a randomized controlled trial (RCT). Dentomaxillofac Radiol 2016;45(2):20150224.

34. Petersen LB, Olsen KR, Matzen LH, et al. Economic and health implications of routine CBCT examination before surgical removal of the mandibular third molar in the Danish population. Dentomaxillofac Radiol 2015;44(6):20140406.

35. Petersen LB, Olsen KR, Christensen J, et al. Image and surgery-related costs comparing cone beam CT and panoramic imaging before removal of impacted mandibular third molars. Dentomaxillofac Radiol 2014;43(6):20140001.

36. Ludlow JB, Davies-Ludlow LE, White SC. Patient risk related to common dental radiographic examinations: the impact of 2007 International Commission on Radiological Protection recommendations regarding dose calculation. J Am Dent Assoc 2008;139(9):1237–43.

37. Ludlow JB, Timothy R, Walker C, et al. Effective dose of dental CBCT-a meta analysis of published data and additional data for nine CBCT units. Dentomaxillofac Radiol 2015;44(1):20140197.

38. Dodson TB. Surveillance as a management strategy for retained third molars: is it desirable? J Oral Maxillofac Surg 2012;70(9 Suppl 1):S20–4.

39. Kinard BE, Dodson TB. Most patients with asymptomatic, disease-free third molars elect extraction over retention as their preferred treatment. J Oral Maxillofac Surg 2010;68(12):2935–42.

40. Blakey GH, Marciani RD, Haug RH, et al. Periodontal pathology associated with asymptomatic third molars. J Oral Maxillofacial Surg 2002;60(11):1227–33.

41. White RP Jr, Madianos PN, Offenbacher S, et al. Microbial complexes detected in the second/third molar region in patients with asymptomatic third molars. J Oral Maxillofac Surg 2002;60(11):1234–40.

42. Shugars DA, Jacks MT, White RP Jr, et al. Occlusal caries experience in patients with asymptomatic third molars. J Oral Maxillofac Surg 2004;62(8):973–9.

43. Shugars DA, Elter JR, Jacks MT, et al. Incidence of occlusal dental caries in asymptomatic third molars. J Oral Maxillofac Surg 2005;63(3):341–6.

44. Stathopoulos P, Mezitis M, Kappatos C, et al. Cysts and tumors associated with impacted third molars: is prophylactic removal justified? J Oral Maxillofac Surg 2011;69(2):405–8.

45. Güven O, Keskin A, Akal UK. The incidence of cysts and tumors around impacted third molars. Int J Oral Maxillofac Surg 2000;29(2):131–5.

46. London: NICE 2000 Guidance on the extraction of wisdom teeth. National Institute for Clinical Excellence. Technology appraisal guidance [TA1]. Published date: 27 March 2000.

47. McArdle LW, Renton T. The effects of NICE guidelines on the management of third molar teeth. Br Dent J 2012;213(5):E8.

48. Mettes TG, Nienhuijs ME, van der Sanden WJ, et al. Interventions for treating asymptomatic impacted wisdom teeth in adolescents and adults. Cochrane Database Syst Rev 2005;(2):CD003879.

49. Mettes TD, Ghaeminia H, Nienhuijs ME, et al. Surgical removal versus retention for the management of asymptomatic impacted wisdom teeth. Cochrane Database Syst Rev 2012;(6):CD003879.

50. Ghaeminia H, Perry J, Nienhuijs ME, et al. Surgical removal verses retention for the management of asymptomatic disease-free impacted wisdom teeth. Cochrane Database Syst Rev 2016;(8):CD003879.

51. Ventä I, Vehkalahti MM, Huumonen S, et al. Signs of disease occur in the majority of third molars in an adult population. Int J Oral Maxillofac Surg 2017;46(12):1635–40.

52. Garaas R, Moss KL, Fisher EL, et al. Prevalence of visible third molars with caries experience or periodontal pathology in middle-aged and older Americans. J Oral Maxillofac Surg 2011;69(2):463–70.

53. Nunn ME, Fish MD, Garcia RI, et al. Retained Asymptomatic Third Molars and Risk for Second Molar Pathology. J Dent Res 2013;92(12):1095–99.

54. Blakey GH, Jacks MT, Offenbacher S, et al. Progression of periodontal disease in the second/third molar region in subjects with asymptomatic third molars. J Oral Maxillofac Surg 2006;64(2):189–93.

55. Matzen LH, Schropp L, Spin-Neto R, et al. Use of cone beam computed tomography to assess significant imaging findings related to mandibular third molar impaction. Oral Surg Oral Med Oral Pathol Oral Radiol 2017;124(5):506–16.

56. Allen RT, Witherow H, Collyer J, et al. The mesioangular third molar–to extract or not to extract? Analysis of 776 consecutive third molars. Br Dent J 2009;206(11):E23 [discussion: 586–7].

57. Falci SG, de Castro CR, Santos RC, et al. Association between the presence of a partially erupted mandibular third molar and the existence of caries in the distal of the second molars. Int J Oral Maxillofac Surg 2012;41(10):1270–4.

58. McArdle LW, McDonald F, Jones J. Distal cervical caries in the mandibular second molar: an indication for the prophylactic removal of third molar teeth? Update. Br J Oral Maxillofac Surg 2014;52(2):185–9.

59. Montero J, Mazzaglia G. Effect of removing an impacted mandibular third molar on the periodontal status of the mandibular second molar. J Oral Maxillofac Surg 2011;69(11):2691–7.

60. Sidlauskas A, Trakiniene G. Effect of the lower third molars on the lower dental arch crowding. Stomatologija 2006;8(3):80–4.

61. Harradine NW, Pearson MH, Toth B. The effect of extraction of third molars on late lower incisor crowding: a randomized controlled trial. Br J Orthod 1998;25(2):117–22.

62. Niedzielska I. Third molar influence on dental arch crowding. Eur J Orthod 2005;27(5):518–23.

63. Camargo IB, Sobrinho JB, Andrade ES, et al. Correlational study of impacted and non-functional lower third molar position with occurrence of pathologies. Prog Orthod 2016;17(1):26.

64. Precious DS, Lung KE, Pynn BR, et al. Presence of impacted teeth as a determining factor of unfavorable splits in 1256 sagittal-split osteotomies. Oral Surg Oral Med Oral Pathol Oral Radiol Endod 1998;85(4):362–5.

65. Doucet JC, Morrison AD, Davis BR, et al. Concomitant removal of mandibular third molars during sagittal split osteotomy minimizes neurosensory dysfunction. J Oral Maxillofac Surg 2012;70(9):2153–63.

66. Inaoka SD, Carneiro SC, Vasconcelos BC, et al. Relationship between mandibular fracture and impacted lower third molar. Med Oral Patol Oral Cir Bucal 2009;14(7):E349–54.

67. Wali GG, Sridhar V, Shyla HN. A study on dentigerous cystic changes with radiographically normal impacted mandibular third molars. J Maxillofac Oral Surg 2012;11(4):458–65.

68. Haidry N, Singh M, Mamatha NS, et al. Histopathological evaluation of dental follicle associated with radiographically normal impacted mandibular third molars. Ann Maxillofac Surg 2018;8(2):259–64.

69. Libersa P, Roze D, Cachart T, et al. Immediate and late mandibular fractures after third molar removal. J Oral Maxillofac Surg 2002;60(2):163–5.

70. Chrcanovic BR, Custódio AL. Considerations of mandibular angle fractures during and after surgery for removal of third molars: a review of the literature. Oral Maxillofac Surg 2010;14(2):71–80.

71. Pires WR, Bonardi JP, Faverani LP, et al. Late mandibular fracture occurring in the postoperative period after third molar removal: systematic review and analysis of 124 cases. Int J Oral Maxillofac Surg 2017;46(1):46–53.

72. Abu-El Naaj I, Braun R, Leiser Y, et al. Surgical approach to impacted mandibular third molars–operative classification. J Oral Maxillofac Surg 2010;68(3):628–33.

73. Pichler JW, Beirne OR. Lingual flap retraction and prevention of lingual nerve damage associated with third molar surgery: a systematic review of the literature. Oral Surg Oral Med Oral Pathol Oral Radiol Endod 2001;91(4):395–401.

74. Precious DS. Removal of third molars with sagittal split osteotomies: the case for. J Oral Maxillofac Surg 2004;62(9):1144–6.

75. Doucet JC, Morrison AD, Davis BR, et al. The presence of mandibular third molars during sagittal split osteotomies does not increase the risk of complications. J Oral Maxillofac Surg 2012;70(8):1935–43.

76. Catherine Z, Scolozzi P. Mandibular sagittal split osteotomy for removal of impacted mandibular teeth: indications, surgical pitfalls, and final outcome. J Oral Maxillofac Surg 2017;75(5):915–23.

77. Bodner L, Brennan PA, McLeod NM. Characteristics of iatrogenic mandibular fractures associated with tooth removal: review and analysis of 189 cases. Br J Oral Maxillofac Surg 2011;49(7):567–72.

78. Bux P, Lisco V. Ectopic third molar associated with a dentigerous cyst in the subcondylar region: report of case. J Oral Maxillofac Surg 1994;52(6):630–2.

79. Tümer C, Eset AE, Atabek A. Ectopic impacted mandibular third molar in the subcondylar region associated with a dentigerous cyst: a case report. Quintessence Int 2002;33(3):231–3.

80. Pogrel MA. Coronectomy: partial odontectomy or intentional root retention. Oral Maxillofac Surg Clin North Am 2015;27(3):373–82.

81. Yeung AWK, Wong NSM, Bornstein MM, et al. Three-dimensional radiographic evaluation of root migration patterns 4-8.5 years after lower third molar coronectomy: a cone beam computed tomography study. Int J Oral Maxillofac Surg 2018;47(9):1145–52.

82. Leung YY, Cheung KY. Root migration pattern after third molar coronectomy: a long-term analysis. Int J Oral Maxillofac Surg 2018;47(6):802–8.

83. Dalle Carbonare M, Zavattini A, Duncan M, et al. Injury to the inferior alveolar and lingual nerves in successful and failed coronectomies: systematic review. Br J Oral Maxillofac Surg 2017;55(9):892–8.

Surgical Exposure of Impacted Teeth

Pamela L. Alberto, DMD*

KEYWORDS

- Impacted central incisor • Impacted canine • Impacted second molar • Impacted premolar
- Surgical exposure • Orthodontic treatment

KEY POINTS

- The management of impacted permanent teeth requires a team effort with input from the orthodontist, general dentist, and surgeon to develop a satisfactory treatment plan.
- It is important to evaluate the 3-dimensional position of the impacted tooth to the roots of the adjacent teeth to determine the proper treatment plan.
- A full orthodontic evaluation is required before any surgical intervention.
- The oral and maxillofacial surgeon must decide whether an open or closed exposure procedure should be performed and provide optimal condition for the orthodontist to apply the correct forces for alignment.
- Bonding position on the impacted tooth depends on the intended direction on traction forces to be applied. The orthodontist should determine this position.

The management of impacted teeth other than third molars is one of the most challenging and complicated types of dento-alveolar surgery. Proper diagnosis and treatment planning requires interdisciplinary care by an orthodontist, general dentist, and oral and maxillofacial surgeon but the orthodontist is responsible for the overall success of the treatment plan.[1]

The most common impacted teeth aside from the third molar are maxillary canines, maxillary second molar, mandibular second premolars, and mandibular second molar (**Fig. 1**). There are systemic and local factors that contribute to the impaction of these permanent teeth. The contributing factors include arch length discrepancy, space deficiencies, ankylosed primary teeth, pathology, trauma, and some systemic and genetic factors.[2] Although the incidence of impacted teeth differs in diverse populations, Dachi and Howell[3] reported the incidence being as low as 0.92% for maxillary canines (with most being unilateral), 0.40% for mandibular premolar, 0.13% for maxillary premolar and 0.09% for mandibular canines.[2] Although the overall incidence of impacted teeth, excluding third molars, is rare, it is important that every oral and maxillofacial surgeon understands all treatment options and their management. The appropriate surgical procedure and orthodontic treatment plan will result in a stable, predictable, and aesthetic result.

Surgical exposure of these impacted teeth is accomplished using various approaches. We discuss surgical techniques used to expose the impacted canine, central incisor, premolar, and second molar.

IMPACTED MAXILLARY CANINE
Etiology

Calcification of the maxillary canine starts at 4 to 5 months and erupts into the oral cavity in 11 to 12 years. It remains high in the maxilla above the root of the lateral incisor until the crown is calcified. The maxillary cuspid erupts along the distal aspect of the lateral incisor. This closes the

Department of Oral & Maxillofacial Surgery, Rutgers School of Dental Medicine, Newark, NJ, USA
* 171 Woodport Road, Sparta, NJ 07871.
E-mail address: alberto@sdm.rutgers.edu

Oral Maxillofacial Surg Clin N Am 32 (2020) 561–570
https://doi.org/10.1016/j.coms.2020.07.008

physiologic diastema present between the maxillary central incisors. The maxillary canine travels almost 22 mm during the time of eruption. It should erupt before 13.9 years for girls and 14.6 years for boys.[4] The etiology of impaction is unclear but most likely multifactorial. Because the maxillary canine has the longest path of eruption in the permanent dentition, alteration in position of the central and lateral incisor may be a factor. Arch length discrepancy and space deficiency may result in the canine becoming labially impacted. Studies have shown a higher incidence of palatally impacted canines in cases with missing lateral or peg-shaped incisors. Failure of the primary canine to resorb may cause palatal movement of the permanent canine (**Fig. 2**). However, Thilander and Jacobassom[2] considered failed of resorption of the primary canine to be a consequence rather than a cause of impaction.[4] A genetic predisposition has been shown in some studies. For example, Pirinen found that palatally impacted canines are genetic and related to incisor-premolar hypodontia and preshaped lateral incisors.[5]

Other possible causes are trauma to the anterior maxilla at an early age, pathologic lesions, odontomas, supernumerary teeth, and ankylosis. There is also a higher incidence of impacted maxillary canine following alveolar bone grafting in the cleft patient.[6]

DIAGNOSIS

Diagnosis of the maxillary canine position is a key factor in the comprehensive assessment of the impacted canine. The position of the impacted canine is important when deciding management options for the patient. Localization requires inspection, palpation and radiographic evaluation. The position of the lateral incisor can also give a clue to the canine position. The crown of the lateral root may be proclined if the canine is lying labial to the lateral incisor. Occasionally the impacted canine can be palpated on the labial or palatal aspect. The surgeon can take a series of periapical radiographs along with a panoramic radiograph to locate its position. When taking the series of periapical radiographs, the cone head is shifted horizontally so Clark's Rule can be used to discern the buccal or lingual position of the canine. The 3-dimensional (3-D) cone beam computed tomography (CBCT) is superior in determining the location of the impacted canine but is costly (**Fig. 3**). If you need to extract the over retained primary canine, the resorption pattern on the root will give you a clue as to localization of the crown of the impacted canine. In some cases, you can feel the crown when giving

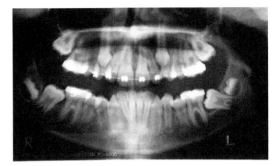

Fig. 1. Impacted maxillary canines with an impacted mandibular second molar.

your infiltration anesthesia on the buccal and palatal mucosa (**Fig. 4**).

TREATMENT OPTIONS

All patients require a thorough clinical evaluation, which should include a visual and tactile examination. The radiographic evaluation should include 2-D radiographs and possibly a 3-D CBCT if the tooth is not palpable, then a comprehensive treatment plan can be developed. An informed consent with discussion of treatment options and alternatives is a must to avoid misunderstanding, which could lead to legal problems. Proper management of the impacted canine can include one of the following treatment options:

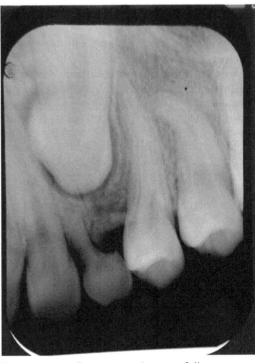

Fig. 2. Failure of primary canine to exfoliate.

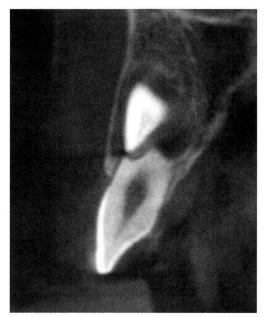

Fig. 3. CBCT of impacted canine resorbing the root of the lateral incisor.

1. No treatment with periodic clinical and radiographic observation.
2. Interceptive removal of the primary canine.
3. Surgical extraction of the tooth
4. Surgical exposure to aid eruption.
5. Surgical exposure with eruption aided by orthodontic guidance.
6. Autotransplantation of the canine

SURGICAL EXPOSURE

There are 3 methods used for surgical exposure and orthodontic alignment[1,7].

1. Open surgical exposure.

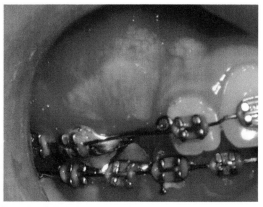

Fig. 4. Canine bulge due to a buccally impacted canine.

2. Surgical exposure with packing and delayed bonding of the orthodontic bracelet.
3. A surgical exposure and bonding of orthodontic bracelet intraoperatively.

If the canine has the correct inclination, the open surgical exposure is the treatment of choice. It has been shown that excision of the gingival over the canine with bone removal is sufficient to allow eruption of the canine.[5]

Chapokas and colleagues[8] introduced a new classification for maxillary canine impactions that included guidelines for selecting the proper surgical approach. The classification included 3 categories. Class I for impactions located palatally, Class II for impactions located labial or center of the alveolar ridge and Class III for impactions located labial to the long axis of the adjacent lateral incisor root. Surgical technique was gingivectomy for Class I, closed exposure for Class II and apically positioned flap for Class III.[9,10]

Flap Design

Flap design is dictated by the location of the impacted canine. If the impacted canine is located buccally, a gingival crest incision can be made in the gingival sulcus. If the impacted canine is high, the incision can be made horizontally above the papillae. Vestibular incisions made at the level of the mucogingival junction should be made only when the impacted canine is above the root apices.

If the impacted canine is palatal, a palatal incision placed in the gingival sulcus can be performed. Palatal incisions placed between the gingival crest and palatal vault should be avoided because trauma to the greater palatine artery could occur. Occasionally, the impacted canine can be positioned transversely in the alveolus. This would require mucoperiosteal flaps on the palatal and labial sides.[11]

SURGICAL EXPOSURE WITH ORTHODONTIC ALIGNMENT

If surgical exposure with orthodontic alignment has been chosen as the method of treatment, 3 surgical approaches can be used. The closed exposure technique replaces the mucoperiosteal flap over the exposed canine after the bracket and chain is applied.[12] The disadvantage of this technique is that bonding can fail and reexposure is necessary. The window technique removes the gingiva overlying the crown of the impacted canine. The apically repositioned flap technique is used to preserve the attached gingival (**Fig. 5**). Vermette and colleagues[13] found that apically repositioned flaps resulted in more esthetic problems than the closed exposure technique.[14–22] The goal is to choose a technique that exposes the canine within a zone of keratinized mucosa without involvement of the cemento-enamel junction. This minimizes potential periodontal and esthetic complications following orthodontic alignment.

If the inclination of the canine to the midline is greater than 45° then the prognosis for alignment worsens. The closer the impacted canine is to the midline the worse the prognosis.[23]

APPLICATION OF ORTHODONTIC TRACTION DEVICES

Many different devices can be applied to the crown of an impacted canine. These include a wire, pins, crown formers, orthodontic brackets, and temporary anchorage devices (TADs). Wires and pins are no longer placed around the crowns of impacted teeth because they can injure the crown or root of the tooth. The use of crown formers placed or cemented over the crown of the impacted tooth was popular for many years. However, the crown formers would also act as a foreign body causing inflammation and eruption. The device of choice is an orthodontic bracket or gold mesh disk with a gold chain bonded onto the canine crown surface (**Fig. 6**).

There are 2 types of bonding agents that can be used. One is a 2-part self-cure bonding agent and the other is a light cure bonding agent. The advantage of the light cure materials is most can work in a partially wet field. The gold mesh disks work much better than the orthodontic brackets or buttons with the light cure bonding agent. The curing light is able to get at all the bonding agent through the mesh. Because it cannot cure the bonding agent under the bracket, a light cure bonding agent that will also self-cure is preferable.

The tooth surface must also be acid etched. Successful bonding of the bracket improves with hemostasis. Once hemostasis is achieved, the bonding agent is placed on the bracket and pressed firmly against the enamel surface of the tooth. If it is a light cure material, it should be light cured for 20 to 40 seconds (**Fig. 7**).

Bonding site preference depends on the direction of the traction forces. The exact bonding site and direction that the gold chain exits the surgical site should be decided in advance. The chain that is attached to the bracket is then ligated to the patient's arch wire (**Fig. 8**). The orthodontist should activate the appliance within a week. It is important to inform the orthodontist of the vector of force to be used to move the canine.

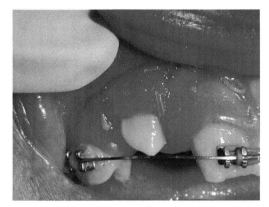

Fig. 5. Apically repositioned flap to preserve attached gingiva.

IMPACTED MANDIBULAR CANINES

Calcification of the mandibular canine starts at 4 to 5 months and erupts into the oral cavity in 9 to 11 years. The mandibular canine is 10 times less frequently impacted as the maxillary canine (**Fig. 9**). It has the largest root of all the teeth and its follicle forms at the level of the inferior border of the mandible. Because the body of the mandible is labial to the alveolus, this may explain why most impacted mandibular canines are labially impacted. Similar to maxillary canines, mandibular canines are 3 times more common in female than male patients.

A treatment plan can be developed once the impacted mandibular canine is localized; assessment of potential damage to adjacent teeth and involvement of the mental nerve is made. The 3-D CBCT enables you to precisely locate the position of the impacted tooth, confirm the integrity of the tooth, and evaluate if there is any resorption on adjacent teeth.

Impacted mandibular canines are usually vertically impacted, close to the labial surface.

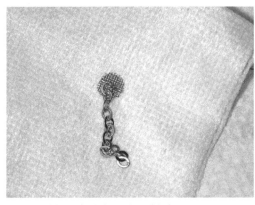

Fig. 6. Gold mesh disk with gold chain.

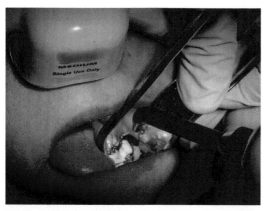

Fig. 7. Light cure for 20 to 30 seconds.

Occasionally, they can be located beneath the apices of the mandibular incisor, but they are rarely found in a horizontal position.[24]

Management of impacted mandibular canine includes the same treatment options as the maxillary canine.

SURGICAL EXPOSURE TO AID ERUPTION

If the mandibular canine impaction is caused by an overlying impediment, this impediment can be surgically removed. Then a bony pathway for eruption can be created.

SURGICAL EXPOSURE WITH ORTHODONTIC GUIDANCE

There are 4 types of incisions, which can be used for exposing the impacted mandibular canine[25]:

1. The labial gingival crevice incision
2. Alternative labial gingival crevice incision
3. Free mucosal incision
4. Lingual gingival crevice incision

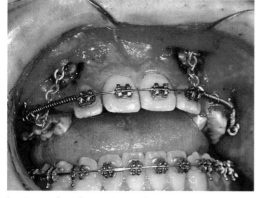

Fig. 8. Brackets ligated to arch wire.

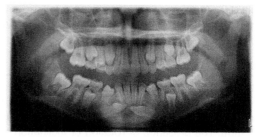

Fig. 9. Impacted mandibular canines in poor position for orthodontic alignment.

The labial gingival crevice incision is in the gingival sulcus from the right first premolar to the left first premolar, preserving the interdental papilla. A vertical releasing incision can be used if additional access is required.

The alternative labial gingival crevice incision is horizontal and made at the base of the interdental papilla, and closure of the incision is more difficult. A vertical releasing incision also can be used if more access is required.

The free mucosal incision is used when the impacted mandibular canine is located at the level of the apices of the incisors or lingual to them. The incision is placed horizontally a few millimeters away from the mucogingival junction in the nonkeratinized mucosa. The incision should remain anterior to the mental foramen to avoid the mental neurovascular bundle.

If the impacted mandibular canine is lingual to the incisors, the lingual gingival crevice incision should be used. The incision is made in the lingual gingival sulcus from the mandibular right first premolar to the mandibular left first premolar. The incision should be extended to provide adequate access. Releasing incisions should not be used. If the lingually impacted mandibular canine is below the level of the apices of the incisors, an extraoral approach may be necessary.

IMPACTED CENTRAL INCISORS

Impacted central incisors occur during the mixed dentition period. Calcification of the central incisor occurs at age 3 to 4 months and erupts at 6 to 9 years. The treatment can be challenging because of its importance to facial esthetics. If the maxillary central incisor has not erupted by age 8, you need to evaluate its position and see if anything is preventing its eruption. Supernumerary teeth cause 47% of all impacted central incisors.[26,27]

Etiology

Eruption failure is caused by supernumerary teeth, odontomas, ectopic position of the tooth bud, ankyloses of the primary tooth, early loss of primary tooth, tooth malformation, and mucosal barrier.

Diagnosis and Radiographs

The clinical examination should evaluate the primary tooth, any bulge or swelling buccal or lingually, and available space for eruption (9 mm). The presence of rotation or inclination of the ipsilateral lateral incisor is pathognomonic for an impacted central incisor.[27]

Radiographic evaluation is needed to verify that it is impacted and determine its location.

Even though the panoramic, occlusal, or periapical radiographs are consider the standard, the 3-D CBCT has proven to be superior to other radiographic methods. The 3-D CBCT enables you to precisely locate the position and evaluate the adjacent teeth for any resorption (**Fig. 10**). This will assist the surgeon on choosing the surgical approach.

Surgical Exposure

Surgical exposure of the central incisor can be performed in 2 ways: the open eruption technique and the closed eruption technique. The open eruption technique is done in 2 ways: the window technique or the apically repositioned flap technique. The window technique involves removal of the

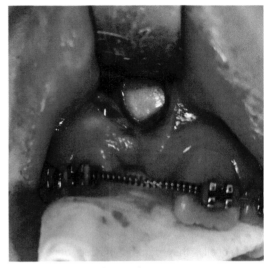

Fig. 11. Exposure of central incisor.

overlying gingiva to allow the eruption of the tooth. If the technique is performed in nonkeratinized gingival mucosa, the tooth will have nonkeratinized labial mucosa around it (**Fig. 11**). Then it will require a gingival graft. Maintenance of the space throughout the treatment is crucial. The apically repositioned procedure involves raising a flap that incorporates 2 to 3 mm of attached gingiva that is apically repositioned to the level of the cemento-enamel junction of the impacted tooth. A gold chain or bracket is bonded to the tooth surface (**Fig. 12**). The closed eruption technique involves raising a labial or palatal flap, bonding a bracket, and replacing the flap. Then orthodontic traction is applied. Many clinicians claim that the closed eruption technique gives esthetic

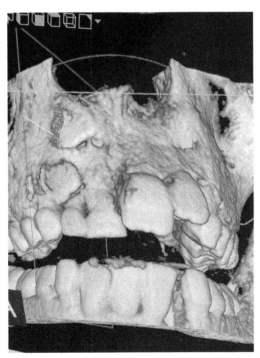

Fig. 10. Three-dimensional CBCT of an impacted incisor.

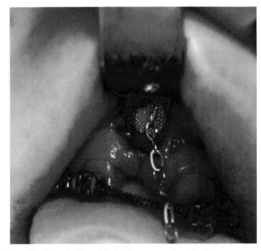

Fig. 12. Bonded gold chain on central incisor.

and periodontal outcomes superior to the apically positioned technique.[27]

When it comes to selecting the procedure, the tooth position will dictate the best exposure method. For labial positioned teeth, low in the alveolus, the window technique or apically repositioned flap can be used. For a palatally positioned tooth, the closed eruption technique or window technique can be used. With the window technique, perio pack will need to be placed to prevent regrowth of soft tissue. If the tooth is coronal to the mucogingival junction, any technique will work. If the impacted tooth is apical to the mucogingival junction, the apically repositioned flap is the procedure of choice. If it is significantly apical to the mucogingival junction, the closed eruption technique is the treatment of choice. Finally, if the impacted tooth is positioned over the root of the lateral incisor, the apically repositioned flap should be used. When considering a procedure, an approach should be chosen that allows the tooth to erupt through attached gingiva.[27]

IMPACTED PREMOLAR

The incidence of impacted premolars is approximately 0.5%. Mandibular premolars have a higher rate of incidence than maxillary premolars.[28] Calcification of the premolar is at 18 or 30 months with eruption in 10 to 13 years (**Fig. 13**).

Etiology

Premolar impactions are usually due to local factors. Mesial drift of teeth is due to premature loss of the primary tooth, pathology, ectopic position of the tooth bud, and ankyloses of the primary tooth. Cleidocranial dysplasia, osteopetrosis, Down's syndrome, hypothyroidism and hypopituitarism can also cause premolar impactions.[29]

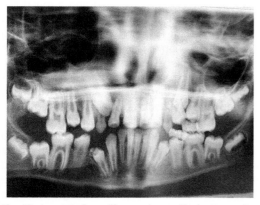

Fig. 13. Impacted maxillary and mandibular premolar.

Diagnosis and Radiographs

It is important to perform a thorough clinical examination and radiographic evaluation. A 3-D CBCT is the best radiograph to see the exact position of the impacted tooth and its proximity to important anatomic structures (mental foramen, maxillary sinus). This will help the surgeon see the best surgical approach to exposing the impacted tooth. It also helps to show the orthodontist the technical difficulty in bringing the tooth into the arch.

Surgical Exposure

The various treatment modalities are the same for impacted premolars. Conservative management with exposure of the crown is advocated even though it is unpredictable and technically difficult. It is best to limit exposure to cases with premolars with no more than 45° tilt of the long axis from normal position. A full-thickness mucoperiosteal flap should be raised either buccally or lingually dependent on position of the tooth. Bone is removed from the buccal or lingual cortex using a #8 round bur until the crown of the tooth is exposed. Then a bracket and chain is bonded to the crown of the tooth. Copious irrigation of the surgical site will prevent any delay in healing and infection. The flap is then sutured back into position. The orthodontist should be apprised of its position so the correct vectors and application of orthodontic forces is applied[28–31].

IMPACTED SECOND MOLARS

The impaction of the second molar is a rare complication in tooth eruption occurring approximately 0.03% to as high as 3%, depending on the study. It occurs unilaterally more commonly than bilaterally and slightly more in men than women (**Fig. 14**). It is more common in the mandible than maxilla.[3]

The management of impacted second molar has always been a challenge for the orthodontist and oral and maxillofacial surgeon. The impacted second molar usually goes unnoticed until the orthodontic treatment is complete and the roots are fully formed. Proper alignment of the second molar into the dental arch is required to complete orthodontic therapy.

ETIOLOGY

There are multiple etiologies for impacted second molar. When the deciduous second molar is lost, the first permanent molar must move forward to accommodate the eruption of the second molar. If this does not occur, the eruption of the second molar is compromised.

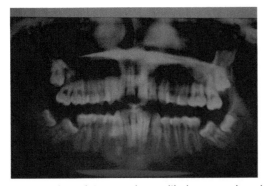

Fig. 14. Bilateral impacted mandibular second and third molars.

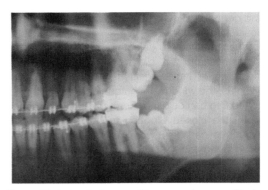

Fig. 16. Impacted maxillary and mandibular second molar due to ortho bands.

This can lead to tipping. If the developing third molar infringes on the space required for the second molar to erupt, mesial tipping occurs (**Fig. 15**). Ill-fitting first molar bands are an iatrogenic cause of the mesial impacted second molar (**Fig. 16**).

Nonextraction treatment has become increasingly common due to the possibility of unpleasing facial aesthetics outcomes. Desnoes[32] has shown that this has also contributed to complications in the eruption of second molar.

RADIOGRAPHS

A panoramic radiograph is the radiograph of choice to evaluate the position of the impacted second molar. When the position of the tooth is horizontal and close to the inferior alveolar nerve, a 3-D CBCT is recommended.

TREATMENT OPTIONS

The location of the second molar and degree of impaction determines the treatment plan.

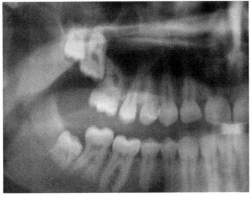

Fig. 15. Impacted maxillary second molar fully developed.

Observation is not an option. Impacted second molars must be treated because they can cause decay and periodontal disease with bone loss.[33] The following treatment options can be used to treat the impacted second molar.

1. Surgical extraction of the impacted second molar.
2. Surgical exposure and uprighting the second molar.
3. Transplantation of the third molar into the impacted second molar site.

SURGICAL EXPOSURE AND UPRIGHTING THE SECOND MOLAR

The decision to upright the impacted second molar is usually made by the orthodontist. The patient is then referred to the oral and maxillofacial surgeon to discuss this combined orthodontic and surgical approach. The treatment plan may not be successful if the second molar root has more than two-thirds root formation. The procedure consists of the following.

After a local anesthetic block, an incision is made along the cervical areas if the first molar is along the external oblique ridge. A full-thickness mucoperiosteal flap is elevated and a round bur is used to expose the crown of the impacted second molar. It is important to avoid exposing the cemento-enamel junction and root surface of the second molar. This exposure will increase the chance of periodontal defects and external resorption.[34] If the third molar is impinging the second molar, it should be removed. Bone grafting is recommended if a defect remains. Then using a 301 elevator, the second molar is gently elevated up. If the second molar can be elevated into proper position, an orthodontic appliance is not required (**Fig. 17**). *Sometimes stabilizing the uprighted second molar can be a problem (**Fig. 17**). If it is not self-stabilizing, an orthodontic bonding material is used to bond the second molar to the first molar. This is not required with maxillary impacted second molar. Luxation of the maxillary impacted second molar will stimulate eruption. In Fig. 15, the second molar is exposed and luxated. Within 6 months, the tooth erupted. After eruption, the third molar was removed (**Fig. 17**).

In most cases, an orthodontic appliance needs to be placed to upright the second molar. Going and Rayes-Lois[34] reports of a technique in which the second molar is bracketed with a band containing a buccal tube. Then a heavy-gauge nickel titanium arch wire is threaded through the tube and the arch wire is ligated to the 2 premolars and canine. The arch wire will then help to upright the second molar.[34] Other appliance can be used instead. For example, segmental springs and nickel titanium coil springs have been successful in uprighting the second molar.[35,36] TADs have been developed that can be placed in the alveolar bone and used as an anchorage device. A 2-week healing period is necessary before elastics are placed. Orthodontic forces of 50 g to 250 g can be placed on the TAD. This method is especially useful when trying to upright lingually tipped lower second molar and buccally tipped upper second molar.[12] In addition, brass wire can be used as a separator when placed below and above the contact point between the first molar and impacted second molar. The wire can be tightened incrementally to upright the second molar. This technique is used infrequently, because it causes pain, swelling, and future periodontal problems.

RISK FACTORS AND COMPLICATIONS

Complications are possible with any surgical procedure. Complications and risk factors should be discussed with the patient before surgery.[23] They include the following:

1. Ecchymosis of the upper lip or lower lip and chin
2. Infection
3. Paresthesia
4. Damage to adjacent structures
5. Noneruption
6. Loss of soft tissue flap/dehiscence
7. Lack of attached gingiva
8. Devitalization of the pulp
9. Pain
10. Early loss of the orthodontic bracket
11. External resorption
12. Loss of tooth

SUMMARY

The exposure of impacted teeth can be challenging but rewarding. The decision to surgically correct these impacted teeth is usually made by the orthodontist. Treatment planning these cases should be multidisciplinary with the oral and maxillofacial surgeon making the final decision on the surgical treatment plan. The risk-to-benefit ratio usually favors the preservation of the impacted tooth. In general, the recommendation is surgical exposure of the impacted tooth with orthodontic alignment into the arch. It is also recommended to upright the second molar with the removal of the impacted third molar. Close follow-up by the orthodontist and surgeon is important to the success of these procedures. Preserving these teeth is an important orthodontic standard of care, so it is imperative that our treatment is based on an appropriate diagnosis made with adequate radiographic localization and consultation with an orthodontist.

DISCLOSURE

The author has nothing to disclose.

REFERENCES

1. Becker A, Chaushu S. Surgical treatment of impacted canines: what the orthodontist would like you to know. Oral Maxfacial Surg Clin North Am 2015;27:449–58.
2. Thilander B, Jacobasson SO. Local factors in impaction of maxillary canines. Acta Odontol Scand 1968;26:145–68.
3. Dachi SF, Howell FV. A Survey of 3874 routine full mouth radiographs. Oral surgery, oral medicine. Oral Pathol 1961;14:1165–309.
4. Stellzig A, Basdra EK, Komposch G. The etiology of canine tooth impaction- a space analysis. Fortschr Kieferorthop 1994;55(3):97–103.

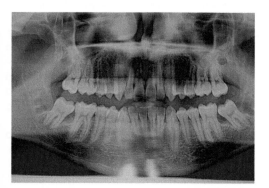

Fig. 17. Impacted second molars surgically uprighted after removal of third molars.

5. Piriren S, Arte S, Apajalahti S. Palatal displacement of canine is genetic and related to congential absence of teeth. J Dental Res 1998;75:1742–6.

6. Thilander B, Myrberg N. The prevalence of malocclusion in Swedish school children. Scand J Dent Res 1973;81:12–20.

7. Jacobs SG. Reducing the incidence of unerupted palatally displaced canines by extraction of deciduous canine. The history and application of this procedure with some case reports. Aust Dent J 1998; 43(1):20–7.

8. Chapokas AR, Almas K, Schincaglia G-P. The impacted maxillary canine: a proposed classification for surgical exposure. Oral Surg Oral Med Oral Pathol Oral Radiol 2012;113:222–8.

9. Bedoya M, Park JH. A review of the diagnosis and management of impacted maxillary canines. J Am Dent Assoc 2009;140:1485–93.

10. Koutzoglou SI, Kostaki A. Effect of surgical exposure technique, age, and grade of impaction on ankylosis of an impacted canine, and the effect of rapid palatal expansion on eruption: a prospective clinical study. Am J Orthod Dentofacial Orthopedics 2013; 143:342–52.

11. Becker A, Chaushu S. Palatally impacted canines: the case for closed surgical exposure and immediate orthodontic traction. Am J Orthod Dentofacial Orthop 2013;143(4):451–9.

12. Park J, Kwon O, Sung J, et al. Uprighting second molars with microimplant anchorage. J Clin Orthod 2004;38(2):100–3.

13. Vermette ME, Kokich VG, Kennedy DB. Uncovering labially impacted teeth: apically positioned flap and closed eruption techniques. Angle Orthodontist 1995;65:23–32.

14. Semb G, Schwartz O. The impacted tooth in patients with alveolar clefts. In: Anderson JO, editor. Textbook and color atlas of tooth impactions. Copenhagen (Denmark): Munksguard; 1997. p. 331–48.

15. Moss JP. The unerupted canine. Dental Pract 1972; 22:241–8.

16. Katsnelson A, Flick WG, Seenu S. Use of panoramic Xray to determine position of impacted maxillary canines. J Oral Maxillofac Surg 2010;68:996–1000.

17. Chaushu S, Chaushu G, Becker A. Reliability of a method for the localization of displaced maxillary canines using a single panoramic radiograph. Clin Orthod Res 1999;2:194.

18. Ericson S, Kurol J. Radiographic examination of ectopically erupting maxillary canines. Am J Orthod Dentofacial Orthop 1987;91:483–92.

19. Haney E, Gansky SA, Lee JS, et al. Comparative analysis of traditional radiographs and cone-beam computed tomography volumetric images in the diagnosis and treatment planning of maxillary impacted canines. Amj Orthod Dentofacial Orthop 2010;137:590–7.

20. Ferguson JW, Pitt SKJ. Management of unerupted maxillary canines where no orthodontic treatment is planned; a survey of UK consultant opinion. J Orthod 2004;31(1):28–33.

21. McSterry PF. The assessment of and treatment options for the buried maxillary canine. Dent Update 1996;23:7–10.

22. Ferguson JW, Pervizi F. Eruption of palatal canine following surgical exposure: a review of outcomes in a series of consecutively treated cases. Br J Orthod 1997;24(3):203–7.

23. Felsenfeld A, Aghaloo T. Surgical exposure of impacted teeth. Oral Maxillofacial Surg Clin N Am 2002;14:187–99.

24. Yavuz M, Aras M. J Contemp Dental Pract 2007;8(7): 925–8.

25. Alling C, Helfrick J, Alling R. Impacted teeth. Philadelphia: W.B. Saunders; 1993. p. 215–6.

26. Smailiene D, Sidlauskas A, Bucinskiene J. Impaction of the central maxillary incisor associated with supernumerary teeth: initial position and spontaneous eruption timing. Stomatologija 2006;8(4):103–7.

27. Borbely P, Watted N, Dubovaka I, et al. Orthodontic treatment of an impacted maxillary central incisor combined with surgical exposure. Inter J Dental Health Sci 2015;2(5):1335–44.

28. Majunatha BS, Chikkaramaiah S, Panja P, et al. Impacted maxillary second premolars: a report of four cases. BMJ Case Rep 2014;2014. bcr2014205206.

29. Abu-Hussein M, Watted NE, Awadi O. Management of lower second premolar impaction. J Adv Dental Res 2015;1(1):1–9.

30. Shastri D, Tandon P, Singh GP, et al. Management of impacted 2nd premolar impaction by buccal approach: a case report. Inter J Dental Health Sci 2014;2(4):1–4.

31. Collett AR. Conservative management of lower second premolar impaction. Aust Dental J 2000;45-4: 279–81.

32. Desnoes H. Abnormalities in the development of the second molars and orthodontic treatment without extraction of premolars. Management of posterior crowding. J Dentofacial Anom Orthod 2014;17:406.

33. Magnusson C, Kjeilberg H. Impaction and retention of second molars: diagnosis, treatment and outcome. Angle orthodontist 2009;79(3):422–7.

34. Going R Jr, Rayes-Lois D. Surgical exposure and bracketing techniques for uprighting impacted mandibular second molars. J Oral Maxillofac Surg 1999;57:209–11.

35. Majourau A, Norton L. Uprighting impacted second molar with segmental springs. Am J Orthod Dentofacial Orthop 1995;107:135–8.

36. McAboy CP, Gruvent J, Siegel EB, et al. Surgical uprighting and reposition of severely impacted second molar. J Am Dent Assoc 2003;134:1459–62.

Current Concepts of Periapical Surgery
2020 Update

Stuart E. Lieblich, DMD[a,b,]*

KEYWORDS

- Apicoectomy • Periapical surgery • Mineral trioxide aggregate • Super EBA
- Complications of apical surgery

KEY POINTS

- Preoperative decision making is vital to determine potential success of periapical surgery.
- Adequate exposure of the root apical region is approached best via a sulcular-type incision.
- Surgical procedures include resection of 2 mm to 3 mm of the apical portion along with root end preparation and seal.
- The surgeon must decide if submission of periapical tissues to pathology is indicated.

PREOPERATIVE PLANNING

Although endodontic care typically is successful, in approximately 10% to 15% of cases,[1] symptoms can persist or spontaneously reoccur. It is known that many endodontic failures are due to the failure to place an adequate coronal seal. Therefore, there is the competing interest of observing the tooth after endodontic treatment to ascertain successful treatment versus placing a definitive restoration with an adequate coronal seal. Many endodontic failures occur a year or more after the initial root canal treatment, often creating a situation where a definitive restoration already has been placed. This creates a higher value for the tooth because it now may be supporting a fixed partial denture. A decision then is needed to determine if orthograde endodontic retreatment can be accomplished, should periapical surgery be recommended or consideration of extraction of the tooth with loss of the overlying prosthesis.

Causes of endodontic failures often can be separated into biologic issues, such as a persistent infection, or technical factors, such as a broken instrument in the root canal system (**Fig. 1**), transportation of the apex, perforation, and ledging of the canal. Failure of endodontic treatment is due most commonly to lack of an adequate coronal seal with the presence of bacteria within the root canal system and apical leakage. Continued infection also may result from debris displaced out the apex during the initial endodontic treatment. Technical factors alone are a less common indication for surgery, comprising only 3% of the total cases referred for surgery,[2] yet it is this author's opinion that there is a higher success rate in these cases.

Prior to surgery, discussions with patients are critical in order for a patient to give appropriate informed consent. The particular risks of surgery based on the anatomic location (sinus involvement or proximity to the inferior alveolar nerve) need to be reviewed and documented. It is important to stress the exploratory nature of periapical surgery to the patient. Depending on the findings at surgery, a limited root resection with retrograde restoration may be placed. The patient and surgeon,

This article has been updated from a version previously published in *Oral and Maxillofacial Surgery Clinics*, Volume 27, Issue 3, August 2015.

[a] Oral and Maxillofacial Surgery, University of Connecticut Health Center; [b] Private Practice, Avon Oral, Facial and Dental Implant Surgery, 34 Dale Road, Suite 105, Avon, CT 06001, USA
* Private Practice, Avon Oral, Facial and Dental Implant Surgery, 34 Dale Road, Suite 105, Avon, CT 06001.
E-mail address: StuL@comcast.net

Oral Maxillofacial Surg Clin N Am 32 (2020) 571–582
https://doi.org/10.1016/j.coms.2020.07.007
1042-3699/20/© 2020 Elsevier Inc. All rights reserved.

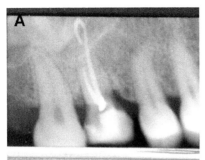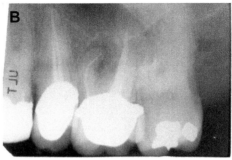

Fig. 1. Two examples of technical factors requiring apical surgery. Although less frequent in occurrence, the success rate usually is high because the canal system likely is well obturated. (*A*) Overfill of gutta percha causing symptoms, including chronic sinusitis. (*B*) Broken endodontic instrument in apical third with pain and drainage. (*From* Lieblich SE. Current concepts of periapical surgery. Oral Maxillofac Surg Clin North Am. 2015;27(3):384; with permission.)

however, also must be prepared to treat fractures of the root and/or the entire tooth. Plans must be made preoperatively on how such situations will be handled should they be noted intraoperatively.

Diagnostic tools, such as a focused periodontal examination of the tooth in question, are necessary to determine if a tooth is worth saving via the apical surgery procedure. Poor prognostic factors, such as significant loss of attachment and mobility, likely would drive a recommendation to extraction with implant placement. Consideration for a localized cone beam radiology examination of the involved area also may provide preoperative evidence of a fracture, which would reduce the likelihood of successful outcomes of the surgery.

Surgical endodontics success rates have dramatically improved over the years with the developments of newer retrofilling materials and the use of the ultrasonic preparation. Previously cited success rates of 60% to 70% now have increased to more than 90% in many studies,[3–5] due to the routine use of ultrasonic retrograde preparation and the use of mineral trioxide aggregate as a filling material. This significant improvement makes apical surgery a more predictable and valuable adjunct in the treatment of symptomatic teeth. Most significantly, studies[6] show that once the periapical bony defect is considered healed (reformation of the lamina dura or cases of healing by scar), the long-term prognosis is excellent. They reported 91.5% of healed cases still successful after a follow-up period of 5 years to 7 years. Therefore, with adequate radiographic follow-up, a surgeon should be able to predict the long-term viability of the tooth and its usefulness to retain a prosthetic restoration.

There is some controversy in the endodontic literature that the use of magnification may improve outcomes in surgical management of

endodontic failures. In a 2-part article by Setzer and colleagues,[7,8] a meta-analysis was reviewed on this subject of endodontic surgery. In part 1 (2010), they compared outcomes with traditional root end preparation with a rotary bur and amalgam filling versus more contemporary surgery with ultrasonic preparation and improved root end filling materials (Super-EBA [Alumina reinforced intermediary restorative material, Bosworth Company, Warwichshire, England] and MTA [Mineral trioxide aggregate ProRoot MTA Dentsply Sirona, Charlotte, North Carolina]). With the more contemporary surgery techniques, the outcomes improved from 59% to 94%. They then divided the literature into 2 groups in 2012: those using no magnification or loupes up to 10×, and those using the operating microscope or an endoscope with magnification greater than 10×. The nonmagnification group had a cumulative success rate of 88% whereas the group with use of magnification had a pooled success rate of 93%. No difference in success was noted for treatment of anterior teeth or premolars with or without magnification but there was some improved success for molars (98% vs 90%, respectively).

The primary option for the treatment of symptomatic endodontically treated teeth is that of conventional retreatment versus the surgical approach. An algorithm for a decision regarding retreatment versus surgery versus extraction is presented in **Fig. 2**. In discussions with patients, the option of conventional retreatment should be discussed. Clinical studies, however, have not shown retreatment to be more successful than surgery and 1 prospective study found surgical treatment to have a higher success rate.[9] Another study found a higher success rate with surgery from 2 years to 4 years (77.8% vs 70.9%, respectively), but from 4 years to 6 years it reversed to a

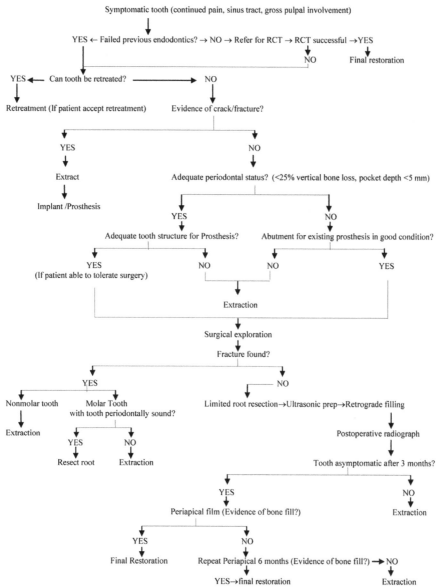

Fig. 2. Algorithm for apical surgery. Prep, preparation; RCT, root canal treatment. (*Adapted from* Lieblich SE. Periapical surgery: clinical decision making. Oral Maxillofac Surg Clin North Am. 2002;14(2):181; with permission.)

success rate of 71.8% with surgery and 83% with conventional retreatment.[10] Although endodontic retreatment seems more conservative, the removal of posts, reinstrumentation of the tooth, and removal of tooth structure increase the chance of fracture. Surgical treatment of failures also provides the opportunity to retrieve tissue for histologic examination to rule out a noninfectious cause of a lesion (**Fig. 3**).

The option of extraction with either immediate or delayed implant placement also must be discussed as an alternative to periapical surgery. There is no debate in dentistry that implants can

outlast tooth supported restorations. It is valuable, therefore, to have data to predict the expected success of the endodontic surgery so that patients can use them in their decision-making process. Factors that improve success are noted in **Box 1**. In cases of an expected poorer success rate, such as the presence of severe periodontal bone loss (especially the presence of furcation involvement), the decision to extract the tooth and place an implant may be a more efficacious and clinically predictable procedure.

There is a body of literature that supports the duration of restorations fabricated on

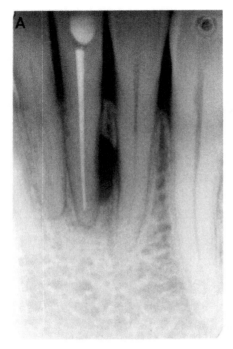
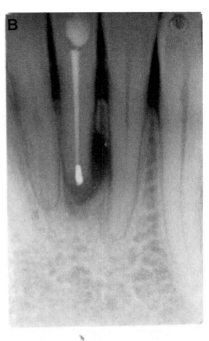

Fig. 3. Atypical radiolucency along the lateral aspect of the root and not truly involving the apex. Although correctly treated at the time of referral due to the nonresolving radiolucency with periapical surgery, the suspicious nature of the lesion warranted submission of the tissue for histologic examination. Confirmation with the original treating dentist revealed the indication for the endodontic treatment was solely the incidental finding of a radiolucency and vital pulp tissue was noted. The final pathology was a cystic ameloblastoma. (A) preoperative radiograph, note lateral radiolucency not associated with the apex. (B) post surgery shows good apical seal but residual lateral pathology. (*From* Lieblich SE. Current concepts of periapical surgery. Oral Maxillofac Surg Clin North Am. 2015;27(3):386; with permission.)

endodontically treated teeth. Blomlof and Jansson[11] found surgically treated molars with healthy periodontal status had a 10-year survival rate of 89% and Basten and colleagues[12] reported a 92% 12-year rate. The factors most associated with failures are long posts in teeth with little remaining coronal structure. Thus, the condemnation of a tooth because it can be replaced with an implant is not that clear.

An economic analysis may be indicated in order to guide a patient's decision. If the tooth has a final prosthetic restoration already in place, it usually is easier to recommend surgical intervention. If the symptoms do not resolve, patients have only expended additional time, operative risk, and expense of the surgical portion of their care because they already have a definitive restoration. The surgeon should review the factors in **Box 1** to help predict the likelihood of the surgical intervention being successful. If a tooth has multiple factors that indicate the success of the surgical intervention would be compromised and/or a tooth has a poor expectation for 10-year survival, then extraction with implant placement is a more efficacious means of care.

The surgeon may be called on to treat teeth that cannot be negotiated for conventional orthograde endodontics. The treatment of teeth with calcified canals may be managed appropriately with apical surgery alone with a retrograde filling if the tooth is critical to a restorative treatment plan. Danin[13] showed at least a 50% rate of complete radiographic healing and only 1 failure in 10 cases over a 1-year observation period in cases treated surgically only and without endodontic treatment. Bacteria still remained in the canals of the tooth in 90% of these cases, which may lead to a later failure.

DETERMINATION OF SUCCESS

More complicated decisions are involved with teeth that have not been definitively restored. In that situation, the surgeon not only has to consider the preoperative potential for the apical surgery to be successful but also often must determine when a case is deemed successful and can proceed to the final restoration. Once a final restoration is placed, considerably more time and expense have been invested and subsequent failure is more troublesome to the patient.

Box 1
Factors associated with success and failures in periapical surgery

Success

Preoperative factors

1. Dense orthograde fill

2. Healthy periodontal status

   a. No dehiscence

   b. Adequate crown:root ratio

3. Radiolucent defect isolated to apical one-third of tooth

4. Tooth treated

   a. Maxillary incisor

   b. Mesiobuccal root of maxillary molars

Postoperative factors

5. Radiographic evidence of bone fill after surgery

6. Resolution of pain and symptoms

7. Absence of sinus tract

8. Decrease in tooth mobility

Failure

Preoperative factors

1. Clinical or radiographic evidence of fracture

2. Poor or lack of orthograde filling

3. Marginal leakage of crown or post

4. Poor preoperative periodontal condition (furcation involvement)

5. Radiographic evidence of post perforation

6. Tooth treated

   a. Mandibular incisor

Postoperative factors

7. Lack of bone repair after surgery

8. Lack of resolution of pain

9. Fistula does not resolve or returns

Adapted from Lieblich SE. Current concepts of periapical surgery. Oral Maxillofac Surg Clin North Am. 2015;27(3):386; with permission.

Rud and colleagues[14] retrospectively reviewed radiographs after apical surgery to determine radiographic signs of success. Their work showed that with a retrospective review of cases over at least 4 years postsurgery, once radiographic evidence of bone fill occurs, noted as successful healing in their classification scheme, that tooth was stable throughout the remainder of their study period (up to 15 years). A waiting period of more than 4 years is not acceptable in contemporary practice, but their classification scheme has been validated over shorter observation times. They found that if radiographic evidence of bone fill of the surgical defect is noted, then the tooth remained a radiographic success over their observation periods. Many of the partially healing cases, noted as "incomplete healing" in their study, tended to move into the complete healing group during the 2 years after surgery, with little change throughout the next 4 years of observation.

An appropriate follow-up protocol is to obtain a repeat periapical film 3 months after surgery with critical comparison with the immediate postoperative film. If significant bone fill has occurred, mobility has decreased, pain is resolved, and no fistula is present, the case can proceed to the final restoration. If significant bone fill has not been noted, however, the patient should be recalled again at 3 months for a new film. Rubinstein and Kim[15] found complete healing in 25.3% of cases in 3 months, 34% in 6 months, 15.4% in 9 months, and 25.3% by 12 months. Small bony defects healed faster than large bony defects, which showed significant differences in their prospective study. In contrast, any increase in the size of the radiolucency or no improvement should caution a dentist about making a final restoration. If the situation is not clear at that time (6 months postsurgically), a temporary restoration, loaded for a least 3 months, often is a good litmus test of the success of the surgery and predictive as to whether the final restoration will last for some time.

THE CRACKED OR FRACTURED TOOTH

Preoperative radiographs and a careful clinical examination should be done with a high index of suspicion of a vertical root fracture (VRF) prior to undertaking surgery. Mandibular molars and maxillary premolars are the teeth that most frequently present with occult VRFs. Although surgical exploration may be needed to definitively show the presence of a fracture (**Fig. 4**), subtle radiographic signs may alert the surgeon that a fracture is present and the surgery is unlikely to be successful. Tamse and colleagues[16] looked at radiographs of maxillary premolars for comparison with the clinical findings at the time of surgery. Few (1 of 15) teeth with an isolated, well corticated periapical lesion had a VRF. In contrast, a halo-type radiolucency almost always was associated with a VRF (**Fig. 5**). This type of radiolucency also is known as a J type, where a widened periodontal

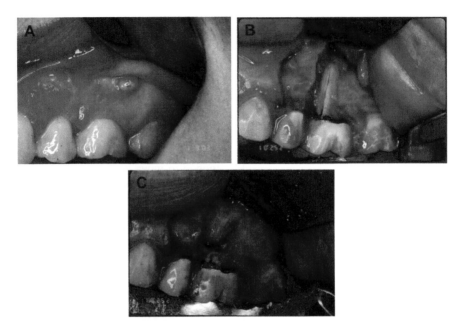

Fig. 4. VRF that was not diagnosed until explored at the time of surgery. The use of a sulcular flap permitted a resection of the mesiobuccal root and preservation of the tooth with its existing restoration. (*A*) preoperative situation appears to be a classic apical pathology with a fistual (*B*) after full thickness sulcular incision a vertical fracture was obvious. (*C*) resected mesial root which allows tooth to be maintained. (*From* Lieblich SE. Current concepts of periapical surgery. Oral Maxillofac Surg Clin North Am. 2015;27(3):388; with permission.)

ligament space connects with the periapical lesion creating the J pattern.

It is critical in patient discussions to review the exploratory nature of the surgery and this author routinely uses that as a descriptor of the planned surgery. In cases of root fracture, a decision during surgery may need to be made either to resect a root or extract a tooth if a fractured root is found. Obtaining appropriate preoperative consent as well as determining how the extracted tooth site will be managed (with or without a temporary removeable partial denture) must be established before surgery commences.

CONCOMITANT PERIODONTAL PROCEDURES

The use of guided tissue regeneration (GTR), alloplastic or allogenic bone grafting, and root planing in conjunction with periapical surgery can be considered. In cases of severe bone dehiscence, the likelihood of success is known to be substantially compromised and may lead to an intraoperative decision to extract the tooth. Periodontal probing, prior to surgery, often detects the presence of significant bony defects. Sometimes the amount of bone loss cannot be appreciated until the area is flapped (**Fig. 6**). Thus, the exploratory

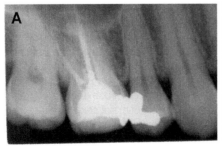 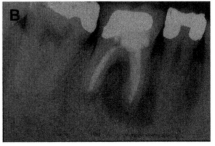

Fig. 5. (*A*) Example of a periapical lesion isolated to the apical one-third of the root. These rarely are associated with a VRF. (*B*) In contrast, this type of radiographic lesion, known as a halo or J-type radiolucency, has ill-defined cortical borders and most likely is associated with VRF. (*From* Lieblich SE. Current concepts of periapical surgery. Oral Maxillofac Surg Clin North Am. 2015;27(3):388; with permission.)

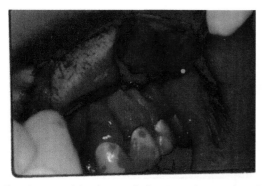

Fig. 6. A combination endodontic and periodontal lesion has a very low likelihood of success. The decision was preoperatively to treat the tooth surgically because an adequate final restoration had already made been placed. Otherwise extraction with consideration of local bone grafting is indicated. (*From* Lieblich SE. Current concepts of periapical surgery. Oral Maxillofac Surg Clin North Am. 2015;27(3):389; with permission.)

nature of the surgery needs to be stressed preoperatively with the patient.

The placement of an additional foreign body, such as a Gore-tex membrane, to an area already infected is more likely to lead to failure of the surgery. Membrane stabilization and adequate mobilization of soft tissues to cover the membrane may increase the complexity of the surgical procedure. Nonresorbable membranes also require a second procedure for membrane removal that may not be tolerated by the patient as well as lead to an increase in scarring. A recent review by Tsesis and colleagues[17] seems to show a trend toward higher success with the use of resorbable membranes in cases of large defects and through and through lesions. This author, however, does not advocate grafting or the use of membranes in conjunction with endodontic surgery. Clinical success, defined as reduction in symptoms and spontaneous bone fill, is demonstrated routinely without the use of allogenic bone or other GTR procedures (**Fig. 7**).

SURGICAL PROCEDURES

Various steps are involved in the periapical surgical procedure. Initial exposure of the apical region is needed. This must allow access to apex for the root resection. Approximately 2 mm to 3 mm of the root apex is resected. The root resection removes the end of the root containing the aberrant canals. Also, the further from the coronal portion of the tooth, the less dense the endodontic filling is likely to be.

Following the root resection, a thorough curettage of the periapical region is accomplished,

with cognizance of local structures, such as the maxillary sinus or the inferior alveolar nerve. Curettage removes periapical debris that may have been forced out the apex during the previous preparation of the root canal system. Tissue may be recovered at this time for histologic examination if indicated (discussed later). A retrograde filling then is prepared with the use of the ultrasonic device. This creates a microapical restoration that is retentive due to the parallel walls. The ultrasonic device creates a very conservative preparation and often finds unfilled canals or an isthmus of retained pulpal tissue connecting 2 canals, particularly in the mesiobuccal roots of maxillary first molars. The ultrasonic preparation has been shown to be advantageous to the rotary drills because it centers the preparation along the long axis of the canal and significantly reduces the tendency to create root perforations.[18]

The retrograde filling is important to hermetically seal the root canal system, preventing further leakage of bacterial into the periapical tissues. Many filling materials have been used throughout the years and many do work well. The most contemporary material is MTA and has been shown histologically to deposit bone around it. Its handling characteristics are somewhat different from those of other dental materials because it is hydrophilic and does not reach a full firm set for 2 hours to 4 hours. This is not clinically significant because the region is not load bearing, at least for quite some time after the apical surgery. MTA has been shown to produce regeneration of cementum, something not seen with other root end filling materials.

SURGICAL ACCESS

Surgical access is a compromise between the need for visibility and the risk to adjacent structures. Many surgeons utilize the semilunar flap to access the periapical region. Although it provides rapid access to the apices of the teeth, it substantially limits the surgery to only a root resection and periapical seal. Proponents of this flap claim that it prevents recession around existing crowns, which could lead to a metal margin showing postoperatively.

The semilunar flap is placed entirely in the nonkeratinized or unattached gingiva. By definition, this tissue is constantly moving during normal oral function, leading to dehiscence and increased scarring. Incisions placed in unattached tissues tend to heal slower and with more discomfort.

Once a semilunar incision is made, the surgeon has access limited to only the periapical region. If the root is noted to be fractured, extraction via this flap may lead to a severe defect. With a

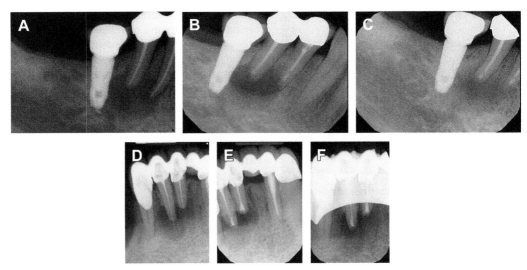

Fig. 7. Large periapical lesion associated with teeth #27 and #28 in proximity with an implant (*A*). Apical surgery was performed (*B*) with MTA seal; no graft or membrane was placed into the defect. (*C*) Shows bone fill after 3 months. (*D*) preoperative periapical showing large periapical defect. (*E*) immediate postoperative radiograph (*F*) 3 month postoperative film showing good bone fill of defect without the use of graft or other guided tissue regeneration procedure. (*From* Lieblich SE. Current concepts of periapical surgery. Oral Maxillofac Surg Clin North Am. 2015;27(3):389; with permission.)

multirooted tooth, a root resection of one of the fractured roots may not be possible. Additionally, localized root planing or other periodontal procedures cannot be accomplished. The size of the bone defect may be greater than that anticipated based on the preoperative radiographs and the possibility of the suture line being over the defect might cause the incision to open up and heal secondarily. Lastly, it is known that many cases of periapical surgery on maxillary molars and premolars involve an opening into the sinus cavity,[19] and the incision line with this type of flap might contribute to a postoperative oral-antral fistula.

In contrast, a sulcular incision with 1 or 2 vertical releases keeps the incision primarily within the attached gingival, promoting rapid healing with less pain and scarring. Healing of the incision is facilitated by curetting the adjacent teeth and any exposed root surfaces prior to closure. The incision permits full observation of the root surface, leading to more accurate apical localization and treatment of a fractured root should it be discovered on flap reflection (see **Fig. 4**). By keeping the incision as far away from the sinus opening as possible and over healthy bone (versus a sulcular incision), the chance of an oral-antral communication is reduced significantly.

Concerns about sulcular incisions have revolved primarily around the concern for an esthetic defect that may be created with the shrinkage or loss of the interdental papilla. Jansson and colleagues[20]

found the greatest predicator of papilla loss was the presence of a continued apical infection and found no difference in the attachment whether a semilunar or trapezoidal flap was used. Recent publications by Velvart[21] proposed the use of a "papilla base incision," in which the triangle of interdental papilla is not incised and not mobilized during reflection of the flap. They report maintenance of the papilla with little to no recession in contrast to mobilization of the papilla. von Arx[3] (**Figs. 8** and **9**) reviewed the papilla-based incision with the intrasulcular type and found less recession with this type of flap design.

The treatment of maxillary molar teeth is noted to be in proximity of the maxillary sinus. By planning an incision at the gingival margin of the tooth, there should be adequate bone for closure of the incision. The surgeon must be careful not to displace root fragments or packing material into the sinus, which can become a nidus of infection. Consideration for preoperative antibiotics and postoperative sinus precautions (use of decongestants, to sneeze with mouth open and no nose blowing) should be reviewed with the patient as well.

In the mandible, treatment of molars and premolars often are more difficult due to the dense cortical bone and surgical view. The location of the inferior alveolar nerve, in particular, the mental foramen, needs to be taken into account. One report[22] noted a relatively high incidence of neurosensory changes in these cases. The investigators

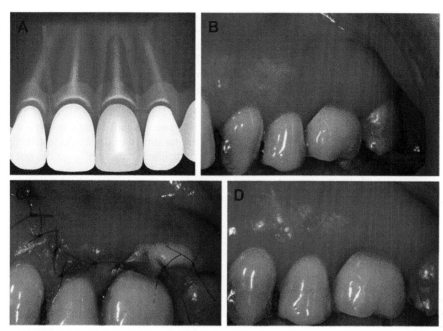

Fig. 8. Papilla-based incision has been shown to have less recession than the intrasulcular incision. (*A*) schematic of the papilla based incision. (*B*) preoperative periodontal status, (*C*) flap sutured in place (*D*) 2 months of healing showing maintenance of the periodontal status without recession. (*From* von Arx T, Vinzens-Majaniemi T, Bürgin W, et al. Changes of periodontal parameters following apical surgery: a prospective clinical study of three incision techniques. Int Endod J. 2007;40(12):959–69; with permission.)

reported an incidence of 38% altered sensation after premolar apical surgery and 14% overall of the pooled mandibular molars and premolars. The proximity of the mental nerve dictates the need for careful surgical procedures and preoperative counseling of patients to advise them of the risk.

TO BIOPSY OR NOT?

A clinical controversy has ensued over the consideration as to whether all periapical lesions treated

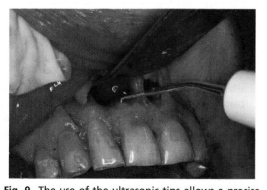

Fig. 9. The use of the ultrasonic tips allows a precise and retentive retrograde preparation. A minimal to no bevel is needed, which exposes less of the dentinal tubules in the apical aspect of the tooth. (*From* Lieblich SE. Current concepts of periapical surgery. Oral Maxillofac Surg Clin North Am. 2015;27(3):390; with permission.)

surgically should have soft tissue removed and submitted for histologic evaluation. An editorial by Walton[23] questioned the rationale of submitting all soft tissue recovered for histologic examination, which then ignited a series of letters to the editor. Organizations such as the American Association of Endodontists, have stated in their standards that if soft tissue can be recovered from the apical surgery, then it must be submitted for pathologic evaluation.

On cursory review, it seems that it is easier to make this recommendation than to have a surgeon determine if there is anything unusual about the case that warrants histologic examination. Walton[23] makes a convincing argument against the submission of all tissues, because similar-appearing radiolucencies that are not treated surgically do not have tissue retrieved for pathologic identification. It also is accepted that the differentiation between a periapical granuloma or periapical cyst has no direct bearing on clinical outcomes and, therefore, cannot be used as a rationalization for the submission of tissue.

The dilemma falls back to the surgeon that if a rare lesion should present itself in the context of a periapical lesion, and is not biopsied in a timely manner, the surgeon may have exposure in a potential malpractice suit. Many surgeons have a case or 2 in their careers that have surprised

Box 2
Indications for nonsubmission of periapical soft tissues for histologic review

1. Clear evidence of preexisting endodontic involvement of a tooth

   a. Pulpal necrosis was present, not just a periapical radiolucency

2. Unilocular radiolucency associated with apical one-third of the tooth

3. Lesion is not in association with an impacted tooth

4. No history of malignancy, which could represent spread of a metastasis

5. Patient returns for follow-up examinations and radiographs

6. No tissue recovered at the time of surgery

From Lieblich SE. Current concepts of periapical surgery. Oral Maxillofac Surg Clin North Am. 2015;27(3):391; with permission.

them based on the final pathologic diagnosis. Careful review of these cases, however, usually depicts a clinical situation inconsistent with a typical periapical infection (see **Fig. 3**).

An approach more logical than a purely defensive one is to set up guidelines on which it is determined submission of tissue was not indicated. These are listed in **Box 2**. It is recommended that a surgeon have documented in the record the rationale for electing not to submit tissue in each specific case. At a recent meeting of the American Association of Oral and Maxillofacial Surgeons, only 8% of those attending a symposium on endodontic surgery "always" submit tissue for histologic examination (Lieblich, personal communication, 2018).

EVIDENCE-BASED REVIEW OF THE VARIABLES

The highest level of information can be determined from evidence-based reviews of the literature. Combing individual clinical studies can give the clinician more robust evidence for choosing a specific recommendation for their patients. A Cochrane review[24] reviewed the literature to determine factors that influenced success for primary outcomes (1-year healing based on radiographs and lack of clinical symptoms) and secondary outcomes (>1-year healing with absence of clinical symptoms). Using these pooled data, some conclusions can be inferred but there were no areas where "strong" evidence for 1 option over another could be determined. Therefore, clinician

judgment and independent decision based on the unique aspect of each patient still need to be determined.

The following issues were reviewed and the reader is directed to the Cochrane article for more details and the specific clinical significance.

1. Root end resection with or without root end filling versus root canal retreatment for secondary treatment of periapical lesions (2 trials, 126 participants): these studies did not show a difference with either technique. As expected, the surgical group had increased pain over the first week but then there were no differences. These data suggest that a decision to undergo surgical treatment is not inferior to conventional endodontic retreatment. In cases of post and core/full coverage restorations, there are data to consider that surgery may have better outcomes even in the absence of a conventional root canal filling.[25]

2. Cone beam radiography versus conventional periapical films: neither of these preoperative diagnostic techniques improved outcome measures. The decision to utilize a higher amount of radiation must be balanced against the specific clinical information that can be gained with the detail from the cone beam.

3. Antibiotic prophylaxis (1 trial, 250 participants): no improved outcomes were noted with antibiotic premedication versus administration of a placebo. Here again the evidence is weak and clinicians may want to consider antibiotics on each specific case

4. Magnification devices: surgical microscope versus endoscope versus surgical loupes (1 trial, 98 participants/150 teeth). In the 2-part study, improved outcomes were not found using 1 type of magnification device over another. Some form of magnification is favored by those performing apical surgery but the type does not seem to be clinically significant.

5. Incision type (2 trials, 52 participants). One study looked at the retention of papilla height with the papilla-based incision versus a full papilla mobilization with a sulcular type incision. With the papilla-based incision, there was weak evidence that less loss of the height was noted 1 year after surgery. A separate study looked at postoperative pain with the 2 types of incision and, other than at day 3 (slightly less pain with papilla-based procedure), there were no differences.

6. Ultrasonic device versus conventional bur for root end preparation (1 trial, 290 participants): this study at risk for high bias did show weak evidence of improved outcomes with the use

of the ultrasonic device. Most clinicians find the use of the ultrasonic to provide more accuracy to prepare the canal for the retrograde restoration and allow the need for less of a bevel, potentially preserving more of the periodontal support for the tooth.

7. Root end filling material (7 trials, 846 participants): probably the area that generates the most controversy in apical surgery is the choice of root end filling materials along with the need for any filling material at all. The review noted no differences with intermediate restorative material versus Super EBA versus MTA. Therefore, these all are acceptable materials. One study does show an increased success with the use of MTA versus smoothing the orthograde endodontic gutta percha material at the apex, leading to the recommendation that a retrograde restoration be placed during apical surgery procedures.

8. Grafting versus no grafting (4 trials, 106 participants): a concern among surgeons is whether there is a need for grafting the defect created by the apical pathology as well as the surgical approach. Various studies of the use of calcium sulfate, GTR (membrane with bovine bone), and platelet-rich fibrin have not shown any improvement in radiographic healing. Some reduction in pain in the 2-hour and 6-hour time points with the use of platelet-rich fibrin and a reduction of swelling up to 5 days postoperatively were the only benefits noted. This information is consistent with a recent report[26] that showed regeneration of the buccal cortical plate with no loss in volume without grafting or GTR.

DISCLOSURE

The author is a paid consultant of Pacira BioSciences, Parsippany, New Jersey.

REFERENCES

1. Kerekes K, Tronstad L. Long-term results of endodontic treatment performed with a standardized technique. J Endod 1979;5:83–90.

2. El-Siwah JM, Walker RT. Reasons for apicectomies. A retrospective study. Endod Dent Traumatol 1996; 12:185–91.

3. Von Arx T, Kurl B. Root-end cavity preparation after apicoectomy using a new type of sonic and diamond-surfaced retrotip: A 1-year follow-up study. J Oral Maxillofac Surg 1999;57:656–61.

4. Von Arx T, Vinzens-Majanemi T, Jensen S. Changes of periodontal parameters following apical surgery. Int Endod J 2007;40:959–69.

5. Zuolo ML, Ferreira MO, Gutmann JL. Prognosis in periapical surgery: a clinical prospective study. Int Endod J 2000;33(2):91–8.

6. Rubinstein RA, Kim S. Long-term follow-up of cases considered healed one year after apical microsurgery. J Endod 2002;28:378–83.

7. Setzer FC, Shah S, Kohli M, et al. Outcome of endodontic surgery: a meta-analysis of the literature—part 1: comparison of traditional root-end surgery and endodontic microsurgery. J Endod 2010;36: 1757–65.

8. Setzer FC, Shah S, Kohli M, et al. Outcome of endodontic surgery: a meta-analysis of the literature—part 2: comparison of endodontic microsurgical techniques with and without the use of higher magnification. J Endod 2012;38:1–12.

9. Danin J, Stromberg T, Forsgren H, et al. Clinical management of nonhealing periradicular pathosis. Surgery versus endodontic retreatment. Oral Surg Oral Med Oral Pathol Oral Radiol Endod 1996; 82(2):213–7.

10. Trobinejad M, Corr R, Handysides R, et al. Outcomes of nonsurgical retreatment and endodontic surgery: A systematic review. J Endod 2009;35(7):930–7.

11. Blomlof L, Jansson L. Prognosis and mortality of root-resected molars. Int J Periodontics Restorative Dent 1997;17:190–201.

12. Basten CH, Ammons WF, Persson R. Long term evaluation of root-resected molars: a retrospective study. Int J Periodontics Restorative Dent 1996;16: 206–9.

13. Danin J, Linder LE, Lundqvist G, et al. Outcomes of periradicular surgery in cases of apical pathosis and untreated canals. Oral Surg Oral Med Oral Pathol Oral Radiol Endod 1999;87(2):227–32.

14. Rud J, Andreasen JO, Jensen JE. A follow-up study of 1,000 cases treated by endodontic surgery. Int J Oral Surg 1972;1:215–28.

15. Rubinstein RA, Kim S. Short term observation of the results of endodontic surgery with the use of a surgical operation microscope and Super-EBA as root-end filling material. J Endod 1999;25:43–8.

16. Tamse A, Fuss Z, Lustig J, et al. Radiographic features of vertically fractured, endodontically treated maxillary premolars. Oral Surg Oral Med Oral Pathol Oral Radiol Endod 1999;88:348–52.

17. Tsesis I, Rosen E, Tamse A, et al. Effect of guided tissue regeneration on the outcome of endodontic treatment: A systematic review and meta-analysis. J Endod 2011;37(8):1039–45.

18. Wuchenich D, Meadows D, Torabinejad M. A comparison between two root end preparation techniques in human cadavers. J Endod 1994;20: 279–82.

19. Feedman A, Horowitz I. Complications after apicoectomy in maxillary premolar and molar teeth. Int J Oral Maxillofac Surg 1999;28:192–4.

20. Jansson L, Sandstedt P, Laftman AC, et al. Relationship between apical and marginal healing in periradicular surgery. Oral Surg Oral Med Oral Pathol Oral Radiol Endod 1997;83:596–601.

21. Velvart P. Papilla base incision: a new approach to recession free healing of the interdental papilla after endodontic surgery. Int Endod J 2002;35:453–60.

22. Mainkar A, Zhu Q, Safavi K. Incidence of altered sensation following mandibular molar and premolar periapical sugery. J Endod 2020;46(1):29–33.

23. Walton RE. Routine histopathologic examination of endodontic periradicular surgical specimens—is it warranted? Oral Surg Oral Med Oral Pathol Oral Radiol Endod 1998;86(5):505.

24. Del Fabbro M, Corbella S, Sequeira-Byron P, et al. Endodontic procedures for retreatment of periapical lesions. Cochrane Database Syst Rev 2016;(10): CD005511.

25. Truschnegg A, Rugani P, Kirnbauer B, et al. Long term follow up of apical microsurgery of teeth with post and core restorations. J Endod 2020;46(2):178–84.

26. Crossen D, Morelli T, Tyndall D, et al. Periapical microsurgery- A 4-dimensional analysis of healing patterns. J Endod 2019;45(4):402–6.

Preprosthetic Dentoalveolar Surgery

Wallace S. McLaurin, DMD, Deepak Krishnan, DDS*

KEYWORDS

- Pre prosthetic • Edentulous • Vestibuloplasty • Tori • Exostoses

KEY POINTS

- Preprosthetic dentoalveolar surgery continues to be an important factor in successful rehabilitation of the oral cavity.
- Anatomic considerations in preprosthetic surgery.
- Hard-tissue preprosthetic surgical techniques.
- Soft-tissue preprosthetic techniques.
- Skin substitutes in preprosthetic surgery.

INTRODUCTION

Rehabilitation of the dentition has been an ongoing process as far back as 700 BC, which often referred to removal of disease and replacement of the lost structures to restore function. Prepros-thetic surgery is a vital component to achieving the goals of restored dentition. Regardless of whether it was the prehistoric times or the era of osseointe-grating implants, most patients require some aspect of preprosthetic surgery when an attempt is made for oral rehabilitation. This rehabilitation of the edentulous patient can pose significant challenges to the restorative dentist and surgeon. The intent of this article is to discuss preoperative patient planning, preprosthetic surgical options, and other relevant considerations.

PREOPERATIVE EVALUATION

Complete or partial edentulism is known to be more common in the aging population. The surgi-cal management of the condition demands a thor-ough preoperative assessment to ensure both medical risk stratification and optimization before rendering safe surgical treatment.[1] Thus, the initial evaluation entails the investigation of any medical comorbidities and a deep dive into the overall health of the patient. During the physical examina-tion, the patient should undergo a standard head and neck evaluation with a focus on the unique anatomic consideration of the edentulous condi-tion, including asymmetries of the maxilla or mandible, gingival type and mucosal quality, pres-ence of maxillomandibular tori and exostoses, high frenum attachments, interarch space, vestib-ular depth, and vertical dimension of occlusion. The use of standardized classification systems such as the one introduced by Cawood and Howell can help standardize the evaluation of the edentulous ridge anatomy.[2] Traditionally, the data collection process required standard stone models for surgical planning and prosthetic fabri-cation. However, current technological advance-ments, such as with cone beam computed tomography scan and intraoral scanner, have modernized data collection processing to an incredibly accurate level, bypassing the need for alginate impressions and stone models.[3,4]

ANATOMIC CHANGES WITH EDENTULISM

Understanding the unique maxillomandibular edentulous anatomy and its differences from its dentate counterpart is vital to the success of sur-gery. Edentulous ridges resorb significantly with

Oral and Maxillofacial Surgery, University of Cincinnati Medical Center, 200 Albert Sabin Way ML 0461, Cincin-nati, OH 45219, USA
* Corresponding author.
E-mail address: gopaladk@ucmail.uc.edu

Oral Maxillofacial Surg Clin N Am 32 (2020) 583–591
https://doi.org/10.1016/j.coms.2020.07.001
1042-3699/20/© 2020 Elsevier Inc. All rights reserved.

time, and with time there is a significant reduction in both bulk and quality of available bone stock, and with resorption, the inferior alveolar canal and foramen are positioned more superiorly in the mandible.[5] The foramen can have variable presentations of its anatomic location.[6] The genial tubercle can become more superiorly positioned. With edentulous, aging, and bony atrophy, the vascular support to the mandible shifts from a centrifugal to a centripetal arrangement.[7]

In the maxilla, there may be little bone between the crest of the ridge and the nasal floor. Similarly, the posterior maxilla in the region of the maxillary sinuses may have minimal bone between the crest of ridge and the sinus cavity. The entire ridge may seem flat and confluent with the palatal shelf in severe and chronic edentulism.

INDICATIONS FOR SURGERY

The edentulous ridge of the maxilla and mandible resorb differently among individuals but generally follows a similar pattern. The maxilla resorbs on the facial surface and the inferior surface of the alveolar ridge. The mandible resorbs in an inferior and anterior pattern.[8] These resorptive patterns can yield a ridge that is unable to accommodate a denture.

The following circumstances can necessitate a surgical procedure to ensure smooth ridges with adequate width and height for denture retention:

- Mandibular tori
- Maxillary palatal torus
- Mandibular or maxillary exostoses
- Overhanging maxillary tuberosities
- Severe bony undercuts
- Knife edge ridges

Alveoloplasty can be completed in order to flatten the bone and allow for a larger "shelf" of bone for the denture. Soft tissue may also require augmentation before restoration fabrication. With conventional dentures, vestibular sulcus depth is of utmost importance. Shallow sulcus depth will require a vestibuloplasty.

Other instances of soft tissue indications may include

- Hyperplastic maxillary tuberosities,
- Epulis fissurata, or
- Unfavorable frenum attachments.

In the patient with dental implants adequate tissue height and thickness is a necessity. Soft tissue augmentation in the form of vestibuloplasty, keratinized tissue augmentation, or lowering of the floor of the mouth may be required.

SURGICAL PROCEDURES

Once the decision has been made to proceed with preprosthetic surgery, the goal is to establish ideal hard and soft tissue contours. The bony ridge should be U-shaped with adequate height and width without undercuts, protuberances, or sharp edges. The oral mucosa should have adequate thickness with appropriate buccal and lingual depth.[9,10]

Mandibular Tori

A common procedure before denture fabrication is mandibular tori removal (**Fig. 1**). The procedure may be completed in the ambulatory setting under general anesthesia or local anesthesia. Excessive tori may pose more of a surgical challenge and be better addressed in the operating theater. Regardless of the setting, establishing profound local anesthesia is imperative. In general, the initial incision involves making a crestal incision and reflecting a full-thickness mucoperiosteal flap. In the case of bilateral mandibular tori, the crestal incision is carried from the posterior right alveolar ridge to the posterior left alveolar ridge. If needed, a buccal hockey-stick releasing incision may be completed to the posterior extent. A full-thickness mucoperiosteal flap is elevated on the lingual surface of the mandible, exposing the tori. Delicate soft tissue management is imperative, as trauma to the lingual mucosa complicates the postoperative recovery. After the tori are exposed and adequately visualized, a Seldin retractor is placed between the exposed lingual surface of the mandible and the lingual mucosal flap in order to protect the lingual tissue.[10]

There are several methods to remove the bony protuberances. A rongeur can be used to snip the exostoses. A drill using a pineapple-shaped bur under copious irrigation may be used instead. Most surgeons prefer to score the superior aspect of the protruding bone with surgical drill and a fissure bur with irrigation. A chisel with mallet is then used to removal the tori. After the initial ostectomy, a bone file or handpiece with bur may be used to level any remaining undercut (**Fig. 2**). Digital palpation of the lingual surface of the mandible is performed to assess the smoothness of the remaining structure and the presence of residual undercuts or projections. After bone removal is completed, the area is thoroughly irrigated to remove unwanted debris. The area is checked for hemostasis. The mucosal flaps are then closed in running fashion with resorbable sutures. This technique, largely reliant on diligent soft tissue management, can be used for any bony protuberance in the maxilla or mandible.

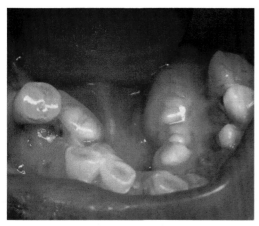

Fig. 1. Mandibular tori: large bilateral mandibular tori.

Maxillary Palatal Torus

A thorough discussion with the restorative dentist is necessary before proceeding with surgical removal. At times, surgery can be avoided with a well-fitting denture in the presence of the tori. The technique for removal of a palatal torus is predominantly based on clinical presentation (**Fig. 3**). As with mandibular tori, these cases can be addressed in the ambulatory or operating room setting under general or local anesthesia depending on the extent of surgery required. Given that this procedure can be highly stimulating and may result in excess bleeding, additional precautions should be undertaken with surgery in the ambulatory setting, especially in the presence of an open-"guarded" airway and the potential respiratory sequelae. A protected airway with endotracheal tube may be necessary when the removal of the torus is suspected to be more demanding than routine.

Following administration of local anesthesia, a #15 blade is used to make a complete incision through the palatal mucosa to bone. The incision is performed along the long axis of the tori in the center of the protuberance. With a larger palatal torus, a "Y" type incision is added to the anterior and posterior extent of the incision for adequate

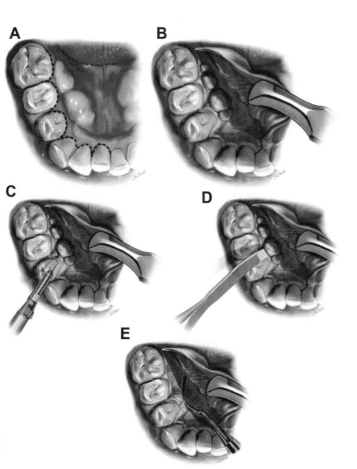

Fig. 2. Mandibular tori removal. (*A*) Scalloped sulcular incision as noted. (*B*) Reflection of the mucosal tissue. (*C*) Rotary instrument use to score bone and create groove at the tori/alveolar bone junction. (*D*) Chisel and mallet use to separate tori. (*E*) Bone file or rotary instrument used to smooth any remaining edges. (*From* Ness GM. Palatal and lingual torus removal. In: Kademani D, Tiwana PS, editors. Atlas of oral and maxillofacial surgery. St. Louis: Elsevier; 2016. p. 124–5; with permission.)

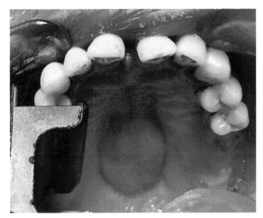

Fig. 3. Palatal torus: large irregular shaped midline palatal torus.

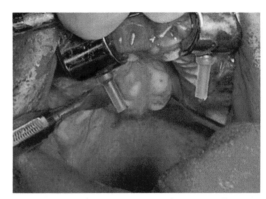

Fig. 5. Palatal torus: exposure of torus with instruments placed to safe-guard the maxillary mucosa. Torus removal may be completed with scoring of the bone and a chisel or rotary instrument.

tissue reflect[10] (Fig. 4). After adequate exposure and visualization, the torus is scored into smaller sections (Fig. 5). A chisel and mallet are then used to remove each section and thus the bulk of the torus. A 4.0-mm oval carbide bur is used under copious irrigation to relieve any irregularities. The mucosal tissues are protected by placing a Seldin retractor or a periosteal elevator in between the bone and the flap. The area is thoroughly irrigated and then closed with resorbable sutures. A variety of alternative techniques exist but are not discussed here.

Maxillary Tuberosity Reduction

Excess tissue in the maxillary tuberosity region can restrict the interarch distance and compromise denture fit and fabrication (Fig. 6). When evaluating this area, imaging or soft tissue probing can help distinguish between soft or hard tissue abnormalities. After determining the nature of this

excess tissue, the surgeon can then choose a surgical technique.

An elliptical incision along the most bulbous portion of the overhanging crest is preferred by most to address excess fibrous tissue. The area is widely undermined, and the fibrous tissue is then removed[10] (Fig. 7). At this point, there is usually excess mucosal tissue, which should be trimmed and primarily closed. Care must be taken to identify and preserve anatomic landmarks, especially the maxillary sinus floor when removing bone.

In the case of excess bone contributing to the hyperplastic tuberosity, a similar crestal incision or elliptical incision can be made to expose this bone. As previously described, the soft tissue is widely undermined with the periosteum adequately reflected to expose the overhanging bone. At this point rongeur or handpiece with bur under irrigation may be used to reduce the bony excess. Primary closure is then achieved via standard suture technique (Fig. 8).

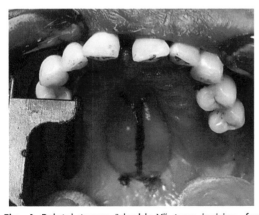

Fig. 4. Palatal torus: "double-Y" type incision for exposure of palatal torus.

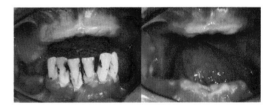

Fig. 6. Tuberosity reduction. (Left) Poor dentition with excessive tuberosities bilaterally. (Right) Postextraction of teeth and bilateral bony tuberosity reduction with crestal incisions. Note the increased interarch space. (Courtesy of Gordon Huntress, DDS, Cincinnati, OH.)

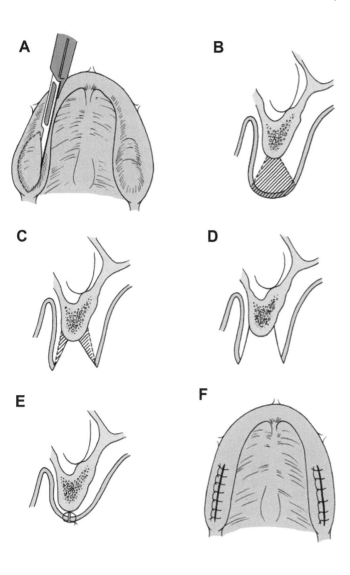

Fig. 7. Maxillary soft tissue tuberosity reduction. (*A*) Elliptical incision around soft tissue to be excised in the tuberosity area. (*B*) Soft tissue area excised with the initial incision. (*C*) Undermining of buccal and palatal flaps to provide adequate soft tissue contour and tension-free closure. (*D*) View of final tissue removal. (*E, F*) Soft tissue closure. (*From* Tucker MR, Bauer RE. Preprosthetic surgery. In: Hupp JR, Ellis E III, Tucker MR, editors. Contemporary oral and maxillofacial surgery. 7th edition. Philadelphia: Elsevier; 2019. p. 234; with permission.)

FRENECTOMY

Although a frenectomy is often not thought to be a preprosthetic procedure, it can be helpful in prepping the oral cavity for a prosthetic rehabilitation. Maxillary and mandibular vestibular or labial frenum can cause the denture bases to become unseated.[9] When evaluating a patient, frenum attachments should be assessed for high attachments on the alveolar ridge, which can distort denture seating. Frenuloplasty or frenectomy should be performed in such scenarios. Many techniques have been described to relieve freni. Diamond excision has been frequently used for maxillary midline and mandibular lingual frenum release. This excision is best used in the presence of ample soft tissue.

However, when the tissue is hyperplastic and short, Z-plasty is a better-suited technique. In the bicuspid region, a local vestibuloplasty may be often necessary to relieve the hyperplastic tissue. In this situation, an incision is made in the area of the mucogingival junction, and a supraperiosteal flap is generated. The resultant flap edges are then sutured in an apical position to the periosteum and thus reestablishing a more appropriate frenum height.

Soft Tissue Vestibuloplasty

Inadequate depth of the vestibule can occur due to many reasons. Most notably, the edentulous bony atrophy causes the muscle attachments of the mandible to become superiorly positioned over time. This reduced vestibular height compromises

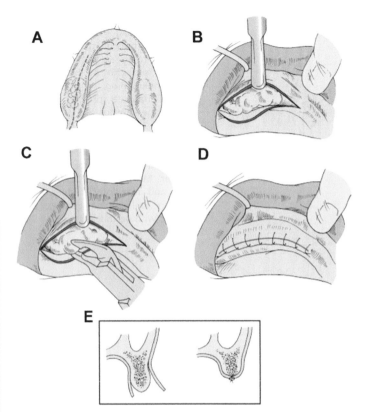

Fig. 8. Bony tuberosity reduction. (*A*) Incision extended along the crest of the alveolar ridge distally to the superior extent of the tuberosity area. (*B*) Elevated mucoperiosteal flap provides adequate exposure to all areas of bony excess. (*C*) Rongeur used to eliminate bony excess. (*D*) Tissue reapproximated with a continuous suture technique. (*E*) Cross-sectional view of the posterior tuberosity area, showing vertical reduction of bone and reapposition of the mucoperiosteal flap. (In some cases removal of large amounts of bone produces excessive soft tissue, which can be excised before closure to prevent overlapping.) (*From* Tucker MR, Bauer RE. Preprosthetic surgery. In: Hupp JR, Ellis E III, Tucker MR, editors. Contemporary oral and maxillofacial surgery. 7th edition. Philadelphia: Elsevier; 2019. p. 226; with permission.)

denture fit and function for the patient. One of the several vestibuloplasty techniques can be performed in order to increase vestibular depth depending on the remaining bone height. The selected method pursued depends chiefly on the remaining bone height.

Transpositional flap vestibuloplasty

Patients with 15 mm or more between the mental foramina are good candidates for transpositional flap vestibuloplasty.[9] The primary intent of this procedure is to increase the vestibular depth along the anterior mandible to assist with denture stability. A horizontal incision is made on the inner surface of the lower lip, and a supraperiosteal dissection is executed superiorly. Once the alveolar ridge is encountered, the superior extent of the dissection is complete. A #15 blade is used to make an incision in the periosteum at the level of the alveolar ridge. The resultant periosteal flap is dissected away from the bone inferiorly; a skin graft is applied and secured to the denuded lip. The raised mucosal bed is then sutured at the depth of the vestibule.

Vestibuloplasty with split-thickness skin graft or collagen or dermal matrix substitutes

When the operator is facing a situation where minimal vestibular depth and mucosal tissue are available, skin grafting or adjunctive grafts may be necessary. The split-thickness skin graft has been shown to provide a stable vestibular depth without significant loss of the gained depth or adverse bone resorption.[11,12] Adjunctive techniques use commercially available dermal or collagen matrices instead of the skin grafts that are now available. Porcine collagen matrices have shown promising results when compared with autogenous grafts.[13–15] One must consider adnexal structures and esthetics when deciding on the best material to use. Given that high success has been demonstrated and that a donor site is spared, a mucosal substitute is a sound option for these procedures. The skin substitutes are gaining in popularity as their function and success has become established over time. In addition to avoiding the second surgical site, it also often reduces the chances of hair growth in the mouth.

The inner thigh or the lateral thigh is considered an ideal location for harvesting split-thickness skin grafts due to the absence of adnexal structures in this region. The graft is usually obtained with a thickness of 0.012 to 0.016 mm^3. The dermatome is set to these dimensions and used to harvest a 5 to 6 cm width graft. The surgical incision is made along the mucogingival junction, and a supraperiosteal plane is dissected to the desired depth of the vestibule. The incisional margin is then sutured to the depth of the vestibule. The graft is trimmed to the desired size and fixed in place either with a surgical stent, circummandibular wiring, or by suturing the graft to the host bed.[16] If using a stent, it is typically left in place for 7 to 10 days.[9] The graft can also be immobilized by anchoring it either to a preexisting implant or to the surgical bed during implant placement.[17]

In similar fashion, a mucosal substitute such as a dermal matrix or a collagen matrix can be applied instead of a harvested autogenous graft. When using such a substitute the procedure is essentially the same. A standard supraperiosteal dissection is created, and once appropriate vestibular depth is achieved, the graft is placed and secured as discussed previously[15] (**Figs. 9 and 10**).

Floor of Mouth Lowering

The practice of most vestibuloplasties have become unnecessary in the era of osseointegrating implants but they continue to be a necessary tool in the armamentarium of a preprosthetic surgeon. Once a very popular and commonly performed procedure, floor of mouth lowering has become a lost art among preprosthetic procedures. As noted previously, when inadequate depth of sulcus prevents prosthesis placement, it may become necessary to alter the depth of the floor of mouth.

When planning for floor of mouth lowering, an incision is carried out in the retromolar region crossing midline anteriorly to the contralateral retromolar region. Care is taken in the area of the retromolar region to avoid incising deeply, as the lingual nerve may be present in the region. Blunt mucosal and supraperiosteal dissection is then completed on the lingual surface. Once the mylohyoid muscle is identified, it must be incised anteriorly from its attachment to the mandible. At this point, the extent of the mylohyoid muscle can be determined, and the posterior attachment is incised freeing the muscle for inferior repositioning. Close attention should be given to the genioglossus attachment to the genial tubercle. In general, half of the genioglossus muscle can be removed at the tubercle in order to gain depth inferiorly.[16] At this point, if a skin graft is planned, your skin graft may be inset and sutured (suturing may require passing transdermal via an awl) (**Fig. 11**). An acellular skin substitute such as a dermal or collagen matrix may also be used and placed over the denuded periosteum in lieu of using a skin graft.[18] Occasionally, the wound is left to allow healing by secondary granulation, and in those instances, 2 weeks should be allowed for such secondary mucosalization.

SOFT TISSUE AUGMENTATION

Keratinized tissue is vital to periimplant tissue health.[11] In today's practice, dental implants are at the forefront of every treatment plan. Although dental implants have lessened the need for pre prosthetic surgery, bone grafting techniques may cause vestibular violation and require additional keratinized tissue or surgical vestibuloplasty. Keratinized tissue may be obtained by completing an autogenous graft from the palate or by using commercial products. Several other skin substitutes are available in the marketplace, and any

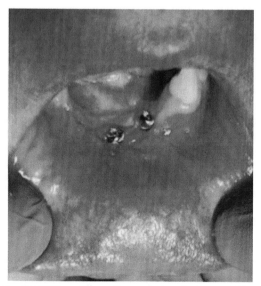

Fig. 10. Tissue alternative: incorporated skin substitute in the mandibular vestibule. Increased keratinized tissue and increased vestibular depth by using mucosal substitute.

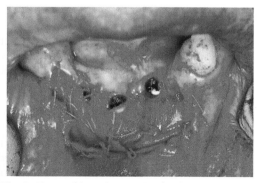

Fig. 9. Tissue alternative: mucosal substitute in place to help aid in vestibular depth and keratinized tissue.

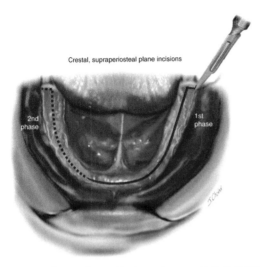

Fig. 11. Floor of mouth lowering: crestal incision completed from retromolar region. Supraperiosteal dissection and hemostat placed under the mylohyoid to help identify the structure and dissect from the lingual surface of the mandible. The posterior dissection occurs slightly medial to help protect the lingual nerve. Dissection of the anterior occurs hugging the lingual cortex of the mandible to protect the lingual nerve C. Suture passed through mucosa and mylohyoid and is passed through the awl allowing for the lingual tissue to be lowered and sutured to the buccal mucosal flap. (*From* Perciaccante VJ, Farish SE. Vestibuloplasty. In: Kademani D, Tiwana PS, editors. Atlas of oral and maxillofacial surgery. St. Louis: Elsevier; 2016. p. 156–9; with permission.)

discussion of such available products are beyond the scope of this article.

BONE GRAFTING

Bone substitutes to increase bone height and width have become commonplace in oral rehabilitation. Bone grafting is a vital component of preprosthetic surgery. Given the complexity of bone grafting and the products available for ridge augmentation, the surgical procedures or products that are available for usage are not discussed in this section. Alveolar ridge augmentation and "preprosthetic" bone grafting are discussed in separate chapter.

COMPLICATIONS

Generalized complications such as significant edema, infection, pain, and others are not discussed here. However, there are specific complications associated with the procedures described earlier.

Neurosensory disturbances can be life changing. When performing these surgeries, one must have sound and delicate technique to preserve the inferior alveolar nerve, lingual nerve, and the mental nerves. Postprocedure, one might expect to have hypoesthesia of the lip and chin. The patient should be monitored for neural recovery on a monthly basis. The standard window of neural intervention is at 3 to 6 months.[19]

Most patients who undergo floor of mouth lowering will have some dysphagia or odynophagia.[20] The patient should be placed on a liquid diet to adequately maintain nutrition and hydration. These symptoms typically resolve after surgical edema subsides. In addition, postoperative hematoma or arterial bleed may elevate the floor of the mouth, thereby compromising the airway. Emergency evacuation in the operating room setting may be necessary in the event of the hematoma including emergency intubation with monitoring. Emergency tracheostomy can be considered if unable to perform a standard intubation.[20]

A major concern for all vestibuloplasties is loss of vestibular depth. Although variable depending on the type of graft, skin graft shrinkage can be as high as 40%.[20] If regression of the depth is noted, a second procedure may be necessary to regain depth.

SUMMARY

Preprosthetic surgery begins with the final goal of ideal prosthetic dental rehabilitation. While evaluating an edentulous patient, preprosthetic surgery should always be considered in order to establish future restorative success.[21] The surgeon must collaborate with the restoring dentist to set forth the best treatment plan possible. Surgery should establish ideal contour, quantity, and quality of the denture bearing field.[10]

DISCLOSURE

The authors have nothing to disclose.

REFERENCES

1. Steele JG, et al. How do age and tooth loss affect oral health impacts and quality of life? a study comparing two national samples. Community Dent Oral Epidemiol 2004;32(2):107–14.
2. Cawood JI, Howell RA. A classification of the edentulous jaws. Int J Oral Maxillofac Surg 1988;17(4):232–6.
3. Al-Rimawi A, et al. Trueness of cone beam computed tomography versus intra-oral scanner derived three-dimensional digital models: an ex vivo study. Clin Oral Implants Res 2019. https://doi.org/10.1111/clr.13434.

4. Papaspyridakos P, et al. Digital versus conventional implant impressions for edentulous patients: accuracy outcomes. Clin Oral Implants Res 2015;27(4):465–72.

5. Polland KE, et al. The mandibular canal of the edentulous Jaw. Clin Anat 2001;14(6):445–52.

6. Matveeva N, et al. Morphological alterations in the position of the mandibular foramen in dentate and edentate mandibles. Anat Sci Int 2017;93(3):340–50.

7. Forman G. Presenile mandibular atrophy: its aetiology, clinical evaluation and treatment by jaw augmentation. Br J Oral Surg 1976;14(1):47–56.

8. Devaki V, et al. Pre-prosthetic surgery: mandible. J Pharm Bioallied Sci 2012;4(6):414.

9. Costello BJ, et al. Preprosthetic surgery for the edentulous patient. Dent Clin North Am 1996;40(1):19–38.

10. Ephros H, et al. Preprosthetic surgery. Oral Maxillofac Surg Clin North Am 2015;27(3):459–72.

11. Ladwein C, et al. Is the presence of keratinized mucosa associated with periimplant tissue health? a clinical cross-sectional analysis. Int J Implant Dent 2015;1(1). https://doi.org/10.1186/s40729-015-0009-z.

12. Landesman HM, et al. Resorption of the edentulous mandible after a vestibuloplasty with skin grafting. J Prosthet Dent 1983;49(5):619–22.

13. Maiorana C, et al. The efficacy of a porcine collagen matrix in keratinized tissue augmentation: a 5-year follow-up study. Int J Implant Dent 2018;4(1). https://doi.org/10.1186/s40729-017-0113-3.

14. Preidl RHM, et al. Collagen matrix vascularization in a peri-implant vestibuloplasty situation proceeds within the first postoperative week. J Oral Maxillofac Surg 2019;77(9):1797–806.

15. Schmitt CM, et al. Long-term outcomes after vestibuloplasty with a porcine collagen matrix (mucograft®) versus the free gingival graft: a comparative prospective clinical trial. Clin Oral Implants Res 2015;27(11):e125–33.

16. Kademani D, Paul ST. Atlas of oral andMaxillofacial surgery. St. Louis: Elsevier; 2016.

17. Heberer S, Katja N. Clinical evaluation of a modified method of vestibuloplasty using an implant-retained splint. J Oral Maxillofac Surg 2009;67(3):624–9.

18. Girod DA, et al. Acellular dermis compared to skin grafts in oral cavity reconstruction. Laryngoscope 2009;119(11):2141–9.

19. Kushnerev E, Yates JM. Evidence-based outcomes following inferior alveolar and lingual nerve injury and repair: a systematic review. J Oral Rehabil 2015;42(10):786–802.

20. Samit A, Kenneth K. Complications associated with skin graft vestibuloplasty. Oral Surg Oral Med Oral Pathol 1983;56(6):586–92.

21. Cillo JE, Richard F. Reconstruction of the shallow vestibule edentulous mandible with simultaneous split thickness skin graft vestibuloplasty and mandibular endosseous implants for implant-supported overdentures. J Oral Maxillofac Surg 2009;67(2):381–6.

Reconstruction of the Extraction Socket
Methods, Manipulations, and Management

Daniel B. Spagnoli, DDS, MS, PhD[a], Christopher C. Niquette Jr, DDS[b,c],*

KEYWORDS

- Socket graft • Ridge preservation • Extraction socket manipulation • Socket management

KEY POINTS

- Each extraction socket presents unique challenges for reconstruction. These should be addressed from an anatomic, biologic, and scientific approach.
- Biologics (PRF, Bone Morphogenetic Protein, plasma) act as adjuncts to already established socket management techniques. As a socket reconstruction becomes more complex, the importance of these grafting agents is magnified.
- Implant planning should begin at the time of tooth extraction. Socket manipulations can increase the quantitative gain and the predictability of bone grafting. These aid in streamlining dental implant reconstruction for patients.

Socket grafting is an attempt to recreate the native bone and soft tissue environment, which subsequently fosters tooth replacement. To facilitate this reconstruction, an understanding of the alveolar bone structural biology, morphology, histology, and the molecular organization of its complex associated tissues is paramount. The lifecycle of alveolar bone is codependent on its relationship with developing or mature teeth. Periodontal ligament–mediated attachments between the developing tooth and alveolar bone proper leads to alveolar bone growth during eruption of primary and permanent teeth.[1] The periodontal ligament is often classified as having supracrestal, crestal, horizontal, apical, and interradicular zones. These are all similar in composition but emphasized because of their role in maintaining bone associated with all aspects of the tooth. A dense layer of bone adjacent to root is delineated as primary alveolar bone. This layer forms the attachment for periodontal ligament fibers and is often referred to as bundle bone because of the thick insertion of Sharpey fibers and collagen bundles.[1,2] For clarity, this is the radiographically identifiable structure referred to as lamina densa. Loss of defined lamina densa radiographically often signals a pathologic or physiologic change within the bone.[3,4] **Fig. 1** illustrates the individual anatomic components of the tooth-bone interface.

Fig. 2 simulates panoramic, axial, cross-sectional, and sagittal views of the maxilla or mandible that correlate with computed tomography images. These images demonstrate the extensive trabecular bone associated with tooth roots.

a Private Practice, Brunswick Oral and Maxillofacial Surgery, 90 Medical Center Drive Southwest, Supply, NC 28462, USA; b Brunswick Oral and Maxillofacial Surgery; c Private Practice, Third Coast Oral and Maxillofacial Surgery, Grand Rapids, MI, USA
* Corresponding author. 2119 64th Street Southwest, Byron Center, MI 49315.
E-mail address: chipniquette@gmail.com

Oral Maxillofacial Surg Clin N Am 32 (2020) 593–609
https://doi.org/10.1016/j.coms.2020.07.010
1042-3699/20/© 2020 Elsevier Inc. All rights reserved.

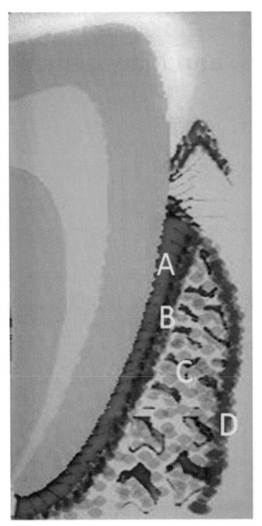

Fig. 1. Alveolar bone, PDL, tooth concept. (*A*) PDL space. (*B*) Alveolar bone proper/bundle bone. (*C*) Trabecular cancellous bone. (*D*) Facial cortical bone. PDL, Periodontal Ligament.

Dental function stimulates bone to develop in an anisotropic orientation of bone trabeculae. These are generally perpendicular to the primary force on the tooth. Bone trabeculae extend from primary alveolar bone to the inner and outer cortical bone and act to fill the interdental or interradicular space.[1–3,5,6]

Anisotropic bone also forms to a dental implant. **Fig. 3** demonstrates implant #30, 4 months post-extraction and placement of immediate molar implant, with healing abutment and with platelet-rich fibrin (PRF).[a] Note maintenance of bone trabeculae with anisotropic orientation between #29 lamina densa and implant surface. Also note the bone trabeculae that have developed between the distal root socket, grafted with PRF, the implant, and #31 lamina densa. Crestal bone height is maintained in association with platform switched crestal aspect of the implant.

Bone adaptation to functional forces through mechanical transduction and remodeling is part of the natural lifecycle of bone and plays an important role in the adaptation of bone to functional demands.[4] Consider trabecular bone as agile with the capacity to rapidly remodel and adapt. Alveolar bone especially in the mandible has one of the highest natural rates of remodeling of all the bones in the body. In contrast to the internal remodeling mediated by tooth functional forces, external remodeling of the inner and outer cortex is mediated as a function of periosteum and muscular attachment.[5,7] The face is not static and continues to change throughout life. For example, the attrition of teeth may lead to occlusal and mesial drift or overt passive tooth eruption. The mandible, in particular, has some potential to respond to this by the deposition of bone along its inferior border.[7] In contrast, the periosteum, especially of the facial surface of the alveolus, is resorptive in nature. Resorptive remodeling of the facial aspect of alveolar bone may lead to root fenestration or dehiscence.

Following tooth extraction, bundle bone or alveolar bone proper especially in the facial and crestal region undergoes rapid regressive remodeling.[2] This is followed by bone loss from the facial and inner cortex of the alveolar bone. Accelerated loss of facial plate is most likely a function of lack of trabecular bone between the tooth root and the facial plate together with a resorptive effect from facial periosteum.[1,5–8] **Fig. 4** highlights the resorptive periosteum of the face, as described by Enlow and coworkers.[7]

Extensive literature is available related to socket grafting, socket preservation, and socket regeneration. Autogenous grafts, allografts, and

---

[a]Platelet-rich fibrin production protocol is as follows. After administration of intravenous antibiotic, the arm opposite the intravenous fluid administration, contralateral extremity used to avoid dilution with concurrently administered intravenous fluids, is palpated for a larger diameter vessel. Once isolated, the vessel is entered with an 18-gauge needle. Venous blood is collected into a 9-mL serum clot activated vaccutainer. This tube is then spun in a centrifuge for 13 minutes at 2750 rpm. PRF is then removed from the tube. It is used compressed or uncompressed depending on the application and clinician preference.

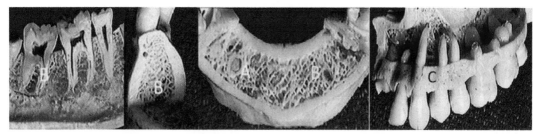

Fig. 2. Maxillary and mandibular root relationships to trabecular and cortical bone. (A) Alveolar bone proper adjacent to root. (B) Trabecular bone anisotropic orientation perpendicular to root forces extending to inner and outer cortex, interradicular, or interdental. (C) Thin facial cortical bone with no trabecular bone prone to dehiscence, fenestration, and rapid resorption.

biologics have been evaluated as sources of socket graft or reconstruction materials. All of these approaches have been shown to preserve or reconstruct socket structural biology and reduce the rate of bone loss following extraction. Extensive reviews have concluded that grafting of the socket reduces bone loss, but it does not eliminate this loss or completely maintain alveolar dimensions.[8–19] Following extraction, areas of the socket, such as the facial cortical environment, devoid of marrow and bone trabeculae seem to be susceptible to rapid bone loss.

This may be a factor of decreased tropic effects and vascular supply. In these areas there is essentially no separation between the primary alveolus and the facial cortex. A basic sequence of socket changes after extraction is detailed in **Fig. 5**.

Recognition of these concepts suggests grafting within the socket alone may be insufficient and grafting the facial socket environment in areas susceptible to rapid bone loss may be necessary for total maintenance of alveolar architecture.[8,12] **Fig. 6** demonstrates a socket that, despite grafting with rhBMP2 the facial cortical wall was not maintained. In addition, when practical it may be

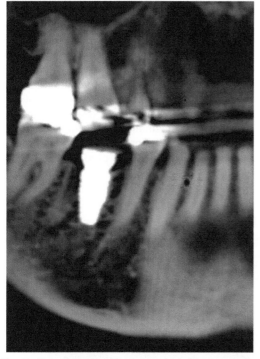

Fig. 3. Note the anisotropic pattern of bone on the mesial of implant #30 that has been maintained and the new anisotropic pattern forming on the distal within the previous extraction socket.

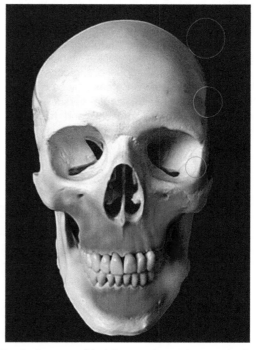

Fig. 4. Concept of facial resorptive periosteum in the areas highlighted in *red* interpreted from Enlow and coworkers.[7]

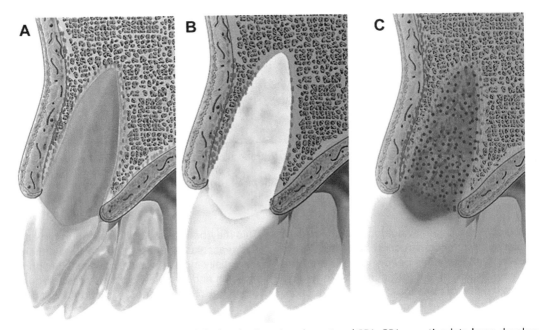

Fig. 5. Sequence of socket remodeling. (*A*) Alveolar bone/tooth root and PDL. PDL can stimulate bone development or maintenance versus resorption, facial periosteum is resorptive (*red*), and palatal periosteum is depository (*green*). (*B*) Extraction socket without graft. Resorptive remodeling especially in crestal facial area devoid of trabecular bone between the socket and facial bone. (*C*) Postextraction grafted socket. Regenerative remodeling with maintenance of socket dimension, but potential loss of transverse dimension because of facial bone resorption by resorptive periosteum especially in crestal areas devoid of trabecular bone.

advisable to place immediate implants together with grafting to accelerate the return of tropic functional forces to the socket environment.

Traditional and modified approaches to management of extraction socket biologic and morphologic preservation or reconstruction should be considered on a case by case basis. Biotype, socket health, acute versus chronic infection, native bone present, and trabecular bone support for cortical bone must all be considered. Patient health factors, including oral hygiene, systemic disease, and inhaled smoke products, may variably affect outcomes. Effective socket reconstruction following tooth extraction may require a variety of approaches depending on the location of the socket, pre-extraction condition of the alveolar bone, disease state, and structural or aesthetic requirements. Biologic agents, such as PRF or Infuse (Medtronic, Minneapolis, MN), the rh-BMP2 product, are used as

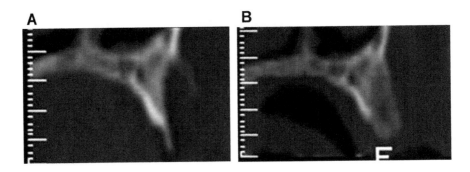

Fig. 6. (*A*) socket grafted with rhBMP-2/ACS at the time of extraction. (*B*) Note the regeneration of socket and facial wall but failure to maintain total transverse alveolar dimension.

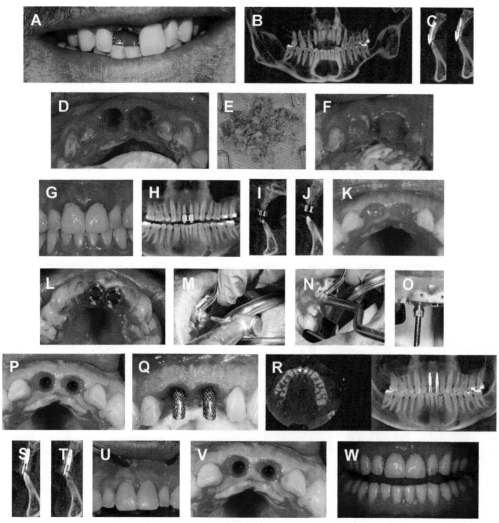

Fig. 7. (*A*) Preoperative photograph of teeth #8 and #9, which are fractured and nonrestorable. (*B*) Panoramic radiograph showing apical radiolucencies. (*C*) Transverse view reveals thin and deficient facial wall anatomy. (*D*) Extraction sockets with crestal facial wall deficiency. (*E*) Graft including Infuse, cancellous allograft, and morcellized PRF. (*F*) Graft material placed into extraction sites. (*G*) Ovate pontic temporaries bonded to adjacent teeth. (*H–J*) Panoramic and transverse views of grafted sockets with implant planning. (*K*) Inspection of extraction sockets after removal of temporaries. Good maintenance of transverse dimension and ovate anatomy is revealed. (*L, M*) Guided implant surgery. (*N*) Secondary socket expansion using osteotome. (*O*) Depth guided and timed implant placement. (*P*) Implant osteotomies with flapless approach. (*Q*) Temporary cylinders attached to the implants. (*R–T*) Postoperative radiographs after implant placement and associated facial wall anatomy preserved. (*U*) Immediate temporaries attached to implant temporary cylinders. (*V*) Socket dimensions and tissue health following removal of temporary teeth. (*W*) Final restoration with preservation of gingival azimuth, papillae, and facial tissue projection.

modulators or additives in the following techniques. They act to upregulate wound healing and maximize predictability. Used in combination with traditional methods, anatomic, systemic, or environmental challenges can be mitigated.[17,18] Several case scenarios are presented next to demonstrate some of the many variations on socket grafting and socket regeneration techniques.

CASE 1

Traditional grafting sequence of teeth #8 and #9 in the esthetic zone with moderate biotype, thin fascial wall, and crestal bone defect. Treatment was by atraumatic extraction of central incisors, graft with Infuse (Medtronic), PRF, and cancellous allograft, covered by PRF membrane, and temporized with bonded ovate politics. There was subsequent guided flapless implant placement with immediate temporization. Photographs of Case 1 are detailed in **Fig. 7**.

CASE 2

Tooth #30 presented with acute infection with fistula and mesial buccal facial wall defect. Treatment was stage 1 extraction, debridement, and placement of PRF. In stage 2 at 12 weeks postextraction implant was placed with simultaneous facial wall graft using titanium membrane, Infuse, local autogenous bone from scrapper procurement, and PRF membrane. Photographs of Case 2 are detailed in **Fig. 8**.

CASE 3

Tooth #8 presented with large apical abscess and facial wall defect. Reconstruction of this scenario often benefits from a two-stage approach. Initially perform tooth extraction and removal of pathology together with facial wall supportive membrane and graft. Second stage includes implant placement, and simultaneous bilayer graft. Graft is formed by a sticky bone allograft deep surface toward the implant and outer surface xenograft to resist excessive facial wall remodeling. Photographs of Case 3 are detailed in **Fig. 9**.

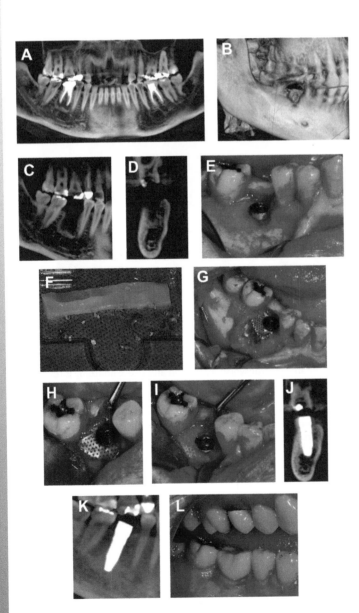

Fig. 8. (*A*) Preoperative Panorex revealing large apical radiolucency on previously endodontically treated tooth #30. (*B*) Three-dimensional reconstruction of the resultant alveolar defect after extraction and grafting with PRF. (*C, D*) Bone fill after stage 1 extraction and grafting with PRF only. (*E*) Secondary implant surgery. After placement of implant in ideal position, there is a resultant vertical bone defect visible along the collar of the implant. (*F*) Bone grafting mixture containing autogenous scrapings from the external oblique ridge and Infuse. (*G*) The graft was positioned adjacent to the implant surface and contained with a mesh, which was fixated using the cover screw of the implant. (*H, I*) After 4 months of healing, the site was reentered, the mesh was removed, and a healing abutment was placed. Note significant vertical bone gain (*I*). (*J, K*) Films at 4 months after implant placement demonstrate good maintenance of the vertical bone gain. (*L*) Restoration in place with good adaptation and height of buccal keratinized tissue.

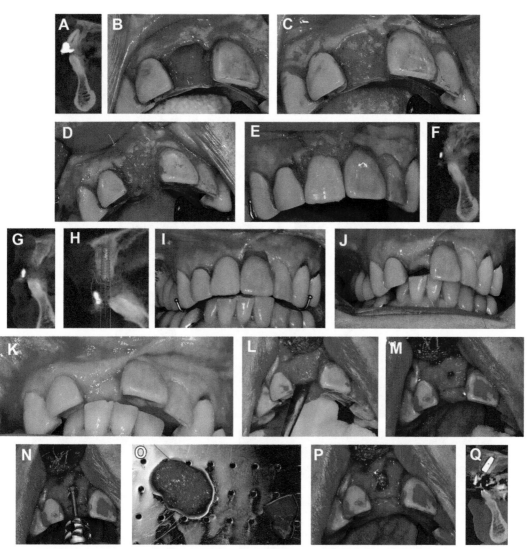

Fig. 9. (*A*) Preoperative radiograph demonstrating large periapical radiolucency with fenestration through the facial cortical palate. (*B*) After atraumatic extraction, note maintenance of the interproximal papilla. (*C*) After thorough debridement of the socket, a graft containing PRF, plasma, Infuse, and corticocancellous mix was placed. (*D*) Bone graft was covered with a PRF membrane and sutured in place. (*E*) Ovate pontic on a transitional partial denture was placed to begin reconstruction of the gingival shape and form. (*F*) Immediate postoperative film demonstrates good fill of the socket with bone graft. (*G*) Three-month postoperative film demonstrates some volume loss especially along the initially absent facial cortex of bone. (*H*) Implant planning. (*I–K*) Clinical photographs with and without the transitional partial denture in place. (*L*) Reentry at 4 months into the site demonstrates good reconstruction of the alveolar bone. (*M*) Initial implant osteotomy. (*N*) Implant with cover screw in place. (*O*) Sticky bone graft containing plasma, PRF, corticocancellous mix, and MinerOss XP (BioHorizons, Birmingham, AL) layered over top. (*P*) Facial enhancement bone graft positioned over buccal and occlusal surface of the implant. (*Q*) Postoperative film demonstrates good implant position, and the dense cortical nature of the MinerOss XP that was used to reconstruct the facial cortical wall of the alveolus.

CASE 4

This case shows external root resorption of tooth #8 with associated large defect in facial wall and alveolar bone. Using the two-stage reconstruction technique, the socket was grafted with Infuse, allograft, and membrane. Subsequently, after 5 months of healing, the site was reentered and an implant was placed using surgical navigation. Photographs of Case 4 are detailed in **Fig. 10**.

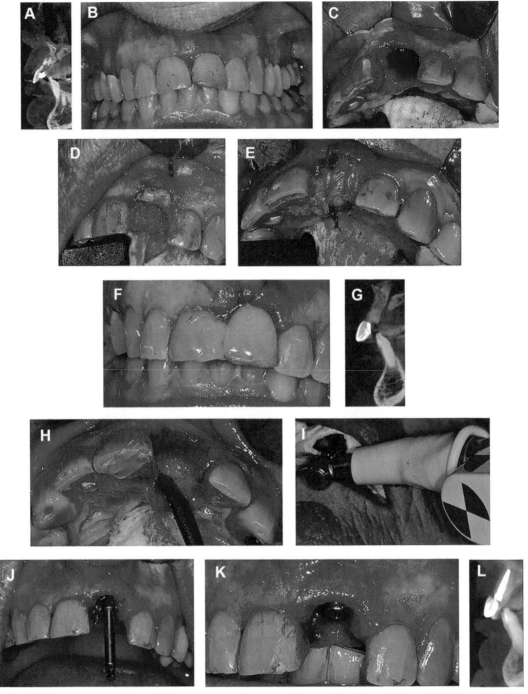

Fig. 10. (*A*) Preoperative radiograph showing extensive external resorption of tooth #8 and facial bone loss from chronic infection. (*B*) Preoperative clinical photograph. (*C*) After atraumatic extraction and grafting of the defect using Infuse, PRF, and corticocancellous. (*D*) A resorbable collagen membrane was positioned apically to reconstruct the facial wall. This membrane was fixated with a suture to tether it to the facial tissue, which is seen apical to grafted site #8. (*E*) PRF membrane positioned over the occlusal aspect of the socket to contain the bone graft and expedite wound healing. (*F*) Temporary bonded into place. (*G*) Four months after extraction and bone graft the alveolus was completely and anatomically reconstructed. (*H*, *I*) At 5 months the socket was reentered for implant placement using surgical navigation. (*J*) After implant placement the implant. (*K*) Implant cover screw in place (*L*) Post op radiograph demonstrating good implant position.

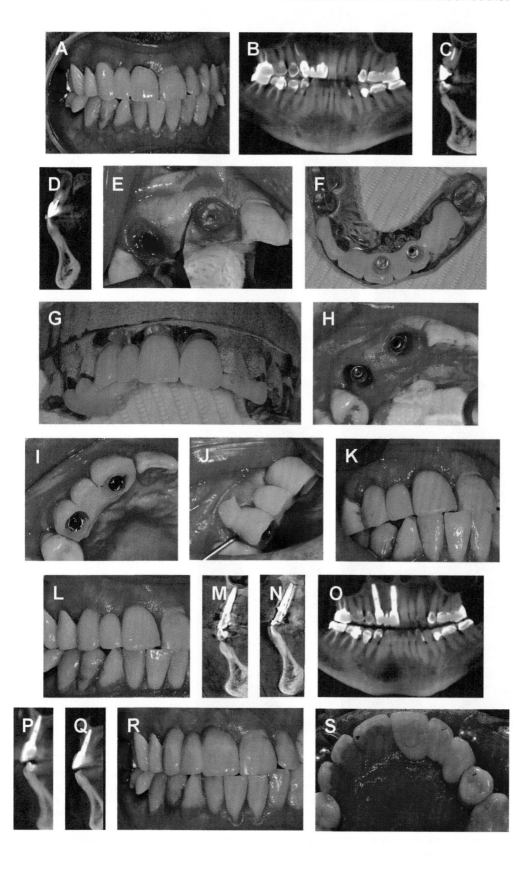

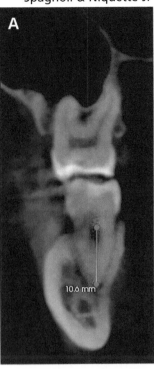

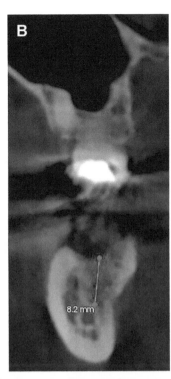

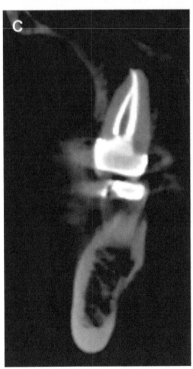

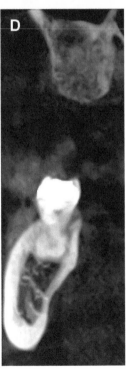

Fig. 12. (*A*, *B*) Extraction of tooth #30 with PRF only and 6-month follow-up; incomplete vertical bone maintenance but shows good bone formation within the socket. (*C*, *D*) Extraction of tooth #2 with removal of periapical pathology and placement of PRF into the socket. Six-month follow-up demonstrates robust wound healing and bone fill.

Fig. 11. (*A*) Preoperative photograph demonstrating three-unit bridge #6 to #8 with previously endodontically treated abutments. (*B–D*) Preoperative radiographs demonstrating periapical pathology, root resorption, and poor long-term prognosis of teeth #6 and #8. (*E*) Atraumatic extraction of teeth #6 and #8 using powertome for PDL expansion and elevation. (*F, G*) Immediate temporary bridge on model. (*H*) Sites #6 and #8 postextraction and immediate implant placement. (*I*) Temporary bridge in place after pickup on temporary cylinders. (*J*) Additional Infuse packed under the facial gingival tissue to maximize wound healing in this area. (*K*) Infuse has been placed as a grout along the facial surface of the extraction sockets and implants. (*L*) Eleven days postoperative photograph demonstrates good maintenance of form and function relating to the keratinized tissue and excellent wound healing. (*M–O*) Implants #6 and #8 with good position, maintenance of the facial cortical plate, and immediate temporaries in place. (*P, Q*) Implants #6 and #8 with final prosthetics in place. (*R, S*) Clinical photographs of final prosthetics in place.

CASE 5

With the esthetic zone failing bridge #6 to #8, the patient requested immediate implants and temporization. Photographs of Case 5 are detailed in **Fig. 11**.

Some sockets are not suitable for immediate graft or patients may defer graft because they are undecided about an implant. These sites were treated with PRF only. In bone grafting, the goal is to create an osteogenic granulation tissue. In general, wound healing upregulates bone forming cytokines and associated cell signaling. The use of biologics alone at these sites combined with the body's own response to insult and healing has contributed to significant bone regeneration as seen in **Fig. 12**.

CASE 6

Fractured #14 requires extraction and has marginal bone height for implant placement. This site is not currently amenable to immediate implant reconstruction. This scenario can benefit from extraction with simultaneous indirect sinus lift of interradicular bone and ridge preservation graft. The aim of this technique is to minimize negative remodeling in the apical portion of the socket and limit the need for formal sinus lift bone grafting. The photographs of Case 6 are detailed in **Fig. 13**. As seen in **Fig. 14**, if no effort is made to combat negative remodeling, loss of grafted bone volume occurs. This process generally begins on the facial cortex at the

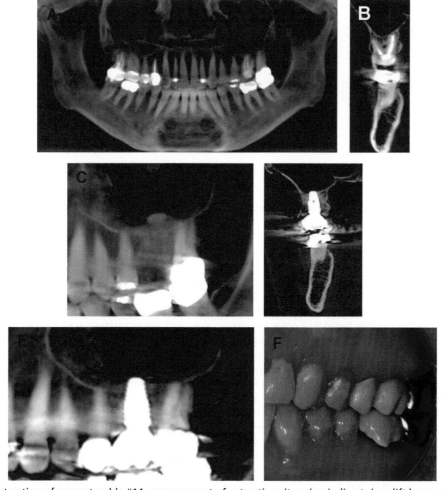

Fig. 13. Extraction of nonrestorable #14, management of extraction site using indirect sinus lift bone graft at the time of tooth removal allows for adequate bone for implant placement at reentry 4 months later. (*A,B*) Pre-op panorex and coronal CBCT slice demonstrating periapical infection and sinus pneumatization above #14. (*C*) Radiograph after extraction shows achievement of indirect sinus lift in combination with socket preservation. (*D, E*) Radiograph after implant placement detailing position of implant as well as bone maintenance at the apical aspect of implant #14. (*F*) Intraoral photograph of restored implant #14.

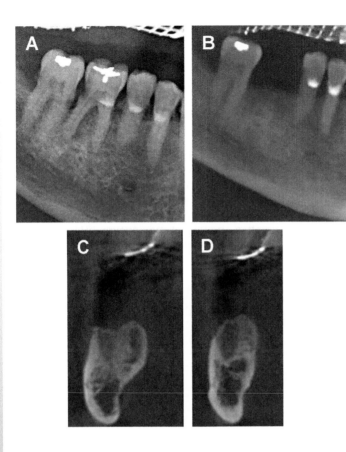

Fig. 14. Extraction of tooth #30 with facial wall intact, and graft with PRF. Simultaneous root planning of adjacent teeth. Note good bone height maintenance and bone regeneration. (A) Pre-extraction of #30 calculus on adjacent roots. (B) Six months postextraction good bone height maintenance and clean adjacent roots. (C) A section midsocket through interradicular bone and distal root alveolus; crestal bone is cortical and visible mineralization present. (D) An additional section through mesial root alveolus cortical crestal bone established, mineralization of bone within the socket is evident, some regressive remodeling of facial crestal area present.

coronal extent of the graft but progresses medially and inferiorly.

CASE 7

This case demonstrates the variations across extraction sockets and their response to bone grafting in view of altered facial wall anatomy. Here we compare existing facial wall defects with an intact facial wall and the subsequent impact on the bone volume changes at 4 months postgrafting. Teeth #6 to #11 were of guarded prognosis because of caries and moderate bone loss. The plan was to remove the teeth and graft using Infuse and corticocancellous allograft in the bony sockets in preparation for future dental implant reconstruction. The 4-month postoperative films are compared with the preoperative film to underscore the differences in bony remodeling when a facial plate is present versus absent. This comparison underscores the importance of the facial plate in extraction socket bone graft reconstruction. It

plays an important role in vascular supply for healthy bone formation, and space maintenance for the management of the resorptive periosteum. Photographs of Case 7 are detailed in **Fig. 15**.

CASE 8

Tooth #7 has a large apical defect and fistula. We plan for extraction and reconstruction. The site is grafted with Infuse, cortical cancellous allograft, and PRF. This is an example of regeneration of facial wall and marrow space trabecular bone. Photographs of Case 8 are detailed in **Fig. 16**.

CASE 9

Recurrent decay in tooth #11, led to plan for immediate implant using the "socket within a socket" technique for apical stabilization of the implant. Using this method, the native palatal bone apical and palatal to the tooth is harnessed

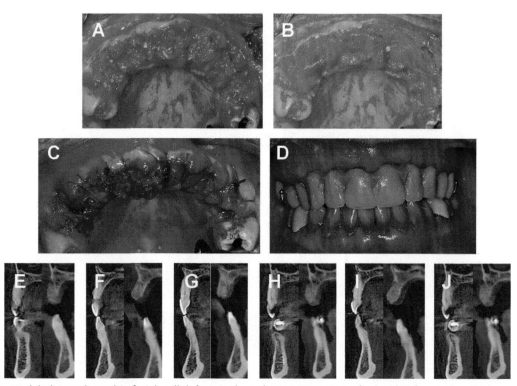

Fig. 15. (*A*) The resultant thin facial wall defects in the esthetic zone were grafted with Infuse and cortical cancellous allograft. (*B*) The facial walls were reinforced with PRF laminated to collagen membranes and bolster sutured to vestibule at the socket base. (*C*) Tissues were reapproximated using horizontal mattress chromic gut sutures and a running monocryl suture. (*D*) At 4 months postextractions and grafting, the effects of the transitional partial denture with ovate pontics are appreciated. The intaglio surface of the prostheses has already begun tissue and papilla training. (*E*) At site #6 there is a facial wall defect preoperatively and at 4 months one can see the adequate, yet incomplete bone fill at this site. (*F, G*) Teeth #7 and #8 have thin, but intact facial walls before extraction. When these sites are grafted, one can see the complete bone fill at 4 months. (*H*) Tooth #9 has loss of facial bone and again it is seen that despite grafting there is incomplete bone, especially in the apical third. (*I*) Area #10 has only mild facial bone loss preoperatively. After reconstruction of the site with bone graft the width of the native alveolar bone is well maintained. (*J*) Tooth #11 has significant facial wall bone loss and as expected, in the 4-month postoperative cone-beam computed tomography film decreased bone fill is seen in the apical and coronal thirds of the extraction socket.

and repositioned more facial to be used for primary stabilization of a dental implant. A dual surgical guide protocol was designed to maximize the accuracy of this method. The first surgical guide is designed to direct an implant pilot bur into the stock of palatal bone. Then, using a series of dilating osteotomes, this bone is repositioned facially to create an osteotomy, or socket, within the tooth extraction socket. A second surgical guide is fabricated for implant placement to ensure accurate position, depth, and angulation. It is well accepted that immediate implants are the preferred method of reconstruction in the esthetic zone. By using this "socket within a socket" method, more sites

are amenable to immediate implant placement. Photographs of Case 9 are detailed in **Fig. 17**.

CASE 10

Ankylosed tooth #27 required extraction and grafting to allow orthodontic movement of tooth #28 anteriorly for canine substitution. The resultant edentulous span between #28 and #29 will undergo dental implant reconstruction when the patient has reached facial maturity. The ability to create a nonremodeling, biologically reinforcing graft to mimic the facial cortical bone is important. In this case, we use dentin milling for this purpose. Demineralized milled autogenous

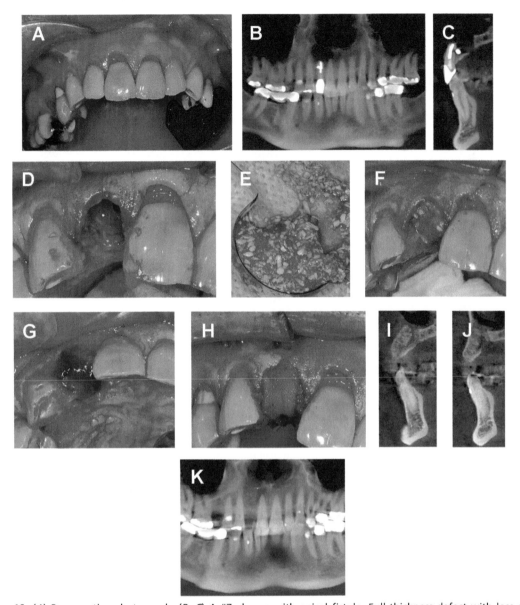

Fig. 16. (*A*) Preoperative photograph. (*B, C*) A #7 abscess with apical fistula. Full-thickness defect with loss of facial wall and nasal floor anatomy. (*D*) Socket debrided and cystic tissue removed but papilla attachment to the adjacent teeth is preserved. (*E, F*) Graft using Infuse, cortical cancellous allograft. (*G*) PRF triple layer membrane inlaid within the socket. (*H*) Collagen membrane over PRF. (*I, J*) Four months post-graft cone-beam computed tomography slices show regeneration of facial wall and establishment of cancellous trabecular bone supporting the facial wall. (*K*) Four-month panoramic view shows good bone maintenance and bone regeneration.

dentin is an antigenically neutral, but osteoinductive graft.[20] In this case, the impacted third molar teeth were removed and processed according to the Kometa Bio parameters for milling. The dentin particulate is finished into 300 to 1200 μm particles. It is then soaked in a cleansing solution, consisting of 0.5 M sodium hydroxide and 20% ethanol, and finally agitated in phosphate-buffered saline for 2 to 3 minutes. Once processed, the dentin was used to graft the facial cortex after a remodeling alveolar bone graft had been placed. This created a bilaminar graft to anatomically reconstruct the right mandible. The photographs of Case 10 are detailed in **Fig. 18**.

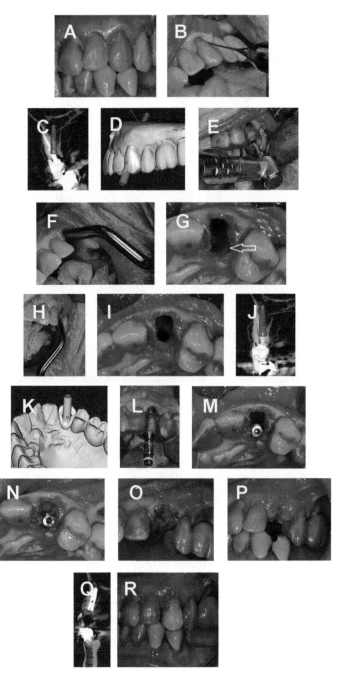

Fig. 17. (*A*) Preoperative photograph demonstrating thin gingival biotype. (*B*) Atraumatic extraction using powertome for PDL space expansion and elevation. (*C*) The first guide directs the pilot burr into the large stock of native palatal bone. (*D*) The angle of the initial implant guide is inappropriate for final implant placement, as illustrated by what would be the screw access of the implant directed out the facial surface of the planned restoration. (*E*) Using the pilot burr, an initial osteotomy is created into the palatal bone. (*F*) Using a series of dilating osteotomes, the initial pilot osteotomy was increased and gradually molded toward an angulation more appropriate for final implant position. (*G*) After dilation and repositioning, the "socket within a socket" begins to take shape. (*H*) Larger diameter osteotome at an improved angulation when compared with *F*. (*I*) Fully developed socket within a socket prepared for implant placement. (*J*) The second surgical guide was planned using the traditional principles of implant planning, screw channel emerging through the cingulum and implant level 2 mm below crestal bone. (*K*) Appropriate screw channel emergence. (*L*) Implant placement through the second surgical guide. (*M*) Implant with cover screw in place. Primary stability was maximized by translating native palatal bone to a more facial position for circumferential bone contact in the apical third of the implant. Also note the intact papilla on the mesial and distal to maximize vascular supply to the site. (*N*) Additional bone graft placed into the remaining extraction socket defect. (*O*) PRF membrane sutured in place over top of implant and bone graft. (*P*) Eleven days after the ovate pontic has begun to shape the papilla and prepare for esthetic emergence profile. (*Q*) Postoperative cone-beam computed tomography slice to demonstrate accurate implant position, complete fill of the extraction socket with bone graft, and bilaminar facial wall enhancement bone graft in the coronal third of the implant. (*R*) Three-dimensional printed composite resin transitional partial denture with ovate pontic in place.

SUMMARY

Alveolar bone and tooth sockets indicated for extraction should be treated with reconstructive concepts. Each extraction site should be evaluated with regards to existing bone and/or existing bone defects. Pathologic and/or physiologic processes that would affect bone or soft tissue wound healing must be considered during the approach to reconstruction. Adjuncts to grafting including graft coverage, facial wall membranes,

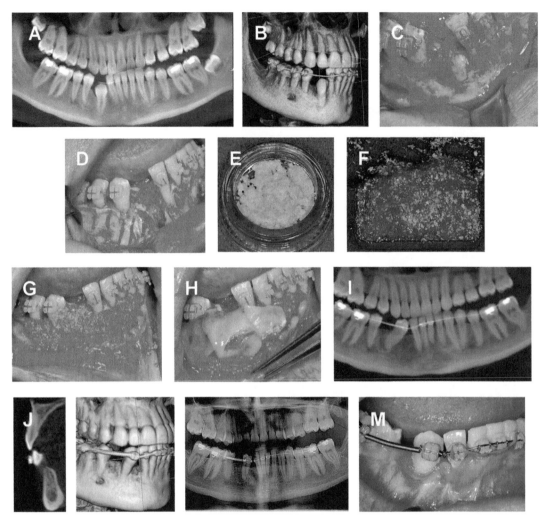

Fig. 18. (*A, B*) Preoperative panorex and three-dimensional reconstruction showing ankylosed tooth #27. (*C*) Flap reflected to reveal tooth #27 in preparation for extraction and surgically facilitated orthodontic therapy of the adjacent teeth. (*D*) Extraction and surgically facilitated orthodontic therapy complete. (*E, F*) Bone grafting mixture containing corticocancellous particulate and Infuse. This was used to reconstruct the alveolar segment of the bone and the extraction socket. (*G*) Once the alveolar bone graft was in place, additional graft of sterile dentin was placed to mimic the facial cortical plate. The dentin graft was created from the milling of teeth #1, #16, and #17 after their extraction. (*H*) PRF was layered over the graft. (*I*) Twelve-month postoperative panorex showing good movement of tooth #28 through the previously grafted site. (*J*) Radiograph demonstrating reconstruction of facial plate in the area of the extraction and alveolar grafting. (*K–M*) Eighteen-month radiograph, three-dimensional reconstruction, and clinical photograph demonstrating movement of tooth #28 through area of previously ankylosed tooth #27.

simultaneous bone expansion, indirect sinus lift, socket within a socket, and facial wall bilaminar grafts should all be considered when evaluating an extraction site for reconstruction. In many cases the immediate placement of an implant forms all or a portion of the graft necessary to maintain a socket and expedite the return of dental function.[2,8] Many types of grafts are used for socket reconstruction. The literature does not clearly support efficacy of any one grafting procedure. Success has been achieved with autogenous bone, allogeneic bone, and various biologics.[9–12,18,21,22] When the goal is to place an implant in an extraction socket the graft should have the potential to remodel completely to biologically natural bone. Without remodeling, mechanical transduction in response to implant loads could be compromised. Biologics, such as Infuse, PRF, or platelet rich plasma, should be considered as a component of the graft, especially when wall defects are present. The goal of reconstructive bone grafting is to create an osteogenic granulation tissue that can mature and remodel into a form that replaces native bone structure. Biologics enhance neovascularization and the population of a wound by vessel-associated pericyte stem cells, which begin the cell lineage responsible for recapitulating alveolar bone and associated tissues.[23] Proper space maintenance contributed by natural anatomy, membranes, or mesh may be necessary to preserve or reconstruct a proper form.

DISCLOSURE

The authors have nothing to disclose.

REFERENCES

1. Pietrokovski J, Massler M. Ridge remodeling after tooth extraction in rats. J Dent Res 1967;46(1):222–31.

2. Mauricio GA, Lindhe J. Dimensional ridge alterations following tooth extraction. An experimental study in the dog. J Clin Periodontol 2005;32(2):212–8.

3. Van der Weijden F, Dell'Acqua F, Slot DE. Alveolar bone dimensional changes of post-extraction sockets in humans: a systematic review. J Clin Periodontol 2009;36(12):1048–58.

4. Yang X, Wang L, Sun Y, et al. Sclerostin is essential for alveolar bone loss in occlusal hypofunction. Exp Ther Med 2016;11:1812–8.

5. Boyne PJ. Osseous repair of the postextraction alveolus in man. Oral Surg Oral Med Oral Pathol 1966;21(6):805–13.

6. Pietrokovski J, Massler M. Alveolar ridge resorption following tooth extraction. J Prosthet Dent 1967;17(1):21–7.

7. Enlow DH, Kuroda T, Lewis AB, et al. The morphological and morphogenetic basis for craniofacial form and pattern. Angle Orthod 1971;41(3):161–88.

8. Kuroda MA, Alsabeeha NH, Payne AG, et al. Interventions for replacing missing teeth: alveolar ridge preservation techniques for dental implant site development. Cochrane Database Syst Rev 2015;(5):CD010176.

9. Alzahrani AA, Murriky A, Shafik S. Influence of platelet rich fibrin on post-extraction socket healing: a clinical and radiographic study. Saudi Dent J 2017;29:149–55.

10. Baniasadi B, Evrard L. Alveolar ridge preservation after tooth extraction with DFDBA and platelet concentrates: a radiographic retrospective study. Open Dent J 2017;11:99–108.

11. Cammack GV, Nevins M, Clem DS, et al. Histologic evaluation of mineralized and demineralized freeze-dried bone allograft for ridge and sinus augmentations. Int J Periodontics Restorative Dent 2005;25(3):231–7.

12. Fiorellini JP, Howell TH, Cochran D, et al. Randomized study evaluating recombinant human bone morphogenetic protein-2 for extraction socket augmentation. J Periodontol 2005;76(4):605–13.

13. Mezzomo LA, Shinkai RS, Mardas N, et al. Alveolar ridge preservation after dental extraction and before implant placement: a literature review. Revista Odonto Ciência 2011;26(1):77–83.

14. Misch CM. The use of recombinant human bone morphogenetic protein-2 for the repair of extraction socket defects: a technical modification and case series report. Int J Oral Maxillofac Implants 2010;25(6):1246–52.

15. Pranskunas M, Galindo-Moreno P, Padial-Molina M. Extraction socket preservation using growth factors and stem cells: a systematic review. J Oral Maxillofac Res 2019;10(3):e7.

16. Simon BI, Zatcoff AL, Kong JJ, et al. Clinical and histological comparison of extraction socket healing following the use of autologous platelet-rich fibrin matrix (PRFM) to ridge preservation procedures employing demineralized freeze dried bone allograft material and membrane. Open Dent J 2009;3:92–9.

17. Spagnoli DB, Choi C. Extraction socket grafting and buccal wall regeneration with recombinant human bone morphogenetic protein-2 and acellular collagen sponge. Atlas Oral Maxillofac Surg Clin North Am 2013;21(2):175–83.

18. Spagnoli DB, Marx RE. Dental implants and use of rhBMP-2. Oral Maxillofac Surg Clin North Am 2011;23:347–61.

19. Vanchit J, Blanchard S. Socket preservation as a precursor of future implant placement: review of the literature and case reports. Compend Contin Educ Dent 2007;28(12):646–53.

20. Kim Y-K, Lee J, Um I-W, et al. Tooth-derived bone graft material. J Korean Assoc Oral Maxillofac Surg 2013;39(3):103–11.

21. Kaku M, Akiba Y, Akiyama K, et al. Cell-based bone regeneration for alveolar ridge augmentation: cell source, endogenous cell recruitment and immunomodulatory function. J Prosthodont Res 2015;59:96–112.

22. Sohn, Huang, Kim, et al. Utilization of Autologous Concentrated Growth Factors (CGF) Enriched Bone Graft Matrix (Sticky Bone) and CGF-Enriched Fibrin Membrane in Implant Dentistry. The Journal of Implant & Advanced Clinical Dentistry 2015;7:11–29.

23. Spagnoli DB. The application of recombinant human bone morphogenetic protein on absorbable collagen sponge (rhBMP-2/ACS) to reconstruction of maxillofacial bone defects. In: Vukicevic S, Sampath KT, editors. Bone Morphogenetic Proteins: From Local to Systemic Therapeutics. Progress in Inflammation Research. Springer Publishing; 2008. p. 43–70.

Oral Soft Tissue Grafting

Janina Golob Deeb, DMD, MS[a], George R. Deeb, DDS, MD[b],*

KEYWORDS

- Soft tissue graft • Allografts • Xenograft • Teeth • Implants

KEY POINTS

- The goal of soft tissue grafting is to improve prognosis, esthetics, and function of teeth and implants.
- New classification systems for soft tissue diagnosis have been developed.
- Allogenic, xenogenic, and biologic materials are increasingly used to compliment or substitute autogenous soft tissue grafts.
- The number of techniques and materials for oral soft tissue grafting is expanding.

Treatment of mucogingival deficiencies has become an integral part in oral and dental rehabilitation. Inadequate keratinized tissue (KT) surrounding teeth and implants can lead to recession.[1,2] Recession refers to the apical displacement of the soft tissue margin including mucosa or gingiva, whichever is present at the site. The presence of healthy tissue at the tooth and implant soft tissue interface correlates to long-term success and stability in function and esthetics. Although KT is not necessary to prevent recession in presence of good plaque control,[1,3] it does decrease recession over time.[4] Implant success is also not absolutely dependent on the presence of gingiva[5]; however, adequate KT is associated with patient comfort and less inflammation around implants.[6–10] Plaque is the primary etiologic factor in periodontal and peri-implant inflammation,[11] and thicker gingiva facilitates its removal and strongly correlates with optimal tissue health around implants.[6] Implants without KT demonstrate increased susceptibility to recession and plaque-induced tissue destruction.[12] Esthetic demands including soft tissue surrounding for natural, restored, or implant-supported dentition have increased. Harmony is expected among teeth, implants, restorations, and adjacent soft tissue (**Fig. 1**).

CAUSE OF RECESSION

Recession around teeth is a result of several predisposing factors including: anatomy; tooth position; orthodontic tooth movement; mechanical and chemical trauma; tooth brushing technique; the quantity, quality, and biotype of surrounding attached gingiva; poorly designed or maintained prosthetic devices; suboptimal restorative margins; high muscle attachment and frenal pull; and calculus and plaque control.[13,14]

Etiologies of soft tissue defects around implants include: poor spatial positioning, excessive abutment contour and implant diameter, horizontal biologic width formation, and periodontal phenotype.[15] Recession around implants may be partially associated with the remodeling of the peri-implant soft tissue barrier following implant placement and restoration.[16]

PAPILLA

Maintenance of papillae height is predictable in healthy periodontium because of tissue rebound based on the height of interproximal bone. Complete papilla fill between teeth is possible with less than or equal to 5 mm distance from the contact point to the bone.[17] Papilla height next to an implant depends on the adjacent tooth's bone

^a Department of Periodontics, School of Dentistry, Virginia Commonwealth University, 521 North 11th Street, Richmond, VA 23298, USA; ^b Department of Oral and Maxillofacial Surgery, School of Dentistry, Virginia Commonwealth University, 521 North 11th Street, Richmond, VA 23298, USA
* Corresponding author.
E-mail address: gdeeb@vcu.edu

Oral Maxillofacial Surg Clin N Am 32 (2020) 611–630
https://doi.org/10.1016/j.coms.2020.07.006
1042-3699/20/© 2020 Elsevier Inc. All rights reserved.

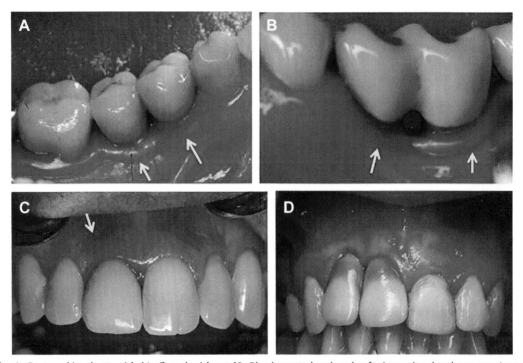

Fig. 1. Restored implants with (*A, C*) and without (*B, D*) adequate hard and soft tissue site development. Arrows are pointing at soft tissue adjacent to restored implants.

height (see **Fig. 1**C).[18] Adjacent implants only average 3.4 mm of soft tissue height over the inter-implant bone crest (see **Fig. 1**A, B, D).[19] Surgical techniques aiming to increase the volume of papillae use platelet-rich fibrin (PRF),[20] injection of hyaluronic acid–based gel,[21] and connective tissue grafts (CTG) with coronally positioned flaps (CAF).[22] To prevent loss of interproximal bone and papilla, implants should be placed 1.5 mm from adjacent teeth,[23] and 3 mm from another implant, because vertical bone loss increases with closer proximity.[24]

CLASSIFICATION OF RECESSION

An early classification of recession was introduced by Sullivan[25] comprising four categories: (I) deep/wide, (II) shallow/wide, (III) deep/narrow, and (IV) shallow/narrow.

Miller Classification System of Marginal Tissue Recession

Miller's[26] classification was introduced in 1985 and it sets realistic expectations for root coverage outcomes. Class I and II groups can achieve almost complete root coverage, class III only partial, and class IV none:

Class I: Recession not passed mucogingival junction, no interdental bone loss

Class II: Recession to/passed mucogingival junction, no interdental bone loss

Class III: Recession to/passed mucogingival junction, some interdental bone loss

Class IV: Recession to/passed mucogingival junction, severe interdental bone loss

Mucogingival Deformities and Conditions Around Teeth

In 1999, the International Workshop by the American Academy of Periodontology proposed a new classification system that comprehensively diagnosed mucogingival deformities and conditions around teeth and on edentulous ridges as two subcategories under developmental or acquired deformities and conditions.[27] This classification was modified at the 2017 World Workshop and now incorporates the interproximal clinical attachment loss measured from cementoenamel junction (CEJ) to the base of the sulcus and the assessment of the exposed root surface.[28,29]

a. Gingival phenotype
b. Gingival/soft tissue recession
c. Lack of gingiva
d. Decreased vestibular depth
e. Aberrant frenum/muscle position
f. Gingival excess
g. Abnormal color
h. Condition of the exposed root surface

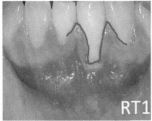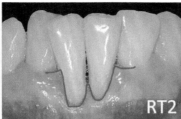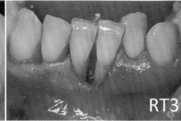

Fig. 2. Recession type according to the 2017 World Workshop Classification.[29]

Recession Type

RT1: Gingival recession with no loss of interproximal attachment (**Fig. 2**)[29]

RT2: Gingival recession associated with interproximal attachment loss that is less or equal to the buccal attachment loss

RT3: Gingival recession associated with interproximal attachment loss that is greater than buccal attachment loss

Gingival Biotype

The thin periodontium has a high incidence of dehiscence and fenestration defects over which recession occurs and continues until the bone margin is reached. Gingival scallop on anterior teeth can reach 4 to 6 mm. The thick biotype is supported by thick bone resisting recession to occur and is characterized by smaller embrasures and flatter 3- to 4-mm anterior gingival scallop. Three biotypes have been described based on gingival thickness, KT width, bone morphotype, and tooth dimension (**Fig. 3**)[29]:

Thin scalloped biotype is characterized by slender triangular teeth, interproximal contacts close to incisal edge, narrow KT, and thin gingiva and alveolar bone.

Thick flat biotype is characterized by square-shaped teeth, prominent cervical convexity, interproximal contacts more apically, broad KT, and thick gingiva and alveolar bone.

Thick scalloped biotype is characterized by slender teeth with pronounced gingival scalloping, narrow KT, and thick fibrotic gingiva.

DEVELOPMENT OF MUCOGINGIVAL SURGERY

The term "periodontal plastic surgery" was introduced by Miller.[30,31] It encompasses regenerative and reconstructive surgical procedures that prevent or correct anatomic, developmental, traumatic, and disease-related defects of oral soft tissue or bone in form and function and enhance soft tissue characteristics around teeth, implants,

and prosthetic restorations.[31,32] Soft tissue manipulation from adjacent or distant donor sites is generally separated into:

1. Pedicle grafts
   a. Flap advancement procedures
      - CAF
      - Semilunar CAF

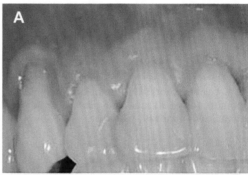

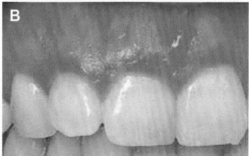

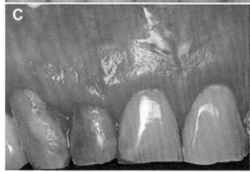

Fig. 3. Thin scalloped biotype (*A*), thick flat biotype (*B*), and thick scalloped biotype (*C*).

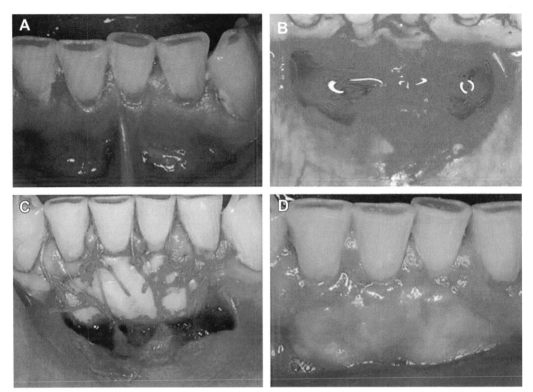

Fig. 4. Lower incisors with frenum pull, minimal KT, and RT1 recession (*A*). Frenectomy and recipient site preparation (*B*). Thick FGG sutured in place (*C*). Healing after 4 weeks shows good KT and recession coverage but suboptimal color match (*D*).

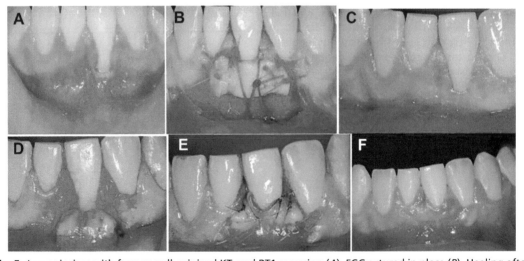

Fig. 5. Lower incisor with frenum pull, minimal KT, and RT1 recession (*A*). FGG sutured in place (*B*). Healing after 2 months shows good color match and KT but suboptimal root coverage (*C*). Second surgery (*D*) to coronally advance KT (*E*) achieved complete root coverage (*F*).

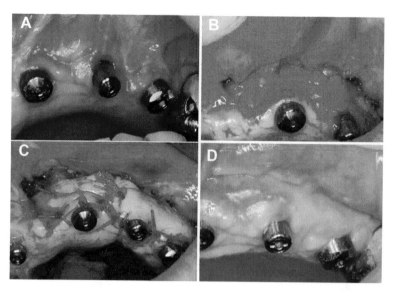

Fig. 6. Free gingival graft. Second-stage implants with multiple freni and deficient KT and vestibule (*A*). Recipient site preparation (*B*). Two thick FGG stabilized by sutures (*C*). Following 6 weeks healing increased KT and vestibular depth are achieved (*D*).

b. Flap rotation procedures
  - Laterally sliding flap
  - Partial-thickness double pedicle graft
  - Rotational flap
  - Transpositioned flap
2. Free soft tissue grafts
   Free gingival grafts (FGG)
   Subepithelial tissue grafts (SCTG), CTG

FREE GINGIVAL GRAFT

FGG was introduced in 1966[33] and it remains the gold standard for augmentation of KT around teeth (**Figs. 4** and **5**) and implants (**Figs. 6** and **7**).[34] Additional indications include elimination of the frenal attachments, increase of vestibular depth, stabilization of progressive gingival recession, and protection of denture-bearing surfaces.[35]

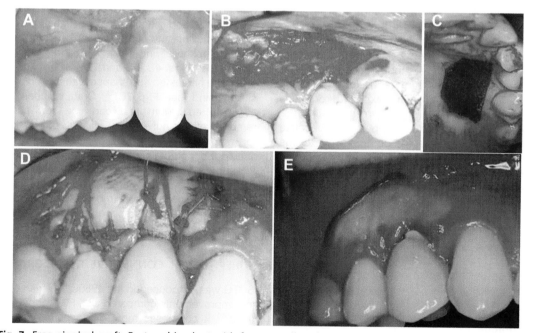

Fig. 7. Free gingival graft. Restored implant with frenum pull and recession (*A*). Recipient site preparation (*B*). Thick FGG harvested (*C*) and sutured (*D*). Following 6 weeks healing increased KT and vestibular depth are achieved (*E*).

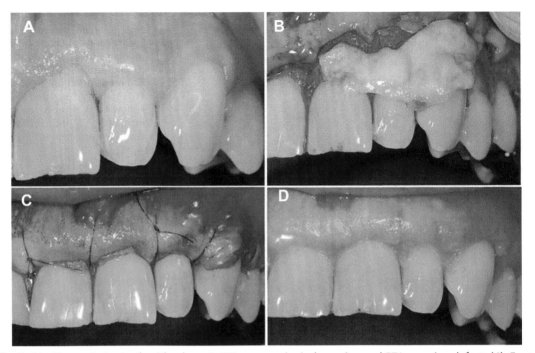

Fig. 8. Maxillary anterior teeth with adequate KT, uneven gingival margins, and RT1 recession defects (*A*). Envelope flap with elevated papillae and an SCTG (*B*) and CAF (*C*) enhanced esthetics and achieved complete root coverage (*D*).

The autogenous FGG is categorized by thickness into thin (0.5–0.8 mm), average (0.9–1.4 mm), and thick (1.5 to >2 mm).

Thin grafts can increase the amount of KT, they provide the best color match, and have to be placed in intimate contact with an intact blood supply to survive (see **Fig. 4**). They heal the fastest and undergo the highest (25%–30%) secondary shrinkage.[25,36] The average thickness graft is suited for all types of grafting, it provides acceptable appearance and better protection against future recession. The thick FGG is used for covering exposed root surfaces, is more resistant to future recession,[37,38] but results in less esthetic appearance because of color and thickness incompatibility to the adjacent gingiva (see **Fig. 4**). Rapid revascularization is expected for uniform thin or intermediate grafts placed on a periosteum, whereas uneven thicker FGGs placed on bone undergo a prolonged period of revascularization and healing.[38,39] FGG can achieve root coverage in 44%[40] and up to 89.9%[41] of the sites or it is used as a two-stage procedure for root coverage with coronal advancement of healed graft (see **Fig. 5**D–F).[42]

Technique

The incision is made at the mucogingival junction along the recipient area extending but not involving the sulcus of adjacent teeth or implants. The initial horizontal incision should be placed at the desired new gingival level (CEJ for Miller class I and II; below the CEJ for class III and IV). Vertical incisions are placed on the lateral aspects of the horizontal incision at 90° or slightly divergent toward mucosa. Recipient site is prepared by a split-thickness dissection leaving intact periosteum, removing any aberrant frenal attachments, and de-epithelializing marginal and papillary gingiva (see **Figs. 4**B, **6**B and **7**B). Gingival grafts should be harvested and shaped with the recipient site in mind (see **Fig. 7**C).[33] Graft includes the overlying epithelium and can use soft tissue removed after gingivectomy, palatal, or masticatory gingiva as autogenous donor sources.[43] Graft should be completely immobilized by sutures. Interrupted sutures on the edges enable good marginal adaptation, whereas sling sutures facilitate intimate contact with the vascular bed and elimination of the dead space between FGG and recipient bed (see **Figs. 4**C, **5**B, **6**C and **7**D).

SUBEPITHELIAL CONNECTIVE TISSUE GRAFT

SCTG was introduced in the 1980s,[44,45] with clinical improvements compared with FGG or pedicle flaps.[46] It comprises most grafts performed for root coverage[37] and augmentation procedures in combination with variety of flap designs and provides long-term stability against recession

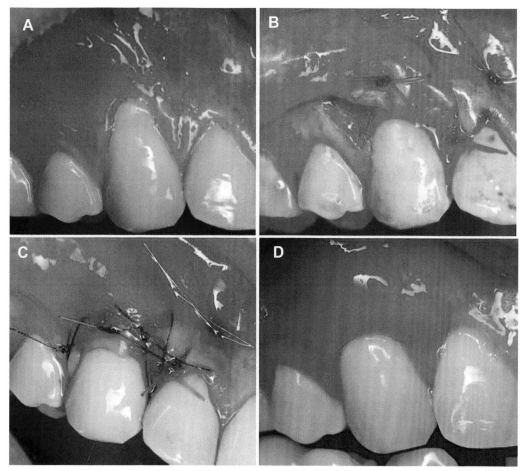

Fig. 9. Maxillary canine with no KT and RT1 recession (*A*). SCTG (*B*) with papilla pedicle flap to reposition KT from adjacent sites (*C*) was performed to enhance thickness of KT and maintain mucogingival junction and vestibular depth (*D*).

relapse.[47] The SCTG is divided by thickness into three categories: thin (0.5–0.8 mm), average (0.9–1.4 mm), and thick (1.5 to >2 mm).

Surface Treatment

Root or implant surface should be smooth and clean before receiving the SCTG. Root surface irregularities and restorations should be removed or reshaped. Root planning and chemical root surface treatment with citric acid,[41] tetracycline, or EDTA are used to remove endotoxins and smear layer exposing dentinal tubules essential for new attachment. Chemical conditioning of dentin can stimulate the attachment of fibroblasts[48] and gingival keratinocytes, facilitating the reformation of a junctional epithelium.[49] Citric acid causes greater morphologic alterations than EDTA[50] or tetracycline,[48,51,52] and is not consistently supported in literature.[53]

Recipient Site Flaps

CAF achieves better root coverage and recession reduction with addition of a graft, which provides superior long-term stability against recession relapse and reduction of KT, especially in cases with suboptimal KT.[47,54] The horizontal incision is made at the level of desired gingival margin, usually at the level of CEJ. The incision extends to the interdental area adjacent to the terminal grafted tooth (**Fig. 8**). Vertical incisions enable increased access, but decrease blood supply and can cause scarring. They should extend beyond mucogingival junction to allow manipulation of the flap in the coronal direction (**Figs. 9**B and **10C**). Graft is sutured in place with resorbable sutures extending to the edges of the recipient bed (see **Fig. 9**B). Flap should be sutured with longer lasting monofilament sutures (**Figs. 9**C and **10E**). Use of CAF is better suited for sites with minimal KT and thinner SCTG, frequently seen in Miller

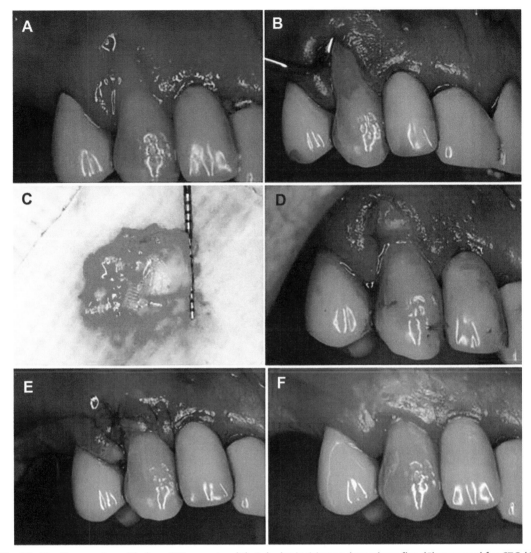

Fig. 10. Maxillary canine with deep RT1 recession (*A*). Sulcular incision and envelope flap (*B*) prepared for CTG (*C*) with retained epithelial collar left exposed (*D*) under CAF (*E*). Recession coverage, increased KT, and stable vestibular depth are achieved (*F*).

class I defects. In the absence of KT, SCTG with CAF results in predictable root coverage and non-keratinized mucosa as the soft tissue margin (**Fig. 9**D).[55]

Envelope flap was introduced with similar success by undermining partial-thickness dissection in the tissues surrounding the defect without reflecting a traditional flap or vertical incisions.[56] Incision is placed in the sulcus and a split-thickness pouch is developed under the surface of the tissue. The recipient bed should extend to undermine papillary tissue coronally to the CEJ. The envelope flap must extend far enough laterally and apically to allow passive placement of the graft (**Fig. 9**; **Fig. 11**). This dissection is difficult

and tactile sensation guides the preparation of the recipient site among periosteum, mucosa, and gingiva. The suturing technique is also more challenging; however, fewer sutures are needed because of good graft stability. The suturing technique is designed to pull the donor tissue into the tunnel. This technique is used for augmentation of deficient soft tissue contours under fixed prosthesis or around implants (see **Fig. 11**). This flap design provides excellent graft stability and maintenance of ample blood supply from the adjacent papillary, overlying mucogingival and underlying mucoperiosteal sides.

Partially covered CTG can achieve root coverage and increase in KT because the exposed

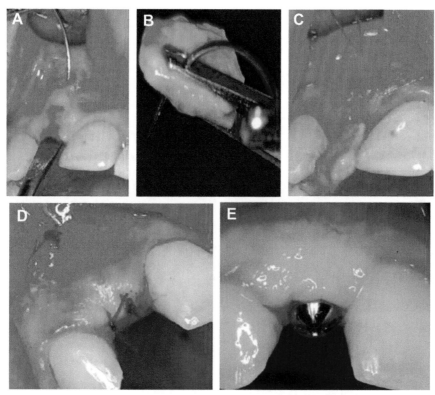

Fig. 11. Implant site with deficient facial soft tissue volume (*A*) prepared with split-thickness envelope flap. SCTG (*B*) is pulled (*C*) and secured into recipient site with a few sutures (*D*) yielding improved soft tissue contours in esthetic zone (*E*).

CTG keratinizes over the exposed graft surface. KT width correlates with the presurgical dimensions plus the height of the exposed graft.[55] It is suitable for Miller class I, II, and III recession defects with deficient KT. Partially exposed CTG must be thick enough to survive over the avascular root surface. It offers the advantage in maintaining the vestibular depth and position of mucogingival junction.[55] Exposed retained epithelial collar yields similar root coverage and better gingival augmentation compared with covered de-epithelialized graft that performs better esthetically (**Fig. 10**).[57]

Double pedicle flap should be considered when the objective includes the increase of KT and maintenance of mucogingival junction position (see **Fig. 10**; **Fig. 12**).[58] Coronally advanced, double pedicle, and tunneling flaps in conjunction with an autogenous SCTG are all effective in obtaining root coverage and improving clinical parameters.[59]

Laterally sliding, semilunar, and rotational flaps and are mostly used without SCTG and are suitable for high vestibules and sites with thick and wide adjacent KT that can be transpositioned. Pedicle flaps from adjacent areas are mobilized

to augment deficient soft tissue components at any stage of implant therapy[60–62] and are often used to develop implant sites (**Figs. 13**A–D). Because of limitations of flap mobility and numerous alternative procedures, these techniques remain in use in specific circumstances around teeth (**Fig. 13**E–H).

Donor Sites

Palatal gingiva between raphae and posterior teeth is the most common donor site for SCTG. It is composed of connective tissue and loosely organized glandular and adipose tissue.[63,64] Maxillary tuberosity presents an alternative donor site with rich connective tissue, minimal fatty and glandular components, and minimal risk for complications.[65,66] Encroaching on neurovascular structures can lead to bleeding and nerve injury (**Fig. 14**I). Greater palatine groove is located at the junction of vertical and horizontal palate with palatal vault depth ranging from 7 to 17 mm from the neurovascular line. The incision should end 2 mm above the neurovascular line, thus the width of donor tissue can vary from 3 to 13 mm, averaging 8 mm.[63]

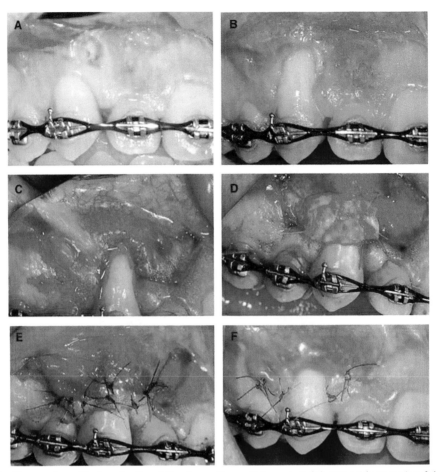

Fig. 12. Maxillary canine with fenestration following orthognathic surgery (*A*). RT1 wide recession following unsuccessful tunneling SCTG procedure (*B*). Bilateral pedicle flaps were used (*C*) to provide blood supply over wide avascular root surface area covered with SCTG (*D*), and to maintain vestibular depth (*E*). Favorable root coverage achieved at 2 weeks (*F*).

Donor sites can experience complications including bleeding, pain, flap necrosis, and recession.[67] Shallow palatal vault results in more bleeding because SCTG contains more medium and large vessels.[68] Donor sites are stabilized by suturing or adding materials promoting hemostasis (oxidized regenerated cellulose, absorbable gelatin sponge, thrombin)[69] and healing (PRF).[70,71] Removable devices for palatal donor sites include polymethylmethacrylate stents, orthodontic retainers, or existing dentures (**Fig. 14**). Palatal stents should be secure and tightly adhering to the palatal tissue. Stents are important for thicker bilateral grafts, patients with bleeding problems, and tendency for slower healing, including smokers.[67,72] Cyanoacrylate tissue adhesive is safe for oral use and is applied over recipient site in a thin layer.[73]

TYPES OF DONOR TISSUE

Autogenous grafts can result in discomfort and bleeding on donor site.[69] Alternative materials have been explored to achieve soft tissue augmentation outcomes comparable with autogenous grafts.[74] Although these alternative materials do not surpass the SCTG, they come in ample supply and provide patient satisfaction, esthetics, reduced morbidity, and surgical time.[75,76]

Allografts

Allografts, such as acellular dermal matrix, are biocompatible, derived from human dermis, processed to remove cellular and epidermal components, and freeze-dried. Graft maintains structural framework with proteins, collagen network, elastin filaments, hyaluronan,

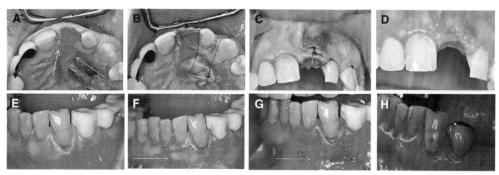

Fig. 13. Rotated pedicle flap (*arrows*) from adjacent palatal donor site (*A*) used over bone graft in socket preservation (*B,C*). Optimal KT and soft tissue volume at implant placement at 3 months (*D*). Abundant gingiva on the lateral incisor (*E*) is used as a lateral sliding flap (*arrows*) to reposition to the deficient adjacent site on the canine (*F,G*). Favorable healing at donor and recipient site at 12 weeks (D).

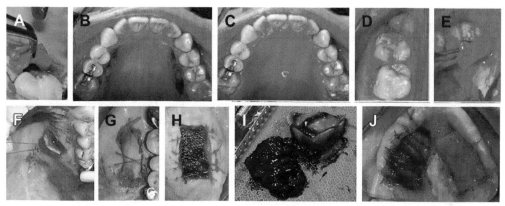

Fig. 14. Palatal donor site for SCTG (*A*) closed with sutures bilaterally (*B*) and custom made palatal acrylic stent (*C*). Alternative donor site is maxillary tuberosity (*D, E*). Palatal donor sites for FGGs (*F*) can be covered with PRF (*G*), oxidized regenerated cellulose (*H*), and for heavy bleeding cases (*I*) collagen sponge with thrombin (*J*).

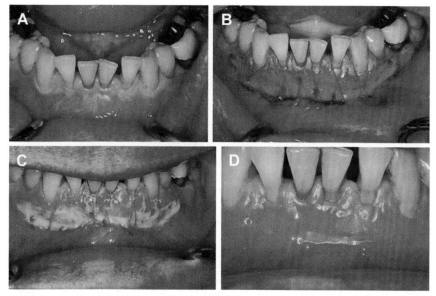

Fig. 15. Allograft as substitute for FGG. Multiple mandibular teeth with RT2 recession and deficient KT (*A*). Allograft sutured to recipient site (*B*). Healing at 2 weeks (*C*) and 8 weeks (*D*).

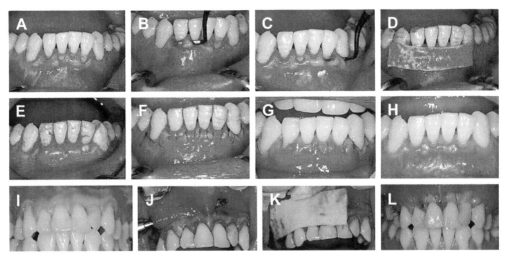

Fig. 16. Allograft as SCTG. Multiple mandibular (*A–H*) and maxillary (*I–L*) teeth with RT1 recession. Sulcular incision (*A*) and envelope flap (*B, C, J*) with lateral portal in maxillary vestibule (*J*) to facilitate placement of plain (*K*) or soaked in PRP (*D*) allograft (*E*) covered by CAF (*F*). At 2 weeks (*G, L*) and 2 months (*H*) healing with improved clinical parameters.

proteoglycans, and basement membrane, and can therefore be used as a soft tissue graft.[77] Allografts have been used in medicine[78] and dentistry for root coverage and soft tissue augmentation.[77,79]

Allografts are used instead of FGG[80] for KT augmentation (**Fig. 15**)[81] or as SCTG for root coverage (**Fig. 16**).[79] Allografts yield overall predictable results but are inferior to autogenous

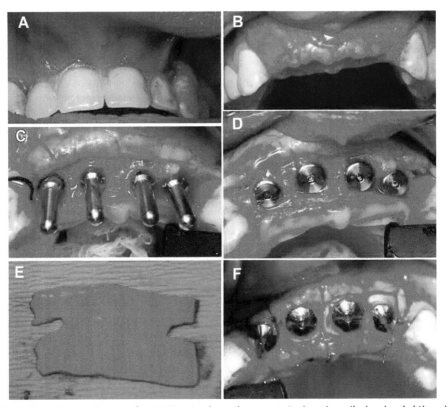

Fig. 17. Allograft used as a substitute for SCTG at implant placement. Reduced vestibular depth (*A*) and facial KT resulted from ridge augmentation procedure (*B*). Existing KT is repositioned facially (*C,D*) and enhanced by allograft (*E*) sutured under the flap (*F*).

grafts in defect coverage, KT gain, attachment gain, and residual probing depth.[74,82,83] In implant therapy, acellular dermal matrix is used at any stage to enhance soft tissue thickness. It is used during ridge augmentation as a barrier over bone graft, as an SCTG under the flap at the time of placement (**Fig. 17**),[84] or at uncovering to increase the width of KT.[85]

Xenografts

Xenografts are a viable alternative to SCTG in the treatment of recession defects with comparable esthetic outcomes and root coverage,[86] but also do not surpass the autogenous SCTG in root coverage and recession reduction.[74–76] Xenogenic thick collagen matrix is used around teeth or implants achieving similar KT gain compared with SCTG (**Fig. 18**).[74] Around implants, xenografts offer good tissue incorporation with similar soft tissue augmentation as SCTG and favorable patient acceptance (**Fig. 19**).[9]

Guided Tissue Regeneration

Guided tissue regeneration (GTR) is based on the different healing potential of various cells.[87] Barrier membranes promote regeneration of all periodontal tissues through cell exclusion during healing. Coverage of exposed roots and implants is achieved with GTR using absorbable and nonabsorbable membranes (**Fig. 20**). Autogenous SCTG results in superior root coverage and KT width,[88–91] and provides better long-term stability and esthetic results compared with GTR on teeth.[92]

Living Cellular Construct

Living cellular constructs (LCS) are 0.75-mm-thick grafts composed of allogenic keratinocytes, fibroblasts, extracellular matrix proteins, and bovine collagen,[74,93] delivered on a semipermeable polycarbonate membrane on an agarose-rich nutrient medium.[94] Histologically and clinically, LCS-treated sites resemble gingiva resulting in a site-

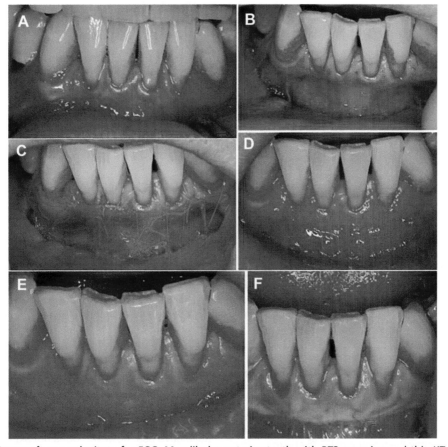

Fig. 18. Xenograft as a substitute for FGG. Mandibular anterior teeth with RT2 recession and thin KT (*A*). Split thickness flap is performed to prepare recipient site (*B*) with Xenograft sutured in place (*C*). Healing at 2 weeks (*D*), 4 weeks (*E*) and 8 months (*F*).

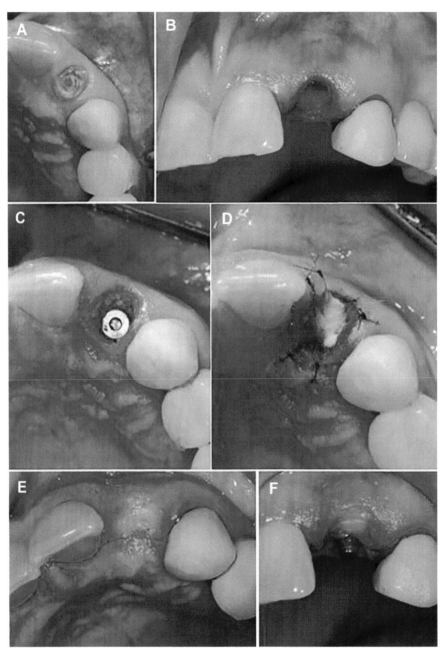

Fig. 19. Immediate implant placement (*A–C*) with bone graft (*C*) and soft tissue xenograft (*D*) allowing secondary intention healing in crestal area (*E*), resulting in enhanced soft tissue volume and KT at 3 months (*F*).

appropriate color matching tissue, absence of scar formation, and a mucogingival junction alignment. They achieve inferior KT gain with superior esthetics and patient satisfaction than FGG.[93]

Tissue-engineered living human fibroblast-derived dermal substitute is used instead of an FGG to increase the amount of KT,[95] and may offer potential as a substitute to an SCTG for Miller class I or II recession defects.[96]

Biologic Agents

Biologic agents are growth factors and signaling molecules able to regulate cellular events involved in wound healing by stimulating cellular proliferation and differentiation in grafted site.[97] Their adjunctive use, however, does not significantly influence mean root coverage and KT gain.[74] They are used in conjunction with CAF, GTR,

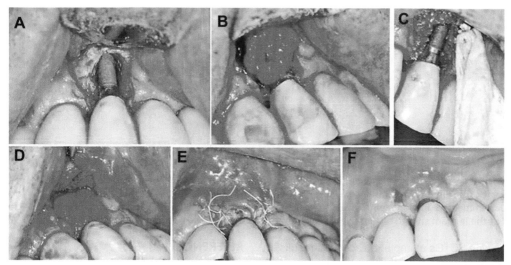

Fig. 20. Facial dehiscence on an implant abutment for large fixed prosthesis (*A*). Chemical decontamination of the implant surface (*B*). Defect grafted with xenogeneic bone graft (*C*) and membrane (*D*) and CAF (*E*). Favorable coverage and KT at 3 weeks (*F*).

autogenous, allogenic, or xenogenic grafts. These agents include enamel matrix derivative (EMD), platelet-derived growth factor (PDGF), platelet-rich plasma (PRP), and PRF.

PDGF stimulates angiogenesis; mitogenesis of mesenchymal cells; chemotaxis of fibroblasts, cementoblasts, osteoblasts, macrophages, and polymorphonucleocytes; and recruitment of osteoprogenitor cells.[98] Recombinant forms of human PDGF are major mitogens for human periodontal ligament cells, promote the synthesis of collagen, and help in wound contraction and remodeling.[99] Addition of rhPDGF-BB to b-trical-cium phosphate and a collagen membrane can achieve comparable root coverage as SCTG.[100]

EMD from developing porcine teeth enhances periodontal regeneration by stimulating angiogenesis and chemotaxis,[101] and influenced activities of cementoblasts and osteoblasts, thus regulating periodontal regeneration.[102] Although the reports on EMD contributions to root coverage outcomes are not consistent,[103–105] EMD has been used successfully in combination with various root coverage procedures, such as laterally[106] and CAF,[103,104] and GTR.[105]

PRP is derived from the autologous blood mixed with thrombin and calcium chloride. It has been used in various surgical fields because it includes high concentration of platelets and fibrinogen.[107] Following activation with thrombin, the platelets release several growth factors including PDGF and transforming growth factor-β, which serve to accelerate the wound healing,[108] hemostasis, and adhesion of graft material.[99] In oral

applications, PRP has produced better results in association with other materials than when used alone (see **Fig. 16**D).[109] In root coverage procedures, PRP enhances vascularity, wound stability, and regenerative potential with superior esthetic outcomes, and decreases patient morbidity.[110]

PRF is a new generation of platelet concentrate from centrifuged blood without any additional agents. The slow polymerization during preparation generates a fibrin network leading to a more efficient cell migration and proliferation.[111] Mechanisms including chemotaxis, angiogenesis, extracellular matrix deposition, and remodeling enhance wound healing and tissue repair (see **Fig. 16**G).[112] The addition of PRF in treatment of recession results in superior root coverage and increase in KT width than CAF alone.[113]

IMPLANTS

Procedures to enhance soft tissue should be incorporated in early phases of implant therapy. Sockets with deficient KT and thin buccal bone favor staged approach to develop implant site with better soft tissue characteristics. Socket preservation allows the site to heal by secondary intention resulting in increased KT compared with CAF to provide primary closure.[114] Bone grafting can implement osseous characteristics of the site, which supports and defines the soft tissue architecture after healing (see **Figs. 13**A–D and **19**).[115] Soft tissue grafting helps maintain tissue stability for immediate implants, sockets with less than 2 mm of buccal plate thickness, thin tissue biotype, and inadequate KT.[116] Enhancing soft

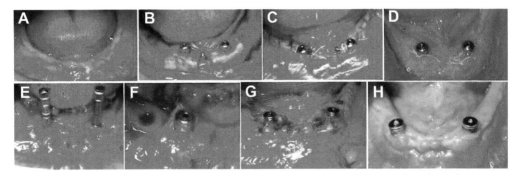

Fig. 21. Augmentation of soft tissue thickness in atrophic mandible (*A*) at the time of implant placement using allograft (*B*) sutured with transalveolar sutures to bony anchorage (*C*) with favorable healing after 2 weeks (*D*). Around immediate implants with alveolar reduction (*E*), autogenous SCTG (*F*) and existing preserved KT can be used at the implant sites (*G*). Transalveolar sutures maintain soft tissue position and vestibular dimensions (*D, H*)

tissue with SCTGs at implant placement results in better aesthetics and thicker peri-implant tissues,[23] and significantly improves maintenance of facial gingival levels in the esthetic zone.[117,118] Techniques using autogenous, allogenic, or xenogenic grafts are used to enhance soft tissue in deficient areas (see **Figs. 11** and **17**).

For full-arch cases requiring osseous reduction, preserving existing gingiva and vestibular depth is achieved by securing flaps in an apical position to a fixed bony anchorage thereby maintaining prosthetic.[119] This technique can also be used in conjunction with SCTG or allograft between the flap and osseous crest (**Fig. 21**).[84] Corrective soft tissue procedures are also performed at one-stage placement or the uncovering of implants, when dividing and repositioning of available gingiva between lingual and buccal aspects of the implant can prevent need for FGG (see **Fig. 17**).[84] Covering recession on buccal aspect of implants can achieve 100% coverage; that gain, however, is not maintained over the 6-month follow-up.[120] When grafting is combined with removal of the crown and reshaping of the prosthetic abutment providing better graft adaptation, the coverage of buccal recession can achieve 96% and a significant increase in KT.[121]

ACKNOWLEDGMENTS

The authors thank the graduate students at Virginia Commonwealth University Department of Periodontics for their contributions of photographs for this publication: Dr Sam Bakuri, Dr Charles Stoianici, Dr Fadi Hassan, Dr Kian Azarnoush, and Dr Peter Lee.

DISCLOSURE

The authors have nothing to disclose.

REFERENCES

1. Kennedy JE, Bird WC, Palcanis KGDH. A longitudinal evaluation of varying widths of attached gingiva. J Clin Periodontol 1985;12(8): 667–75.
2. Wennström J, Lindhe J. Role of attached gingiva for maintenance of periodontal health. Healing following excisional and grafting procedures in dogs. J Clin Periodontol 1983;10(2):206–21.
3. Wennström J. Lack of association between width of attached gingiva and development of soft tissue recession. A 5-year longitudinal study. J Clin Periodontol 1987;14(3):181–4.
4. Dorfman HS, Kennedy JE, Bird W. Longitudinal evaluation of free autogenous gingival grafts. A four year report. J Periodontol 1982;53(6):349–52.
5. Renvert S, Quirynen M. Risk indicators for peri-implantitis. A narrative review. Clin Oral Implants Res 2015;26:15–44.
6. Block MSKJ. Factors associated with soft- and hard-tissue compromise of endosseous implants. J Oral Maxillofac Surg 1990;28(11):1153–60.
7. Pranskunas M, Poskevicius L, Juodzbalys G, et al. Influence of peri-implant soft tissue condition and plaque accumulation on peri-implantitis: a systematic review. J Oral Maxillofac Res 2016;7(3):1–9.
8. Ladwein C, Schmelzeisen R, Nelson K, et al. Is the presence of keratinized mucosa associated with periimplant tissue health? A clinical cross sectional analysis. Int J Implant Dent 2015;1(1) 2–6.
9. Thoma DS, Naenni N, Figuero E, et al. Effects of soft tissue augmentation procedures on peri-implant health or disease: a systematic review and meta-analysis. Clin Oral Implants Res 2018 29:32–49.
10. Romanos G, Grizas E, Nentwig GH. Association of keratinized mucosa and periimplant soft tissue stability around implants with platform switching. Implant Dent 2015;24(4):422–6.

11. Salvi GE, Aglietta M, Eick S, et al. Reversibility of experimental peri-implant mucositis compared with experimental gingivitis in humans. Clin Oral Implants Res 2012;23(2):182–90.

12. Warrer K, Buser D, Lang NP, et al. Plaque-induced peri-implantitis in the presence or absence of keratinized mucosa. An experimental study in monkeys. Clin Oral Implants Res 1995;6(3):131–8.

13. Leichter JW, Monteith BD. Prevalence and risk of traumatic gingival recession following elective lip piercing. Dent Traumatol 2006;22(1):7–13.

14. Tugnait A, Clerehugh V. Gingival recession. Its significance and management. 2001;29.

15. Chu SJ, Tarnow DP. Managing esthetic challenges with anterior implants. Part 1: midfacial recession defects from etiology to resolution. Compend Contin Educ Dent 2013;34(7):26–31.

16. Bengazi F1, Wennström JL, Lekholm U. Recession of the soft tissue margin at oral implants. A 2-year longitudinal prospective study. Clin Oral Implants Res 1996;7(4):303–10.

17. Tarnow DP, Magner AW, Fletcher P. The effect of the distance from the contact point to the crest of bone on the presence or absence of the interproximal dental papilla. J Periodontol 1992;63(12):995–1006.

18. Kan JYK, Rungcharassaeng K, Umezu K, et al. Dimensions of peri-implant mucosa: an evaluation of maxillary anterior single implants in humans. J Periodontol 2003;74(4):557–62.

19. Tarnow D, Elian N, Fletcher P, et al. Vertical distance from the crest of bone to the height of the interproximal papilla between adjacent implants. J Periodontol 2003;74(12):1785–8.

20. Arunachalam LT, Merugu SSU. A novel surgical procedure for papilla reconstruction using platelet rich fibrin. Contemp Clin Dent 2012;3:467–70.

21. Becker W, Gabitov I, Stepanov M, et al. Minimally invasive treatment for papillae deficiencies in the esthetic zone: a pilot study. Clin Implant Dent Relat Res 2010;12(1):1–8.

22. Jaiswal P, Bhongade M, Tiwari I, et al. Surgical reconstruction of interdental papilla using subepithelial connective tissue graft (SCTG) with a coronally advanced flap: a clinical evaluation of five cases. J Contemp Dent Pract 2010;11(6):49–57.

23. Esposito M, Maghaireh H, Grusovin MG, et al. Soft tissue management for dental implants: what are the most effective techniques? A Cochrane systematic review. Eur J Oral Implantol 2012;5(3):221–38. Available at: http://www.ncbi.nlm.nih.gov/pubmed/23000707.

24. Tarnow DP, Cho SCWS. The effect of inter-implant distance on the height of inter-implant bone crest. J Periodontol 2000;7(4):546–9.

25. Sullivan HCAJ. Free autogenous gingival grafts. 3. Utilization of grafts in the treatment of recession. Periodontics 1968;6(4):152–60.

26. Miller PD. A classification of marginal tissue recession. Int J Periodontics Restorative Dent 1985;5(2):8–13. Available at: http://www.ncbi.nlm.nih.gov/pubmed/3858267.

27. Armitage G. Development of a classification system for periodontal diseases and conditions. Ann Periodontol 1999;4(1):1–6.

28. Caton J, Armitage G, Berglundh T, et al. A new classification scheme for periodontal and peri-implant diseases and conditions: introduction and key changes from the 1999 classification. J Clin Periodontol 2018;45(March):S1–8.

29. Cortellini P, Bissada NF. Mucogingival conditions in the natural dentition: narrative review, case definitions, and diagnostic considerations. J Periodontol 2018;89:S204–13.

30. Miller PD. Regenerative and reconstructive periodontal plastic surgery. Dent Clin North Am 1988;32:287–306.

31. Miller P. Concept of periodontal plastic surgery. Pract Periodontics Aesthet Dent 1993;5(5):15–20.

32. Miller PD. Periodontal plastic surgery. Curr Opin Periodontol 1993;136–43.

33. Nabers JM. Free gingival grafts. Periodontics 1966;4(5):243–5.

34. Zucchelli G, Tavelli L, McGuire MK, et al. Autogenous soft tissue grafting for periodontal and peri-implant plastic surgical reconstruction. J Periodontol 2020;91(1):9–16.

35. Langer B, Calagna L. The alteration of lingual mucosa with free gingival grafts. Protection of a denture bearing surface. J Clin Periodontol 1978;49(12):646–8.

36. Rateitschak KH, Egli U, Fringeli G. Recession: a 4-year longitudinal study after free gingival grafts. J Clin Periodontol 1979;6(3):158–64.

37. Jahnke PV, Sandifer JB, Gher ME, et al. Thick free gingival and connective tissue autografts for root coverage. J Periodontol 1993;64(4):315–22.

38. Miller PD. Root coverage with the free gingival graft. Factors associated with incomplete coverage. J Periodontol 1987;58:674–81.

39. Mörmann W, Schaer FFA. The relationship between success of free gingival grafts and transplant thickness. Revascularization and shrinkage–a one year clinical study. J Periodontol 1981;52(2):74–80.

40. Holbrook T, Ochsenbein C. Complete coverage of the denuded root surface with a one-stage gingival graft. Int J Periodontics Restorative Dent 1983;3(3):8–27.

41. Miller PD. Root coverage using the free soft tissue autograft following citric acid application. III. A successful and predictable procedure in areas of

deep-wide recession. Int J Periodontics Restorative Dent 1985;5(2):14–37.

42. Bernimoulin JP, Lüscher B, Mühlemann HR. Coronally repositioned periodontal flap. Clinical evaluation after one year. J Clin Periodontol 1975; 2(1):1–13.

43. Pennel BM, Tabor JC, King KO, et al. Free masticatory mucosa graft. J Periodontol 1969;40(3):162–6.

44. Langer BCL. The subepithelial connective tissue graft. J Prosthet Dent 1980;44(4):363–7.

45. Langer B, Calagna LJ. The subepithelial connective tissue graft. A new approach to the enhancement of anterior cosmetics. Int J Periodontics Restorative Dent 1982;2(2):22–33.

46. Chambrone L, Prato GPP. Clinical insights about the evolution of root coverage procedures: the flap, the graft, and the surgery. J Periodontol 2019;90(1):9–15.

47. Cairo F, Cortellini P, Tonetti M, et al. Coronally advanced flap with and without connective tissue graft for the treatment of single maxillary gingival recession with loss of inter-dental attachment. A randomized controlled clinical trial. J Clin Periodontol 2012;39(8):760–8.

48. Babay N. Attachment of human gingival fibroblasts to periodontally involved root surface following scaling and/or etching procedures: a scanning electron microscopy study. Braz Dent J 2001; 12(1):17–21.

49. Vanheusden AJ, Goffinet G, Zahedi S, et al. In vitro stimulation of human gingival epithelial cell attachment to dentin by surface conditioning. J Periodontol 1999;70(6):594–603.

50. Prasad SS, Radharani C, Varma S, et al. Effects of citric acid and EDTA on periodontally involved root surfaces: a SEM study. J Contemp Dent Pract 2012;13(4):446–51.

51. Balos K, Bal B, Eren K. The effects of various agents on root surfaces (a scanning electron microscopy study). Newsl Int Acad Periodontol 1991;1(2):13–6.

52. Labahn R, Fahrenbach WH, Clark SM, et al. Root dentin morphology after different modes of citric acid and tetracycline hydrochloride conditioning. J Periodontol 1992;63(4):303–9.

53. Caffesse RG, De LaRosa M, Garza M, et al. Citric acid demineralization and subepithelial connective tissue grafts. J Periodontol 2000;71(4): 568–72.

54. Pini-Prato G, Franceschi D, Rotundo R, et al. Long-term 8-year outcomes of coronally advanced flap for root coverage. J Periodontol 2012;83(5):590–4.

55. Cordioli G, Mortarino C, Chierico A, et al. Comparison of 2 techniques of subepithelial connective tissue graft in the treatment of gingival recessions. J Periodontol 2001;72(11):1470–6.

56. Raetzke PB. Covering localized areas of root exposure employing the "envelope" technique. J Periodontol 1985;56(7):397–402.

57. Bouchard P, Etienne D, Ouhayoun JPNR. Subepithelial connective tissue grafts in the treatment of gingival recessions. A comparative study of 2 procedures. J Periodontol 1994;65(10):929=36.

58. Harris RJ. Connective tissue grafts combined with either double pedicle grafts or coronally positioned pedicle grafts: results of 266 consecutively treated defects in 200 patients. Int J Periodontics Restorative Dent 2002;22(5):463–71.

59. Harris RJ, Miller LH, Harris CR, et al. A comparison of three techniques to obtain root coverage on mandibular incisors. J Periodontol 2005;76(10): 1758–67.

60. AL-Juboori MJ. Rotational flap to enhance buccal gingival thickness and implant emergence profile in the esthetic zone: two cases reports. Open Dent J 2017;11(1):284–93.

61. Saade J, Sotto-Maior BS, Francischone CE, et al. Pouch roll technique for implant soft-tissue augmentation of small defects: two case reports with 5-year follow-up. J Oral Implantol 2015;41(3): 315–9.

62. Park S-H, Wang H-L. Pouch roll technique for implant soft tissue augmentation: a variation of the modified roll technique. Int J Periodontics Restorative Dent 2012;32(3):e116–21.

63. Reiser GM, Bruno JF, Mahan PELL. The subepithelial connective tissue graft palatal donor site: anatomic considerations for surgeons. Int J Periodontics Restorative Dent 1996;16(2):130–7.

64. Harris RJ. Histologic evaluation of connective tissue grafts in humans. Int J Periodontics Restorative Dent 2003;23(6):575–83.

65. Tavelli L, Barootchi S, Greenwell H, et al. Is a soft tissue graft harvested from the maxillary tuberosity the approach of choice in an isolated site? J Periodontol 2019;90(8):821–5.

66. Amin PN, Bissada NF, Ricchetti PA, et al. Tuberosity versus palatal donor sites for soft tissue grafting: a split-mouth clinical study. Quintessence Int 2018; 49(7):589–98.

67. Griffin TJ, Cheung WS, Zavras AI, et al. Postoperative complications following gingival augmentation procedures. J Periodontol 2006;77(12): 2070–9.

68. Tavelli L, Barootchi S, Namazi SS, et al. The influence of palatal harvesting technique on the donor site vascular injury: a split-mouth comparative cadaver study. J Periodontol 2019;83–92. https://doi.org/10.1002/jper.19-0073.

69. Rossmann JA, Rees TD. A comparative evaluation of hemostatic agents in the management of soft tissue graft donor site bleeding. J Periodontol 1999; 70(11):1369–75.

70. Jain V, Triveni MG, Kumar AB, et al. Role of platelet-rich-fibrin in enhancing palatal wound healing after free graft. Contemp Clin Dent 2012;3(Suppl S2): 240–3.

71. Kulkarni MR, Thomas BS, Varghese JM, et al. Platelet-rich fibrin as an adjunct to palatal wound healing after harvesting a free gingival graft: a case series. J Indian Soc Periodontol 2014;18(3):399–402.

72. Silva CO, Ribeiro ÉDP, Sallum AW, et al. Free gingival grafts: graft shrinkage and donor-site healing in smokers and non-smokers. J Periodontol 2010;81(5):692–701.

73. Inal S, Yilmaz N, Nisbet C, et al. Biochemical and histopathological findings of N-butyl-2-cyanoacrylate in oral surgery: an experimental study. Oral Surgery, Oral Med Oral Pathol Oral Radiol Endodontology 2006;102(6):14–7.

74. Fu JH, Su CY, Wang HL. Esthetic soft tissue management for teeth and implants. J Evid Based Dent Pract 2012;12(3 SUPPL):129–42.

75. Tonetti MS, Cortellini P, Pellegrini G, et al. Xenogenic collagen matrix or autologous connective tissue graft as adjunct to coronally advanced flaps for coverage of multiple adjacent gingival recession: randomized trial assessing non-inferiority in root coverage and superiority in oral health-related. J Clin Periodontol 2018;45(1):78–88.

76. Atieh MA, Alsabeeha N, Tawse-Smith A, et al. Xenogeneic collagen matrix for periodontal plastic surgery procedures: a systematic review and meta-analysis. J Periodontal Res 2016;51(4): 438–52.

77. Allen EP. AlloDerm: an effective alternative to palatal donor tissue for treatment of gingival recession. Dent Today 2006;25(1):50–2.

78. Wainwright DJ. Use of an acellular allograft dermal matrix (AlloDerm) in the management of full-thickness burns. Burns 1995;21(4):243–8.

79. Harris R. HarrisA comparative study of root coverage obtained with an acellular dermal matrix versus a connective tissue graft: results of 107 recession defects in 50 consecutively treated patients. Int J Periodontics Restorative Dent 2000; 20(1):51–9.

80. Yukna RA, Sullivan WM. Evaluation of resultant tissue type following the intraoral transplantation of various lyophilized soft tissues. J Periodontal Res 1978;13(2):177–84.

81. Scarano A, Barros RRM, Iezzi G, et al. Acellular dermal matrix graft for gingival augmentation: a preliminary clinical, histologic, and ultrastructural evaluation. J Periodontol 2009;80(2):253–9.

82. Hirsch A, Goldstein M, Goultschin J, et al. A 2-year follow-up of root coverage using subpedicle acellular dermal matrix allografts and subepithelial connective tissue autografts. J Periodontol 2005;76(8): 1323–8.

83. Wei P-C, Laurell L, Geivelis M, et al. Acellular dermal matrix allografts to achieve increased attached gingiva. Part 1. a clinical study. J Periodontol 2000;71(8):1297–305.

84. Deeb GR, Deeb JG, Kain NJ, et al. Use of transalveolar sutures in conjunction with grafting to preserve vestibular depth and augment gingival thickness around mandibular implants. J Oral Maxillofac Surg 2016;74(5):940–4.

85. Park JB. Increasing the width of keratinized mucosa around endosseous implant using acellular dermal matrix allograft. Implant Dent 2006;15(3): 275–81.

86. McGuire MK, Scheyer ET. Xenogeneic collagen matrix with coronally advanced flap compared to connective tissue with coronally advanced flap for the treatment of dehiscence-type recession defects. J Periodontol 2010;81(8):1108–17.

87. Melcher A. On the repair potential of periodontal tissues. J Periodontol 1976;47(5):256–60.

88. Al-Hamdan K, Eber R, Sarment D, et al. Guided tissue regeneration-based root coverage: meta-analysis. J Periodontol 2003;74(10):1520–33.

89. Rosetti EP, Marcantonio RAC, Rossa C, et al. Treatment of gingival recession: comparative study between subepithelial connective tissue graft and guided tissue regeneration. J Periodontol 2000; 71(9):1441–7.

90. Tatakis DN, Trombelli L. Gingival recession treatment: guided tissue regeneration with bioabsorbable membrane versus connective tissue graft. J Periodontol 2000;71(2):299–307.

91. Oates TW, Robinson MGJ. Surgical therapies for the treatment of gingival recession. A systematic review. Ann Periodontol 2003;8(1): 303–20.

92. Nickles K, Ratka-Krüger P, Neukranz E, et al. Ten-year results after connective tissue grafts and guided tissue regeneration for root coverage. J Periodontol 2010;81(6):827–36.

93. Scheyer ET, Nevins ML, Neiva R, et al. Generation of site-appropriate tissue by a living cellular sheet in the treatment of mucogingival defects. J Periodontol 2014;85(4):e57–64.

94. McGuire MK, Scheyer ET, Nevins ML, et al. Living cellular construct for increasing the width of keratinized gingiva: results from a randomized, within-patient, controlled trial. J Periodontol 2011;82(10): 1414–23.

95. McGuire MK, Nunn ME. Evaluation of the safety and efficacy of periodontal applications of a living tissue-engineered human fibroblast-derived dermal substitute. I. Comparison to the gingival autograft: a randomized controlled pilot study. J Periodontol 2005;76(6):867–80.

96. Wilson TG, McGuire MK, Nunn ME. Evaluation of the safety and efficacy of periodontal applications

of a living tissue-engineered human fibroblast-derived dermal substitute. II. Comparison to the subepithelial connective tissue graft: a randomized controlled feasibility study. J Periodontol 2005; 76(6):881–9.

97. Anusaksathien O, Giannobile WV. Growth factor delivery to re-engineer periodontal tissues. Curr Pharm Biotechnol 2002;3(2):129–39.

98. Hollinger JO, Hart CE, Hirsch SN, et al. Recombinant human platelet-derived growth factor: biology and clinical applications. J Bone Joint Surg Am 2008;90(SUPPL. 1):48–54.

99. Carlson NE, Roach RB. Platelet-rich plasma: clinical applications in dentistry. J Am Dent Assoc 2002;133(10):1383–6.

100. McGuire MK, Todd Scheyer E. Comparison of recombinant human platelet-derived growth factor-BB plus beta tricalcium phosphate and a collagen membrane to subepithelial connective tissue grafting for the treatment of recession defects: a case series. Int J Periodontics Restorative Dent 2006; 26(2):127–33.

101. Schlueter SR, Carnes DL, Cochran DL. In vitro effects of enamel matrix derivative on microvascular cells. J Periodontol 2007;78(1):141–51.

102. Tokiyasu Y, Takata T, Saygin E, et al. Enamel factors regulate expression of genes associated with cementoblasts. J Periodontol 2000;71(12):1829–39.

103. Hägewald S, Spahr A, Rompola E, et al. Comparative study of Emdogain A. J Clin Periodontol 2002; 29:35–41.

104. Castellanos TA, de la Rosa RM, de la Garza M, et al. Enamel matrix derivative and coronal flaps to cover marginal tissue recessions. J Periodontol 2006;77(1):7–14.

105. Trabulsi M, Oh T-J, Eber R, et al. Effect of enamel matrix derivative on collagen guided tissue regeneration-based root coverage procedure. J Periodontol 2004;75(11):1446–57.

106. Kuru BE. Treatment of localized gingival recessions using enamel matrix derivative as an adjunct to laterally sliding flap: 2 case reports. Quintessence Int 2009;40(6):461–9. Available at: http://www.ncbi.nlm.nih.gov/pubmed/19587887.

107. Marx R. Platelet-rich plasma (PRP): what is PRP and what is not PRP? Implant Dent 2001;10(4):225–8.

108. Marx RE, Carlson ER, Eichstaedt RM, et al. Platelet-rich plasma: growth factor enhancement for bone grafts. Oral Surg Oral Med Oral Pathol Oral Radiol Endod 1998;85(6):638–46.

109. Albanese A, Licata ME, Polizzi B, et al. Platelet-rich plasma (PRP) in dental and oral surgery: from the wound healing to bone regeneration. Immun Ageing 2013. https://doi.org/10.1186/1742-4933-10-23.

110. Bashutski JD, Wang HL. Role of platelet-rich plasma in soft tissue root-coverage procedures: a review. Quintessence Int 2008;39(6):473–83. Available at: http://www.ncbi.nlm.nih.gov/pubmed/19057743.

111. Dohan DM, Choukroun J, Diss A, et al. Platelet-rich fibrin (PRF): a second-generation platelet concentrate. Part I: Technological concepts and evolution. Oral Surg Oral Med Oral Pathol Oral Radiol Endodontology 2006;101(3):E37–44.

112. Rožman P, Bolta Z. Use of platelet growth factors in treating wounds and soft-tissue injuries. Acta Dermatovenerol Alp Pannonica Adriat 2007;16(4): 156–65.

113. Padma R, Shilpa A, Kumar PA, et al. A split mouth randomized controlled study to evaluate the adjunctive effect of platelet-rich fibrin to coronally advanced flap in Miller's class-I and II recession defects. J Indian Soc Periodontol 2013;17(5): 631–6.

114. Barber HD, Lignelli J, Smith BM, et al. Using a dense PTFE membrane without primary closure to achieve bone and tissue regeneration. J Oral Maxillofac Surg 2007;65(4):748–52.

115. Le B, Burstein J. Esthetic grafting for small volume hard and soft tissue contour defects for implant site development. Implant Dent 2008;17(2): 136–41.

116. Hsu YT, Shieh CH, Horn-Lay W. Using soft tissue graft to prevent mid-facial mucosal recession following immediate implant placement. J Int Acad Periodontol 2012;14(3):76–82.

117. Yoshino S, Kan JYK, Rungcharassaeng K, et al. Effects of connective tissue grafting on the facial gingival level following single immediate implant placement and provisionalization in the esthetic zone: a 1-year randomized controlled prospective study. Int J Oral Maxillofac Implants 2014;29(2): 432-40.

118. Grunder U. Crestal ridge width changes when placing implants at the time of tooth extraction with and without soft tissue augmentation after a healing period of 6 months: report of 24 consecutive cases. Int J Periodontics Restorative Dent 2011;31(1):9–17.

119. Deeb GR, Deeb JG, Agarwal V, et al. Use of transalveolar sutures to maintain vestibular depth and manipulate keratinized tissue following alveolar ridge reduction and implant placement for mandibular prosthesis. J Oral Maxillofac Surg 2015;73(1) 48–52.

120. Burkhardt R, Joss A, Lang NP. Soft tissue dehiscence coverage around endosseous implants: a prospective cohort study. Clin Oral Implants Res 2008;19(5):451–7.

121. Zucchelli G, Mazzotti C, Mounssif I, et al. A novel surgical-prosthetic approach for soft tissue dehiscence coverage around single implant. Clin Oral Implants Res 2013;24(9):957–62.

Dental Trauma

Lewis C. Jones, DMD, MD[a,b,]*

KEYWORDS

- Dentoalveolar trauma • Avulsed tooth • Dental trauma • Root fracture • Alveolar fracture
- Mouthguard

KEY POINTS

- Dentral trauma can result from a wide variety of insults to the face, and although the mechanism injury varies depending upon the demographic, the results can often be devastating and costly.
- Injuries to the dentition often do not occur in isolation, and trauma to the dentoalveolar structures can lead to significant injury to adjacent tissues, such as the gingiva, and lower third of the facial soft tissues including the chin and lips.
- Dentoalveolar injuries often require a "team" mentality including many of the dental subspecialties to attain an optimal outcome of restoration of form and function.
- The aim of this article is to describe appropriate treatment modalities to accomplish this restoration based on the stage of the dentition, age of the patient, and nature of the injury.

EPIDEMIOLOGY

Dental injuries are difficult to study because many injuries go unreported or are minor enough to go untreated (eg, a fracture within enamel) or may be treated in settings, such as a private clinic, where the incidence is not studied or followed. However, a 2016 review of the literature demonstrated that despite low reporting, studies found that up to 5% of the population is affected by dental trauma. The prevalence of injuries to the dentition ranges from 6% to 59% and in pediatric patients presenting with craniofacial trauma, one large study demonstrated 76% of patients had dentoalveolar injuries.[1,2] It is no surprise that male patient populations tended to have consistently higher rates of dental trauma than female cohorts; this may be attributed to involvement with contact sports with or without proper protective gear.[2,3] Additionally, there are differences in protective gear worn by males and females even within the same sport type; in softball and lacrosse, facial protection in female competitors is consistently increased over the male counterpart in baseball and lacrosse.

Developmentally speaking, an infant begins to have eruption of the anterior dentition from 6 months and continues until around age 2. During this time, they are also learning to walk/run and play. It is therefore not uncommon to sustain injuries in the anterior primary dentition from falls in the toddler patient.[4] Once they have learned to walk, they walk to playgrounds, where an array of dental-injuring devices exist. School-aged children exhibit many injuries to primary and succedaneous dentition. Once the upper central incisors erupt into the oral cavity, they are large targets that can tend to absorb energy poorly. Then, once the permanent dentition has replaced the primary dentition (around age 12–14) involvement with sports and other activities that put the face at risk of injury (including newly licensed drivers) increases and so the mechanism of injury changes, but the patterns of teeth that are injured do not.[5,6]

In general the anterior maxillary dentition, followed closely by the lower anteriors, are injured more frequently than the posterior dentition. This is logical. Additionally, those with malocclusions, such as a class II division I with increased

a Private Practice, Oral and Maxillofacial Surgery, Elizabethtown OMFS, Louisville, KY, USA; b Oral and Maxillofacial Surgery, University of Louisville, Louisville, KY, USA
* 3935 Dupont Circle, Ste D, Louisville, KY 40407.
E-mail address: joneslewisc@gmail.com

Oral Maxillofacial Surg Clin N Am 32 (2020) 631–638
https://doi.org/10.1016/j.coms.2020.07.009

protrusion to the maxillary dentition (especially those with significant overjet and lip incompetence), have increased tendency to be traumatized.[7] And often the dental structures are not injured in isolation, and concomitant injuries to the soft tissues overlying the dentition abound.[8] Additional injuries seen with dental trauma include facial bone fractures; nasal trauma; and head injuries, such as concussion.[9]

All of this leads to the conclusion that the dental community (pediatric dentist, orthodontist, endodontist, oral surgeon, and periodontist) must be well versed in the proper treatment of dental trauma to be able to deliver appropriate treatment to the injured patient.

DENTAL INJURIES

Injuries to the primary dentition are treated differently from that of the permanent dentition. For this reason, this article is organized with each injury and the appropriate treatment based on the phase of dentition.

Avulsion

A tooth avulsion is a traumatic event (pun intended). Primary teeth that are avulsed should not be replaced because it could lead to problems with the developing dentition.[10] Permanent teeth should be placed in an appropriate medium and transported with the patient for replantation.

The treatment of choice for an avulsed tooth is to have it immediately cleansed (if debris is present) and replaced in the socket.[11] A dental professional can then be sought to help maintain this tooth. If it cannot be replaced in the socket, but the patient has full faculty and is able to transport it in their vestibule in saliva, this is also an appropriate method of transportation. Often this is not possible and the tooth is transported in liquid (to avoid desiccation). Note that in a study of 400 replanted permanent incisors, four factors weighed in greatest in relationship to periodontal ligament healing: (1) stage of root development, (2) length of the dry extra-alveolar storage period, (3) immediate replantation, and (4) length of the wet period (saliva or saline storage).[11] The authors also noted that nonphysiologic storage in some solutions inevitably led to root resorption (homemade saline or sterilizing solutions). For this reason, particular attention should be payed to transport medium if the tooth cannot be placed into the socket immediately (because this is always the treatment of choice if the patient is able).[11]

The transport medium should be of the appropriate pH, and provide nutrients to the periodontal cells (**Table 1**). Hank's Balanced Salt Solution, with its neutral pH and glucose for the periodontal

cells, is the best solution for transport. It is purchased online for around $14. The shelf life of Hank's solution is 2 years and can therefore be kept by a team doctor on the sideline of sports where dental injuries are not infrequent. The other solutions listed are less than ideal because of their acidity, tonicity, or lack of nutrients (glucose).

The tooth should be debrided of any necrotic tissue, the socket irrigated with saline, and the tooth should then be replanted and restored to its original position within the arch form with firm digital pressure. Once an avulsed tooth has been replanted, it should be splinted to the adjacent teeth (nonrigid) for 2 to 3 weeks. Splinting times have been studied with inconclusive effects in regards to duration of splinting and its correlation with restored periodontal health.[11,12] Vitality should be monitored by an endodontist in open apex/partially developed teeth. Closed apex teeth should have a root canal performed within 7 to 10 days following replantation. Problems with replanted teeth include ankylosis (especially in cases where extraoral time of tooth exceeds 60 minutes, or storage in nonphysiologic medium is more than 20–30 minutes), external resorption, internal resorption, and infection.[11] These teeth should be monitored radiographically and clinically following treatment until form and function are restored and then periodically for the first year following replantation. Finally, the patient should be prescribed a 7-day course of broad-spectrum antibiotics and tetanus immunization should be ensured if there is risk based on location of injury.[13]

Patients should also be explained that although many teeth go on to heal, there is a risk of need for future extraction if the tooth does not heal properly. In the study by Andreasen and coworkers[11] of 400 replanted permanent incisors, the need for

Table 1
Transport mediums for avulsed teeth with their averaged respective pH, osmolality, and presence of glucose for cellular metabolism

Medium	pH	Osmolality	Glucose +/−
Saline	7.0	295	-
Tap water	7.5	12	-
Saliva	6.3	115	+
Gatorade	3.0	320	+
Milk	6.75	275	+
Hank's Balanced Salt Solution	7.0	280	+

extraction approached 30% over the period of observation (average observation was 5 years). Additionally, the risk of ankylosis increases with an increase in extraoral time, but several case reports indicate retention of the tooth, even in cases of prolonged extraoral times, such as 15 and 27 hours, is possible.[14,15] In these instances, the informed consent should include the likelihood of ankylosis and its implications, although in the growing patient, this may serve as an interim fix until skeletal maturity is reached and treatments, such as dental implants, are a desirable option.

Intrusion

The timing of addressing the intruded tooth is not as critical as in that of the avulsed tooth, but should be addressed as soon as possible. The first step in treating the intruded tooth is to note the degree to which the tooth is intruded, because this plays an important part in the overall prognosis of the tooth and the treatment. When intact, the adjacent teeth can serve as the point from which to measure as to the millimeters that the tooth appears intruded. However, because many of these injuries occur during adolescence with mixed dentition, this is difficult at times.[16] Teeth that are intruded up to 3 mm should be initially monitored for re-eruption, but if there is no movement in the first month, the patient should be advised to have surgical extrusion or orthodontic extrusion before the possibility of replacement resorption/ankylosis that would render coronal movement of the tooth impossible. Either surgical repositioning or orthodontic extrusion is used to manage moderate cases of 3 to 7 mm, and surgical movements should be performed on all patients with severe intrusion (7 mm or greater). Primary teeth that have been intruded should have closely inspected radiographs and if the tooth remains buccal can be left in place to passively erupt and be monitored for any sign of ankylosis. If the tooth does not re-erupt in the first month it should be extracted to avoid the possibility of ankylosis and impeding the eruption of the permanent dentition. If the tooth appears to disrupt the developing follicle on radiograph, it should also be extracted to avoid undue inflammation/trauma at the follicle of the developing tooth.

Permanent teeth that are intruded less than 3 mm tend to have a better prognosis in terms of replacement resorption, and those with no concomitant coronal fractures resulting in exposed dentin have a decreased incidence of pulpal necrosis.[17]

The vitality of the tooth should be monitored closely because these teeth have a high incidence of pulpal necrosis.[18] These patients should be followed closely by either the general dentist or orthodontist for appropriate treatment of nonvital teeth. Finally, unless a clear portal of entry for bacteria exists with concern for infection, there is no clear indication for the administration of antibiotics in the patient with an intruded tooth.[19]

Extrusion

Primary dentition that has experienced a minor injury (<3 mm) resulting in extrusion can be reduced provided this does not impinge on the developing dentition. Once reduced, they should be splinted for 2 weeks and monitored for infection in the 4 to 6 weeks to follow the injury (**Figs. 1–3**). The patient's primary dentist (pediatric or general/family dentist) should be made aware of the injury so that it, and the apical tooth buds, are appropriately monitored.

Permanent teeth that have extrusive injury are difficult to reduce into their socket if this is not performed within a short period of time of the injury. Accumulated blood product at the apex of the socket is difficult to displace, which must be accomplished if the tooth is to reside fully within its socket. A periapical image of the reduced tooth should be taken to confirm that the tooth has been fully reduced. Splinting (nonrigid) should be placed for 2 weeks, and the tooth monitored for pulpal necrosis, root resorption, and/or infection following the injury.

Lateral Luxation

A tooth that is displaced facially or lingually indicates that the supporting alveolar structure has

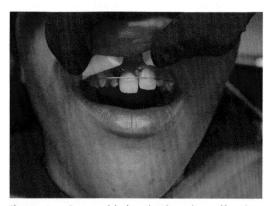

Fig. 1. An 18-year-old cheerleader who suffered an elbow to tooth #8 resulting in extrusion of tooth #8. This tooth was reduced into position and bonded to the adjacent teeth with a flexible splint with 24-gauge wire and composite. The tooth was difficult to reduce because she presented for treatment approximately 24 hours after injury.

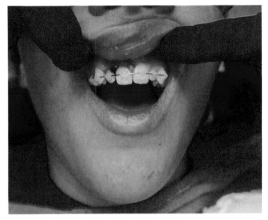

Fig. 2. Tooth is reduced and bonded.

been compromised/injured. These injuries are treated conservatively in the primary dentition with allowance for passive repositioning if there are no significant occlusal interferences. If interferences exist, the luxated teeth are repositioned with digital pressure and left in place. For severe displacement, or if there are suspected injuries to the underlying developing dentition, the tooth/teeth should be extracted.

Permanent teeth that have sustained an injury resulting in lateral luxation should be splinted for 4 to 6 weeks following reduction, because the practitioner is by definition also treating a fracture of alveolar bone. Maxillary teeth most often have fractures to the facial aspects of the periodontium. Small, isolated defects of the alveolus that are fractured and allow for tooth displacement are treated with tooth reduction and nonrigid splinting, whereas large alveolar fractures are treated differently and are addressed in a separate section of this article. These teeth too can be reduced, imaged for documentation of reduction, and monitored for vitality with treatment as deemed

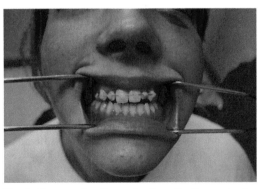

Fig. 3. One week after reduction. Tooth received a root canal treatment and remained splinted for 3 weeks.

appropriate by either the primary dentist or endodontist. The overall prognosis for these teeth is among the poorest prognosis of the luxated teeth (along with extrusive injuries).[20,21]

Subluxation/Concussion

Teeth that have been struck/injured but are not displaced at the time of examination should be checked for mobility and vitality. These teeth have signs of trauma, which can include sensitivity, increased mobility, coronal trauma, and/or bleeding from the adjacent periodontium. Primary teeth should require no treatment acutely, but the teeth involved need to be monitored for signs of pulpal necrosis. In the permanent dentition, if grossly mobile, the practitioner should consider splinting the mobile teeth to the adjacent stable dentition. This should be done for 2 to 3 weeks and then splinting can be removed. As with any of the luxated teeth, these teeth should be monitored and referred for endodontic therapy/bleaching for discoloration to avoid poor cosmesis and infection. The practitioner can expect a period of time that the traumatized tooth will test "nonvital," but more than half of these teeth can return to test positive (with the more minor injuries carrying the better prognosis for doing so).[1]

Root Fracture

Fractures of tooth roots are described as vertical or horizontal. Vertical root fractures extending into the pulp of the tooth should be treated with extraction. The prognosis of these teeth is abysmal and often leads to further bone loss. If left untreated, the additional bone loss may compromise the feasibility of dental implant placement for restoration of the tooth.

Horizontal root fractures require reduction of the fractured segment, followed by splinting and monitoring for tooth vitality. Prolonged splinting (up to 4 weeks) is required for teeth that have been displaced and allows for hard tissue midhealing.[22] Serial examinations help delineate which of the following has occurred: fusion of hard tissue for re-establishment of single unit of the tooth, interposition periodontal ligament formation, or interpositional bone formation. The overall prognosis of the tooth correlates to the level of the fracture: the more apical the fracture, the better the prognosis. Andreasen studied 492 root fractures and found the 10-year survival rate for root fractures were 89% in the apical portion of the root, 67% to 78% at midroot, and only 33% at the cervical portion of the root.[23] These teeth should also be monitored by a general dentist or endodontist for vitality and root canal therapy initiated if pulpa

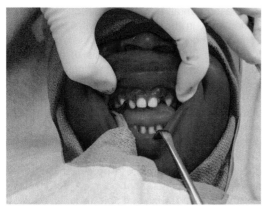

Fig. 4. Alveolar fracture in pediatric dentition.

necrosis becomes evident. Factors that have been found to correlate with overall healing in horizontal root fractures include age (younger patients with immature teeth tend to exhibit better healing of hard tissue between segments) and mobility/dislocation of the coronal fragment (the more the pulpal tissues were traumatized, the poorer the prognosis).[24]

Alveolar Segment Fractures

Pediatric alveolar segment fractures that can be reduced and are stable are left in place to heal with a soft diet. However, larger or more severe fractures may require treatment with a Risdon cable and the developing teeth and bone monitored for proper growth and development (**Figs. 4–6**).

Fractures involving the alveolus are treated to immobilize the bone and allow for bony healing. This requires reduction of the alveolar segment, which is difficult to accomplish if several/many teeth are also involved. Reduction of the segment requires replacement of each tooth into its respective socket and reduction of the bone. All efforts should be made to avoid reflection of periosteum

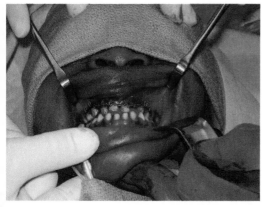

Fig. 5. Risdon cable used for reduction of alveolar fracture.

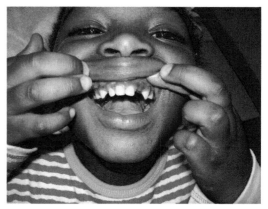

Fig. 6. Healed alveolus approximately 4 weeks after application of risen cables.

over the fracture because this often leads to devitalization of the alveolar segment involved. The bone derives its blood supply from the periosteum. Therefore, if the bone is fractured and cannot derive its blood supply through the adjacent bone, and then the periosteum is reflected and does not allow for blood flow, the bone that is without vascularity and undergoes necrosis. Alveolar segment reduction is often best accomplished with an initial move coronally to allow for the roots of displaced teeth to be repositioned over their sockets and then placed into those sockets with gentle pressure (the amount of pressure required with an increased amount of time between injury and treatment). Once reduced, rigid immobilization allows for bony healing.

Rigid immobilization that does not require reflection of periosteum is accomplished through the use of arch bars. Erich arch bars with the use of 24- and 26-gauge circumdental wires allow for rigid immobilization. Some injuries with concomitant fracture to the maxilla and mandible necessitate more aggressive approaches including the elevation in subperiosteal planes to treat the fractures of the facial bones; the alveolar segment may also be plated if necessary. External fixation can also be used to immobilize and allow for healing in instances where comminution may prevent an open reduction with internal fixation. Although it is rarely used because of the inconvenience and poor cosmesis and necessity of extraoral incisions, it is an effective way to treat otherwise devastating injuries if there is a concern for loss of bone volume because of an open reduction.

Complications with dentoalveolar fractures include pulpal necrosis, which occurs in almost one-half of the involved teeth, and infection and malocclusion.[25] Each of these complications are best managed with a multidisciplinary approach and may include each of the dental specialties.

Splinting

It should be noted that in the previous discussion, the concept of "splinting" was left as vague as rigid (arch bar/plates and screws) versus nonrigid. This was done by intent because there exist a wide variety of splinting techniques that are used depending on the setting, what is available, and what the situation dictates. The important factors are to keep in mind the goal of splinting. These goals are listed next as noted in an article in the *Australian Dental Journal* by Kahler and colleagues,[26] which were modified from Andreasen's original 1972 article.[27]

1. Allow periodontal ligament reattachment and prevent the risk of further trauma or swallowing of a loose tooth.
2. Be easily applied and removed without additional trauma or damage to the teeth and surrounding soft tissues.
3. Stabilize the injured tooth/teeth in its correct position and maintain adequate stabilization throughout the splinting period.
4. Allow physiologic tooth mobility to aid in periodontal ligament healing.
5. Not irritate soft tissues.
6. Allow pulp sensibility testing and endodontic access.
7. Allow adequate oral hygiene.
8. Not interfere with occlusal movements.
9. Preferably fulfill aesthetic appearance.
10. Provide patient comfort.

Keeping this in mind aids the practitioner in making a decision in regards to the methodology for splint placement. The durations noted are helpful, although there does exist a tendency to splint longer than the previously mentioned recommendations.[28]

EXCEPTIONS

The treatments previously described assume a healthy patient with no contraindications to the treatments listed. In cases where patients have existing absolute or relative contraindications to treatment (eg, a history of intravenous bisphosphonates), the treatment plan should be modified accordingly. The well-trained oral and maxillofacial surgeon is equipped to make these decisions and should do so with the view of the patient as a whole and not as an injury in isolation.

ADJUNCTIVE THERAPIES

Adjunctive therapies in the setting of dentoalveolar trauma include the use of chlorhexidine mouth rinse and antibiotics. Because of the nature of the oral cavity, an abundance of bacteria exists. Despite decreased overall use of prophylactic antibiotics in dentistry, in the setting of dental trauma, it is common to prescribe a short course of antibiotics to improve the overall prognosis of the maintenance of dentition.[29] Prolonged infection in this setting can lead to loss of the tooth or segment that was traumatized. Therefore, if the injury includes a definitive portal of entry and/or the host is susceptible because of immunocompetence (eg, diabetes, transplant patients), it is prudent to prescribe a 7-day course of broad-spectrum antibiotics and the patient should be evaluated for the need for a tetanus shot/booster. Additionally, topical use of a "swish and spit" regimen of chlorhexidine oral rinse (0.012%) can decrease the overall infection of traumatized teeth.[30] It should be explained to the patient that although chlorhexidine, used locally in oral solution, has no systemic effects (as compared with the antibiotic regimens), temporary tooth discoloration (plaque staining) and changes in taste can occur with the use of this oral rinse. However, these are short-lived side effects and are easily managed.

Finally, all patients should be advised to follow a strict soft diet to avoid overmanipulation of the recently traumatized tooth. This soft diet can last from 2 to 6 weeks depending on the severity of the injury and extensiveness of the treatment involved.

CONCOMITANT INJURIES

It should be noted that although some dentoalveolar injuries occur in isolation, many have concomitant injuries that occur in the setting of facial trauma, including the maxilla, mandible, or other facial bones (**Fig. 7**). In relationship to fractures of the gnathic skeleton, it should be noted that the re-establishment of premorbid occlusion to

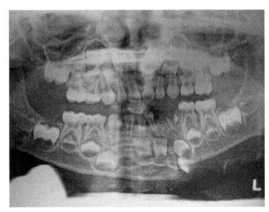

Fig. 7. Pediatric left mandibular body fracture with dentoalveolar trauma including disruption of tooth buds.

the best of the surgeon's ability sets the framework for the rest of the repair. Once the dentition is set into place, it guides the proper reduction and plating of the associated bones. It is rare for a patient to complain of a 1-mm irregularity in the inferior border of their mandible, but 1-mm of discrepancy of occlusion is definitely noticeable and gives a suboptimal result in the patient and the astute practitioner's eyes.

PREVENTION

The most obvious methods for prevention of dentoalveolar injuries are the use of proper proactive equipment including mouthguard and, in some sports, helmets with faceguards. Mouthguards have been shown to significantly decrease the prevalence of dentoalveolar trauma and concussions.[31,32] Mouthguards can and should be worn for all sporting events with a risk of impact to the head and neck region, but as of now seem to be worn with a frequency that parallels perceived risk. Thus, higher-risk sports have higher rates of compliance with mouthguard use.[33] Although a cross-country runner would have no need for a mouthguard, such sports as soccer, volleyball, field hockey, football, lacrosse, and hockey should all require mouthguards for participation. Properly constructed mouthguards do not prevent speaking/communication during a game, but can prevent injuries to the dentition. Additionally, recreational activities, such as skiing, skateboarding, and any other extreme or recreational sport with potential for significant falls or facial impact, can have catastrophic injuries including dentoalveolar insults, some of which could have been mitigated with proper wearing of a mouthguard.[8,34]

SUMMARY

The oral and maxillofacial surgeon is often called on to coordinate the efforts of rehabilitation after a dentoalveolar injury. A comprehensive understanding of the ideal treatments and use of endodontic, orthodontic, periodontal, and pediatric dental colleagues leads to the best possible results with regards to a restoration of form and function. Finally, when in doubt, the following Web site is a great resource, which can be used as a quick reference guide for injuries to permanent and primary dentition: https://dentaltraumaguide.org.

DISCLOSURE

The author has nothing to disclose.

REFERENCES

1. Lam R. Epidemiology and outcomes of traumatic dental injuries: a review of the literature. Aust Dent J 2016;61(1 Suppl):4–20.
2. Gassner R, Tuli T, Hächl O, et al. Craniomaxillofacial trauma in children: a review of 3,385 cases with 6,060 injuries in 10 years. J Oral Maxillofac Surg 2004;62(4):399–407.
3. Kaste LM, Gift HC, Bhat M, et al. Prevalence of incisor trauma in persons 6 to 50 years of age: United States, 1988-1991. J Dent Res 1996;75:696–705.
4. Rezende FM do C, Guajac C, Rocha AC, et al. A prospective study of dentoalveolar trauma at the Hospital das Clinicas Sao Paulo University Medical School. Clinic 2007;62(2):133–8.
5. Lam R, Abbott P, Lloyd C, et al. Dental trauma in an Australian rural centre. Dent Traumatol 2008;24:663–70.
6. Diaz JA, Bustos L, Brandt AC, et al. Dental injuries among children and adolescence aged 1-15 years attending public hospital in Temuco, Chile. Dent Traumatol 2010;26:254–61.
7. Dosdogru EY, Gorken FN, Erdem AP, et al. Maxillary incisor trauma in patients with class II division 1 dental malocclusion: associated factors. J Istanbul Univ Fac Dent 2017;51(1):34–41.
8. Gassner R, Garcia JV, Leja W, et al. Traumatic dental injuries and alpine skiing. Dent Traumatol 2000;16(3):122–7.
9. Gassner R, Bösch R, Tuli T, et al. Prevalence of dental trauma in 6000 patients with facial injuries: implications for prevention. Oral Surg Oral Med Oral Path, Oral Rad, Endo 1999;87(1):27–33.
10. Flores MT, Holan G, Anreasen JO, et al. Chapter 22: injuries to the primary dentition. In: Andreasen JO, Andreasen FM, Andersson L, editors. Traumatic injuries to the teeth. 5th edition. Singapore: Wiley; 2019. p. 576.
11. Andreasen JO, Borum MK, Jocobsen HL, et al. Replantation of 400 avulsed permanent incisors. 4. factors related to periodontal healing. Endod Dent Traumatol 1995;11:76–89.
12. Hinckfuss SE, Messer LB. Splinting duration and periodontal outcomes for replanted avulsed teeth: a systematic review. Dent Traumatol 2009;25:150–7.
13. Sae-Lim V, Wang CY, Trope M. Effect of systemic tetracycline and amoxicillin on inflammatory root resorption of replanted dog, teeth. Endod Dent Traumatol 1998;14:216–20.
14. Sardana D, Goyal A, Gauba K. Delayed replantation of avulsed tooth with 15-hours extra-oral time: 3 year follow up. Singapore Dent J 2014;35:71–6.
15. Savas S, Kucukyilmaz E, Akcay M, et al. Delayed replantation of avulsed teeth: two case reports. Case Report/Open Access 2015;2015:197202.

16. Andreasen JO, Bakland LK, Matras RC, et al. Traumatic intrusion of permanent teeth. Part 1. An epidemic logic study of 216 intruded permanent teeth. Dent Traumatol 2006;22(2):83–9.

17. Andreasen JO, Bakland LK, Andreasen FM. Traumatic intrusion of permanent teeth. Part 2. A clinical study of the effect of preinjury and injury factors, such as sex, age, stage of root development, tooth location, and extent of injury including number of intruded teeth on 140 intruded permanent teeth. Dent Traumatol 2006;22(2):90–8.

18. Andreasen FM. Pulpal healing after lunation injuries and root fracture in the permanent dentition. Endod Dent Traumatol 1989;5(3):111–31.

19. Andreasen JO, Bakland LK, Andreasen FM. Traumatic intrusion of permanent teeth. Part 3. A clinical study of the effect of treatment variables such as treatment delay, method of repositioning, type of splint, length of splinting and antibiotics on 140 teeth. Dent Traumatol 2006;22(2):90–8.

20. Cho WC, Nam OH, Kim MS, et al. A retrospective study of traumatic dental injuries in primary dentition: treatment outcomes of splinting. Acta Odontol Scand 2018;76(4):235–56.

21. Rock WP, Grundy MC. The effect of lunation and subluxation upon the prognosis of traumatized incisor teeth. J Dent 1981;9(3):224–30.

22. Andreasen JO, Ahernsburg SS, Tsilingaridis G. Root fractures: the influence of type of healing and location of fracture on tooth survival rates — an analysis of 492 cases. Dent Traumatol 2012;28(5):404–9.

23. Cvek M, Andreasen JO, Borum MK. Healing of 208 intraalveolar root fractures in patients aged 7-17 years. Dental Traumatol 2001;17(2):53–62.

24. Andreasen JO, Andreasen FM. Healing of 400 intra-alveolar root fractures. 1. Effect of pre-injury and injury factors such as sex, age, stage of root development, fracture type, location of fracture and severity of dislocation. Dental Traumatol 2004; 20(4):192–202.

25. Marotti M, Ebeleseder KA, Schwarzer G, et al. A retrospective study of isolated fractures of the alveolar process in the permanent dentition. Dent Traumatol 2017;33(3):165–74.

26. Kahler B, Hu JY, Marriot-Smith CS, et al. Splinting of teeth following trauma: a review and a new splinting recommendation. Aust Dent J 2016;61(Suppl 1): 59–73. Available at: https://onlinelibrary.wiley.com/doi/full/10.1111/adj.12398. Accessed February 29, 2020.

27. Andreasen JO. Traumatic injuries of the teeth. Copenhagen (Denmark): Munksgaard; 1972. p. 154.

28. Steward C, Kinirons M, Delaney P. Clinical audit of children with permanent tooth injuries treated at a dental hospital in Ireland. Our Arch Padiatr Dent 2011;12(1):41–5.

29. Andersson L, Andreasen JO, Day P, et al. International Association of Dental Traumatology Guidelines for the management of traumatic dental injuries: 2- Avulsion of permanent teeth. Dent Traumatol 2012; 28(2):88–96.

30. DiAngelis AJ, Andreasen JO, Ebeleseder KA, et al. International Association of Dental Traumatology Guidelines for the management of traumatic dental injuries: 1–Fractures and luxation of permanent teeth. Dental Traumatol 2012;28:2–12.

31. Fernandes LM, Neto JCL, Lima TFR, et al. The use of mouthguard and prevalence of dent alveolar trauma among athletes: a systematic review and meta-analysis. Dent Traumatol 2019;35(1):54–72.

32. Chisholm DA, Black AM, Palacios-Derflingher L, et al. Mouthguard use in youth ice hockey and the risk of concussion: nested case-control study of 315 cases. Br J Sports Med 2020;54(14):866–70. Accessed February 28, 2020.

33. Galic T, Kuncic D, Poklepovic Pericic T, et al. Knowledge and attitudes about sports-related dental injuries and mouthguard use in young athletes in four different contact sports-water polo, karate, taekwondo, and handball. Dent Traumatol 2018;34(3) 175–81.

34. Knapik JJ, Marshall SW, Lee RB, et al. Mouthguards in sport activities: history, physical properties and injury prevention effectiveness. Sports Med 2007 37(2):117–44.

Endoscopic Management of Maxillary Sinus Diseases of Dentoalveolar Origin

Justin P. McCormick, MD[a], Melanie D. Hicks, MD[a], Jessica W. Grayson, MD[a], Bradford A. Woodworth, MD[a,b], Do-Yeon Cho, MD[a,b],*

KEYWORDS

- Maxillary sinusitis • Chronic rhinosinusitis • Odontogenic • Odontogenic cyst
- Endoscopic sinus surgery

KEY POINTS

- A wide array of maxillary sinus diseases are from dentoalveolar origin owing to anatomic proximity.
- Advancement of endoscopic instruments and intraoperative navigation systems have allowed maxillary sinus disorders to be managed through endoscopic surgical approaches without a need for open or transoral approaches.
- Endoscopic techniques used in the treatment of maxillary sinus diseases from dentoalveolar origin include balloon sinuplasty, maxillary antrostomy, endoscopic maxillary mega-antrostomy, endoscopic medial maxillectomy, prelacrimal approach to the maxillary sinus, and the endoscopic Caldwell-Luc approach.

INTRODUCTION

The maxillary sinus, first identified by ancient Egyptians, has been well-studied, particularly in relation to its structure, vasculature, and relationship with the dentition.[1,2] The maxillary sinus begins to form during the 10th week of embryonic development as a result of invagination of ethmoid infundibulum mucosa.[1] The sinus continues to enlarge throughout embryonic development and continues ossification up to the 37th week of gestation. Growth progresses throughout childhood until the maxillary sinus reaches its adult size between 18 and 21 years of age.[3]

Anatomically, the alveolar and palatine processes of the maxilla form the floor of the maxillary sinus where the roots of the posterior maxillary dentition lie in close proximity to the floor of the sinus, with the molars having a closer relationship than the premolars.[1] As such, a wide array of maxillary sinus diseases are of dentoalveolar origin.[4,5] When medical therapy fails to control maxillary sinusitis or inflammation, or in cases of neoplasm, surgery is frequently required. The advancement of endoscopic instruments and intraoperative navigation systems has allowed endoscopic approaches using rigid nasal endoscopes to be used frequently to manage maxillary sinus diseases. In this article, we review the minimally invasive endoscopic approaches used by otolaryngologists to manage diseases of the maxillary sinus originating from dentoalveolar pathologies.

Funding: This work was supported by National Institutes of Health (NIH)/National Institutes of Allergy and Infectious disease (K08AI146220), Triological Society Career Development Award, and Cystic Fibrosis Foundation K08 Boost Award (CHO20A0-KB) to D-Y. Cho. The content is solely the responsibility of the authors and does not necessarily represent the official views of the NIH.

[a] Department of Otolaryngology–Head & Neck Surgery, University of Alabama at Birmingham, 1155 Faculty Office Tower, 510 20th Street South, Birmingham, AL 35233, USA; [b] Gregory Fleming James Cystic Fibrosis Research Center, University of Alabama at Birmingham, Birmingham, AL, USA

* Corresponding author. Department of Otolaryngology–Head and Neck Surgery, University of Alabama at Birmingham, 1155 Faculty Office Tower, 510 20th Street South, Birmingham, AL 35233.

E-mail address: dycho@uabmc.edu

Oral Maxillofacial Surg Clin N Am 32 (2020) 639–648
https://doi.org/10.1016/j.coms.2020.07.011
1042-3699/20/Published by Elsevier Inc.

MAXILLARY SINUSITIS
Odontogenic Maxillary Sinusitis Episode

Case study

A 49-year-old woman presented to otolaryngology clinic complaining of left maxillary sinusitis (facial pain and pressure, purulent drainage, and posterior nasal drip with a foul smell). She had received multiple courses of oral antibiotics (at least 6 months) from her local dentist, who was planning to perform a bone graft to close the bony defect between the maxillary sinus and oral cavity. She had a remote history of nasal surgery (inferior turbinate resection) about 30 years ago for her nasal congestion. On examination, purulence was noted in the left middle meatus, with culture returning as the oral anaerobic bacteria *Streptococcus anginosus*. This was treated with culture-directed antibiotics (clindamycin 300 mg 4 times per day) for 2 weeks and saline sinus rinse (240 mL) before a sinus computed tomography (CT) scan (**Fig. 1**A). Based on her CT findings (complete blockage of left maxillary sinus ostium and bony defect), left maxillary endoscopic sinus surgery (opening the maxillary sinus ostium) was recommended to provide an adequate sinus opening for drainage and saline rinse (for irrigation and potential topical drug delivery). The patient wished to avoid any procedure under general anesthesia; therefore, the decision was made to perform in-office balloon sinuplasty of the left maxillary sinus using local anesthesia (topical injection). Upon balloon dilation of the maxillary sinus ostium, thick purulent mucus was expressed. Postoperatively, antibiotics were prescribed in addition to saline sinus rinse. The post-procedure sinus CT (**Fig. 1**B) was obtained 6 months after the in-office procedure to confirm the resolution of left maxillary sinusitis. The post-procedure CT scan showed complete resolution of the left maxillary sinus disease and the patient was able to undergo bone grafting for closure of the bony defect. This technique is advantageous for situations where general anesthesia needs to

be avoided or patient preference is to perform in the clinic under topical and local anesthesia. However, many experts agree that this technique should only be used in a select cohort of sinusitis patients based on their phenotype, anatomy, and comorbidities.[6,7]

Scheme: Balloon sinuplasty (balloon catheter dilation of the paranasal sinuses)

Balloon catheter dilation (BCD) of the paranasal sinuses was initially introduced in 1993, and approved by the US Food and Drug Administration in 2005.[8] BCD has the potential advantages of causing less mucosal disruption and distortion of anatomy, less need for postoperative debridement, and faster returning to regular activities because it can be performed awake in the office under local anesthesia.[9] Several small studies have shown noninferiority of BCD when compared with traditional functional endoscopic sinus surgery.[10–12] Complications have been reported from BCD, so this seemingly less invasive procedure is not without risks.[13] Performing in-office BCD of the maxillary sinus begins with appropriate patient selection and preparation. Indications for BCD are similar to those for standard functional endoscopic sinus surgery, and patients should have a trial of medical therapy before being considered for BCD. Once the decision has been made to proceed with BCD, a thorough review of the patient's CT scan should be performed to identify extent of disease while making note of any anatomic variants that may affect the ease with which BCD can be performed, such as deviation of the septum, concha bullosa, or silent sinus. Achieving adequate anesthesia is imperative when performing in-office BCD. Numerous local anesthetic protocols have been reported in the literature,[14–16] all of which combine topical and infiltrative methods. Typically, we use a combination of 4% tetracaine with oxymetazoline on pledgets placed in the middle meatus and medial to the inferior turbinate, followed by infiltration of 1% lidocaine with 1:100,000 epinephrine along the

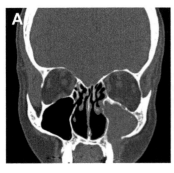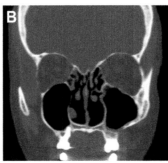

Fig. 1. Odontogenic maxillary sinusitis. (*A*). Coronal CT scan showing complete opacification of unilateral left maxillary sinus with loss of bone, representing oroantral fistula. (*B*) A postprocedure sinus CT (6 months after the balloon sinuplasty) shows complete resolution of the left maxillary sinusitis.

uncinate process and the middle turbinate (**Fig. 2**A). Following adequate anesthesia, an endoscope is used to visualize the middle meatus. The middle turbinate is gently medialized and the free edge of the uncinate is palpated and gently retracted anteriorly (**Fig. 2**B). The balloon catheter device is then inserted into the infundibulum and the natural ostium is palpated (**Fig. 2**C). The wire device is introduced through the natural ostium and placement is confirmed with transillumination. The wire should easily slide into the maxillary sinus, it is important to not force the wire to avoid injury, particularly to the lamina papyracea. After confirmation of appropriate position, the balloon device can then be advanced and inflation may be initiated. Visual confirmation of dilation is evidenced by anterior and medial bulging of the uncinate process and purulent drainage from the maxillary sinus (**Fig. 2**D).[16]

Fungal Maxillary Sinusitis Episode

Case study

A 56-year-old woman who had a history of heart transplantation and currently on immunosuppressant therapy presented to otolaryngology clinic with symptoms of recurrent acute sinusitis every 3 months (purulent drainage, facial pain and pressure, and nasal congestion). A sinus CT scan was obtained after maximal medical therapy (2 weeks of oral antibiotics, saline rinse, and topical steroid spray), which demonstrated moderate to severe mucosal thickening involving the right maxillary sinus without bony erosive or destructive changes

(**Fig. 3**A). However, subtle hyperdense foci were noted within the right maxillary sinus, indicative of likely inspissated superimposed fungal colonization. Based on the CT findings and her immunocompromised status, the decision was made to perform a right endoscopic maxillary antrostomy to clean out the sinus (removing all fungal elements and creating a well-aerated cavity). The patient tolerated the procedure well under general anesthesia with the pathology returning as a fungal mycetoma (fungus ball) (**Fig. 3**B). Odontogenic factors have been reported to increase the risk of developing fungal maxillary sinusitis owing to the close relationship between the molar dentition and the maxillary sinus floor, particularly patients undergoing endodontic procedures.[17–19] Tomazic and colleagues[18] demonstrated that the risk of developing a fungal mycetoma is 2.7-fold higher in patients with odontogenic disease compared with unaffected sinuses. Odontogenic procedures are thought to induce fungal inoculation into the maxillary sinus when the sinus mucosa is penetrated during the procedure.[19,20] Additionally, materials that contain heavy metals (eg, zinc), such as root canal sealers, silver cones, or amalgam, may enter the sinus and provide favorable environment for the growth of fungal species.[21] This patient did have a remote history of dental procedures in her right maxillary molars, although the specific procedural information was not available. Furthermore, any dental procedures that penetrate through the sinus epithelial lining can (1) cause mucociliary dysfunction, (2) deteriorate the natural drainage

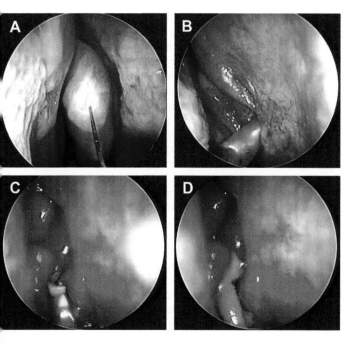

Fig. 2. Balloon sinuplasty (BCD) of the maxillary sinus. (*A*) Local anesthesia. Infiltration of 1% lidocaine with 1:100,000 epinephrine along the uncinate process and the middle turbinate. (*B*) Palpation of the natural ostium of the maxillary sinus with the BCD device. (*C*) After confirmation of placement with transillumination the balloon is advanced, and the sheath is retracted. Upon inflation of the balloon device, the uncinate process is seen bulging medially. (*D*) Purulent secretions are expressed from the maxillary sinus during ostial dilation.

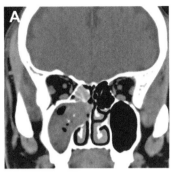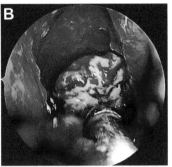

Fig. 3. Fungal maxillary sinusitis. (*A*) Sinus CT scan. Complete opacification of right maxillary sinus with subtle foci of hyperdensity, indicating inspissated superimposed fungal colonization. (*B*) Intraoperative view of fungal ball (mycetoma) within the maxillary sinus.

of sinus mucus, (3) create an anaerobic environment associated with local tissue hypoxia, and (4) allow proliferation of fungal species in the maxillary sinus.[19,20] Therefore, directed endoscopic maxillary antrostomy to enlarge the natural sinus opening (improving ventilation and aeration) and extract the fungus ball is highly effective in managing fungal sinusitis.

Scheme: endoscopic maxillary antrostomy

The endoscopic maxillary antrostomy, introduced in the United States in the 1980s, is the initial step in endoscopic sinus surgery and considered by most to be the (relatively) easiest portion of endoscopic sinus surgery. However, failure to understand the anatomy and natural drainage pathway of the maxillary sinus can lead to technical failure and the need for revision surgery. The key in endoscopic maxillary antrostomy surgery is identifying and incorporating the natural ostium of the maxillary sinus into the surgical antrostomy. Identification and complete removal of the uncinate process is the first step in identifying the natural ostium (**Fig. 4**A, B).[22] Uncinectomy can be performed in an anterior to posterior fashion by incising the uncinate process with a sickle knife just posterior to the maxillary line, a curvilinear mucosal eminence that corresponds to the junction of the uncinate process and the maxilla.[23] Alternatively, the uncinate process may be removed in a posterior to anterior fashion and is the authors' preference because one is less likely to injure or penetrate the lamina papyracea, particularly with hypoplastic maxillary sinuses or cases of very narrow infundibulums. To complete this procedure, an angled ball-tipped probe is used to reflect the free edge of the uncinate process anteriorly. Cutting instruments can then be used to remove the uncinate process from posterior to its anterior attachment to the lacrimal bone. Switching to a 30°, 45°, or 70° endoscope angled laterally, one can then visualize the natural ostium of the maxillary sinus (**Fig. 4**C).[24] Once complete

uncinectomy has been performed and the natural ostium of the maxillary sinus is identified, the antrostomy can be enlarged with cutting instruments and incorporated into a posterior fontanelle if present (**Fig. 4**D). **Fig. 4** demonstrate the important steps in the completion of the endoscopic maxillary antrostomy.

ODONTOGENIC CYST EPISODE
Case Study

A 23-year-old woman with symptoms of right facial pressure was referred to otolaryngology by an oral surgeon. She has a history of odontogenic keratocyst, which was surgically removed twice, most recently 3 years before this presentation. Other than right facial pressure, she did not report any other sinus symptoms. The preoperative sinus CT scan demonstrated an expansile cystic appearing lesion within the right maxillary alveolar recess, representing an odontogenic cyst (**Fig. 5**A). Multiple endoscopic techniques have been used in the treatment of odontogenic cysts, including maxillary antrostomy, endoscopic mega-antrostomy (modified endoscopic medial maxillectomy), medial maxillary sinus wall transposition, and prelacrimal (modified endoscopic Denker's) approach.[25–28] All of these techniques have been used successfully and when reviewing this patient's specific case, a wide maxillary antrostomy (mega-antrostomy) would allow for effective decompression and marsupialization of the lesion without external or transoral approach. Studies have demonstrated that the enucleation and curettage of odontogenic keratocyst have been associated with recurrence, although this finding may be related to the transoral approach.[25,29] Marino and colleagues[25] recently published a case series that no recurrence of odontogenic keratocyst was noticed with endoscopic extended maxillary antrostomy. During the surgery of this specific patient, once the medial wall of maxillary sinus was removed, the

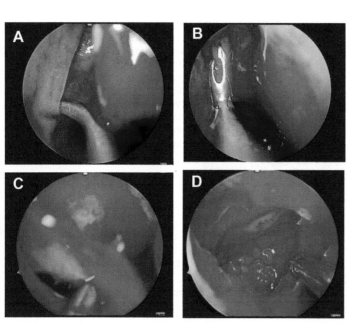

Fig. 4. Endoscopic maxillary antrostomy (*right*). (*A*) Identification of the space behind the uncinate process (infundibulum) using a seeker. (*B*) Complete removal of the uncinate process using 90° grasping forceps. (*C*) Identification and enlargement of the natural ostium of the maxillary sinus. (*D*). Completion of endoscopic maxillary antrostomy (*right*).

odontogenic keratocyst was opened and widely marsupialized into the maxillary sinus (**Fig. 5**B). Therefore, the lesion can continue to drain and avoid cyst reformation.

Scheme: Endoscopic Maxillary Mega-Antrostomy (Modified Endoscopic Medial Maxillectomy)

Despite aggressive medical therapy and adequate resection of the uncinate process with enlargement of the natural ostium, recalcitrant maxillary sinusitis can occur. Additionally, some diseases affecting the maxillary sinus require wide endoscopic exposure for management. Several techniques have been reported for management of persistent maxillary sinus disease to improve drainage and drug delivery, as well as improving endoscopic exposure. The modified endoscopic

medial maxillectomy was first described by Woodworth and colleagues[30] in 2006. In 2008, Cho and Hwang[28] described the endoscopic maxillary mega-antrostomy. The 2 techniques are very similar, with the exception of a more aggressive removal of the inferior turbinate in the modified endoscopic medial maxillectomy and extension of the antrostomy anterior and inferior to Hasner's valve. In both techniques, a portion of the inferior turbinate is resected and the antrostomy is extended down to the floor of the nose. In the cohort by Cho and colleagues,[28] 74% of patients reported complete resolution of symptoms, with no revision surgeries required up to 2 years out.[28] **Fig. 6** shows preoperative and postoperative CT scans of a patient with refractory chronic sinusitis in cystic fibrosis who underwent endoscopic maxillary mega-antrostomy.

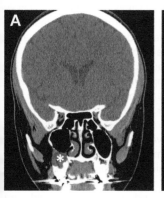
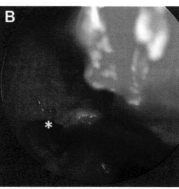

Fig. 5. Odontogenic cyst. (*A*). An expansile cystic appearing lesion (*asterisk*) within the right maxillary alveolar recess, representing an odontogenic cyst. (*B*) Intraoperative view of odontogenic keratocyst (*asterisk*), which was opened and widely marsupialized into the maxillary sinus.

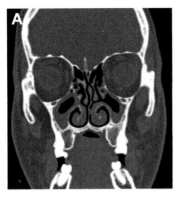
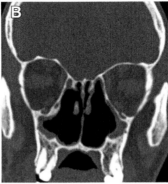

Fig. 6. Pre and post sinus CT scan after endoscopic maxillary mega-antrostomy. (*A*). Coronal CT scan demonstrating recalcitrant bilateral maxillary sinusitis despite prior maxillary antrostomy in a patient with cystic fibrosis. (*B*) Postoperative coronal CT scan after endoscopic maxillary mega-antrostomy and demonstrating nasalization of the maxillary sinuses.

Both the modified endoscopic medial maxillectomy and the endoscopic maxillary mega-antrostomy are performed after a standard maxillary antrostomy has already been completed. Next, the posterior portion of the inferior turbinate is resected after a curved hemostat is used to clamp the inferior turbinate to aid in hemostasis. The turbinate is then resected with endoscopic scissors, including its attachment to the lateral nasal wall. A posterior stump of the turbinate attached to the lateral wall is left and cauterized to avoid bleeding in the region of the sphenopalatine and posterior lateral nasal arteries. The inferomedial wall of the maxillary sinus can then be resected down to the floor of the nose with cutting instruments. Alternatively, a J-curette can be used to puncture the medial wall, after which straight through-cutting forceps can be used to remove the remainder of the medial wall. If needed, drilling the inferior aspect with a 15° diamond burr can be performed; however, care should be taken to prevent trauma to the greater palatine neurovascular bundle, which may result in palatal numbness.[31] A medially based nasal floor mucosal flap has also been described to decrease the amount of exposed bone after resection of the medial maxillary wall.[30]

BENIGN TUMOR EPISODE
Case Study

A 63-year-old man initially presented at the otolaryngology clinic with complaints of rhinorrhea, left nasal congestion with intermittent bloody secretions, and a diminished sense of smell. Nasal endoscopy demonstrated a mass originating from the middle meatus (lateral to the middle turbinate). The preoperative sinus CT and MRI scans showed a heterogeneously enhancing tumor expanding the left maxillary sinus and extending into the nasal cavity and upward into the ethmoid cells and inferior aspect of the left frontal sinus,

suggestive of a slow-growing tumor (**Fig. 7**). The biopsy demonstrated a solid type of ameloblastoma (follicular, plexiform, and acanthomatous pattern). To remove this benign tumor endoscopically with adequate resection margin along the attachment site, the decision was made to perform the extended maxillary antrostomy combining endoscopic maxillary mega-antrostomy (modified medial endoscopic maxillectomy) and prelacrimal approach (as discussed elsewhere in this article). During the surgery, the tumor was attached to the posterior wall of maxillary sinus, which was removed using endoscopic drills and with the addition of the prelacrimal approach complete resection was able to be achieved without the need for external approaches in clearing the adequate margins (at least 1 cm). The patient tolerated the procedure well and remained tumor-free in his recent 4-year follow-up.

Scheme: Prelacrimal Approach to the Maxillary Sinus

Despite these extended approaches to the maxillary sinus, there are still areas that remain difficult to access, particularly when approaching tumors of the anterior or anterolateral walls the maxillary sinus. A transseptal approach has been described to improve exposure[32]; however, this has largely been supplanted by prelacrimal approaches. Morrissey and colleagues[33] described a modification to the prelacrimal approach that was initially reported by Zhou and colleagues[34] in 2013. This technique allows improved access to the anterior and antero-lateral walls of the maxillary sinus and is primarily used for tumor resection as opposed to management of chronic rhinosinusitis. **Fig. 8** shows intraoperative photos of the prelacrimal approach for treatment of an ameloblastoma. It is important to consider the feasibility of achieving adequate margin status when planning for endoscopic resection, and surgeons should not

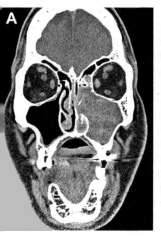
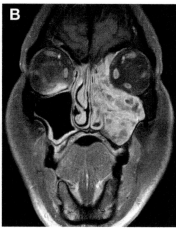

Fig. 7. Ameloblastoma (originating from the left maxillary sinus). (*A*). Coronal sinus CT scan. Extensive mass-like opacification of the left maxillary sinus with expansion and extension into left nasal cavity. (*B*) Coronal T1 contrast-enhanced MRI. Heterogeneously enhancing tumor expanding the left maxillary sinus and extending into the nasal passages.

compromise oncologic principles during attempts to complete endoscopic resection.

The technique described by Morrissey and colleagues[33] begins with uncinectomy and maxillary antrostomy. Although not required for the prelacrimal approach, the authors advocate for improved ease of surveillance postoperatively. A mucosal incision is then made along the lateral nasal wall above the level of the inferior turbinate and carried anteroinferiorly in a curvilinear fashion anterior to the inferior turbinate and into the pyriform aperture. The mucoperiosteum is then elevated to expose the bone of the inferior turbinate and its lateral attachment. A horizontal osteotomy is

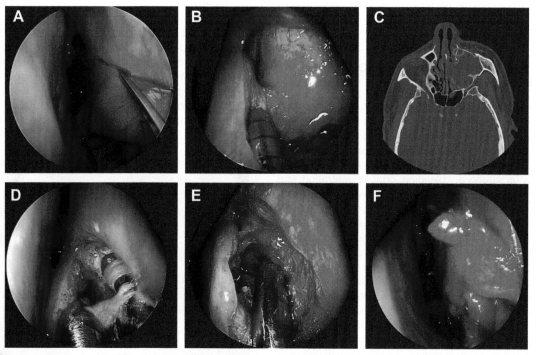

Fig. 8. Prelacrimal approach to the maxillary sinus. (*A*) Mucosal incision along the superior edge of the inferior turbinate turning inferiorly at the anterior head. (*B*) The mucosa is reflected down, exposing the anterior bone of the inferior turbinate and the ridge of the piriform aperture where the drilling will be performed. (*C*) Axial CT scan with red circle outlining the bone removed to complete the prelacrimal approach. (*D*) A powered drill was used to remove the bone. (*E*) Exposure of the maxillary sinus through the prelacrimal window. (*F*) The mucosal incision is sutured at the end of the procedure.

then performed at the inferior edge of the pyriform aperture, followed by a vertical osteotomy extending superiorly and ultimately connecting to another horizontal osteotomy at the level of the maxillary ostium until the nasolacrimal duct is exposed. Alternatively, as depicted, powered drills can be used to remove this prelacrimal bone. The nasolacrimal duct is then retracted medially to allow for a final osteotomy of the posterior bone of the duct that allows removal of the head of the inferior turbinate and bone around the nasolacrimal duct providing access to the maxillary sinus. Once the procedure has been concluded, the inferior turbinate is lateralized and the mucosal incision is sutured.[33]

Additionally, modified perilacrimal approaches have been described by multiple surgeon.[35,36] In one of these modified approaches, an incision is initiated above the axilla of the middle turbinate and continued anteriorly to the piriform aperture. The lateral nasal wall mucosa is elevated and the nasolacrimal duct is elevated superiorly. The lacrimal bone is then removed with cutting instruments and the flap is elevated until it can be tucked posteriorly. The inferior portion of the bone below the nasolacrimal duct system is then drilled and opened. Care should be taken to avoid injury to the medial superior alveolar nerve to prevent numbness of the teeth.

COMPLICATIONS OF ENDOSCOPIC MAXILLARY SINUS SURGERY

With endoscopic surgical techniques, it is critical for the endoscopic surgeon to have thorough knowledge of the anatomy and be capable of recognizing and managing potential complications. The majority of complications with maxillary sinus surgery are bleeding, orbital penetration, and nasolacrimal duct injury.[37] Bleeding complications from isolated maxillary sinus surgery are relatively rare. Mucosal bleeding can typically be controlled with adequate preoperative injection of local anesthesia with epinephrine and topical administration of vasoconstrictive agents during the surgery. Total intravenous anesthesia has also been reported to improve intraoperative visualization with no adverse effects on hemodynamic parameters.[38] Named vascular structures are not frequently encountered with endoscopic approaches to the maxillary sinus; however, the greater palatine neurovascular bundle and posterior lateral nasal branches of the sphenopalatine artery may be injured with extended posterior and inferior dissection of the medial maxillary wall.[39] Therefore, once exposed, these arteries should be well-controlled before finishing the surgery to avoid major postoperative bleeding.

The rate of orbital injury during endoscopic sinus surgery is reported to be less than 0.5%.[37] However, orbital injury during endoscopic sinus surgery can have severe visual consequences (**Fig. 9**). The thin roof of the maxillary sinus separates the sinus from the orbit superiorly. Additionally, the lamina papyracea, is intimately associated with the uncinate process and is at risk of being violated when performing uncinectomy (the first step in opening the maxillary sinus during endoscopic sinus surgery). Disruption of the bony framework of the orbit increases the risk of injury to (1) extraocular muscles, (2) oculomotor nerve, and (3) ophthalmic vessels (which could lead to blindness and orbital hematoma, more commonly during endoscopic ethmoidectomy than maxillary antrostomy). By carefully reviewing the preoperative imaging to recognize anatomic variants and identifying anatomic landmarks during the surgery, surgeons can avoid iatrogenic injury to the orbital contents. BCD of the maxillary sinus is not without risk either. A recent review found 211 adverse events associated with BCD between 2008 and 2018 with 30 patients having orbital complications, 26% of which required decompression with lateral canthotomy.[40]

The nasolacrimal duct courses along the antero medial aspect of the maxillary sinus and is thus at risk when approaching the maxillary sinus endoscopically. It has been reported that up to 20% of nasolacrimal ducts have bony dehiscence. Additionally, previous reports have suggested occult injury to the nasolacrimal duct in 15% of a cohort of patients undergoing endoscopic sinus

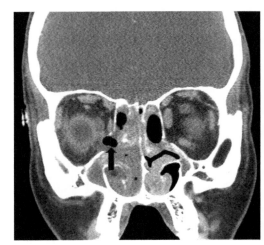

Fig. 9. Orbital complication. A coronal sinus CT image showing a lamina papyracea defect after endoscopic sinus surgery, which resulted in medial rectus injury.

surgery; however, in long-term follow-up, none of these patients developed symptomatic sequelae.[41] If epiphora develops, it will usually present within the first 2 weeks following injury, but may resolve spontaneously after postoperative inflammation subsides.[42] Cases that do not resolve spontaneously may require dacrocystorhinostomy if the obstruction is proven to be within the nasolacrimal duct.[41]

Mucus recirculation is another problem caused by inadequate maxillary sinus surgery. Cilia within the maxillary sinus naturally propel mucus toward the natural ostium, where it is subsequently swept toward the nasopharynx where it can be swallowed.[43] When there is an accessory ostium or surgical antrostomy that fails to connect with the natural ostium, recirculation may occur. This may result in symptoms of sinus pressure, nasal congestion, or recurrent sinusitis.[44] Correction of this recirculation is relatively straightforward and involves connecting the natural ostium with the surgically created antrostomy.[44] For this reason, the importance of adequate antrostomy during the initial surgery should not be underscored, because recirculation can result in significant morbidity and ultimately subject the patient to revision surgical intervention.

SUMMARY

Endoscopic surgery on the maxillary sinus has experienced significant advances in technique and approaches since the maxillary antrostomy was introduced in the 1980s. Disease processes that previously required open surgical approaches to the maxillary sinus can now be treated endoscopically while preserving form and function of the sinus without injuring the maxillary sinus mucosa or disrupting normal mucociliary clearance. Understanding the techniques described in this article will allow surgeons to appropriately plan treatment strategies for patients with a variety of maxillary sinus diseases from dentoalveolar origin.

DISCLOSURE

B. A. Woodworth is a consultant for Olympus and Cook Medical and J. W. Grayson serves on the advisory board for GlaxoSmithKline plc.

REFERENCES

1. Iwanaga J, Wilson C, Lachkar S, et al. Clinical anatomy of the maxillary sinus: application to sinus floor augmentation. Anat Cell Biol 2019;52:17–24.

2. Mavrodi A, Paraskevas G. Evolution of the paranasal sinuses' anatomy through the ages. Anat Cell Biol 2013;46:235–8.

3. Nuñez-Castruita A, López-Serna N, Guzmán-López S. Prenatal development of the maxillary sinus: a perspective for paranasal sinus surgery. Otolaryngol Head Neck Surg 2012;146:997–1003.

4. Bell GW, Joshi BB, Macleod RI. Maxillary sinus disease: diagnosis and treatment. Braz Dent J 2011; 210:113–8.

5. Kim SM. Definition and management of odontogenic maxillary sinusitis. Maxillofac Plast Reconstr Surg 2019;41:13.

6. Piccirillo JF, Payne SC, Rosenfeld RM, et al. Clinical consensus statement: balloon dilation of the sinuses. Otolaryngol Head Neck Surg 2018;158: 203–14.

7. Cingi C, Bayar Muluk N, Lee JT. Current indications for balloon sinuplasty. Curr Opin Otolaryngol Head Neck Surg 2019;27:7–13.

8. Ference EH, Graber M, Conley D, et al. Operative utilization of balloon versus traditional endoscopic sinus surgery. Laryngoscope 2015;125:49–56.

9. Jensen BT, Holbrook EH, Chen PG, et al. The intraoperative accuracy of maxillary balloon dilation: a blinded trial. Int Forum Allergy Rhinol 2019;9: 452–7.

10. Levy JM, Marino MJ, McCoul ED. Paranasal sinus balloon catheter dilation for treatment of chronic rhinosinusitis: a systematic review and meta-analysis. Otolaryngol Head Neck Surg 2016;154:33–40.

11. Bikhazi N, Light J, Truitt T, et al. Standalone balloon dilation versus sinus surgery for chronic rhinosinusitis: a prospective, multicenter, randomized, controlled trial with 1-year follow-up. Am J Rhinol Allergy 2014;28:323–9.

12. Cutler J, Bikhazi N, Light J, et al. Standalone balloon dilation versus sinus surgery for chronic rhinosinusitis: a prospective, multicenter, randomized, controlled trial. Am J Rhinol Allergy 2013;27: 416–22.

13. Alam ES, Hadley JA, Justice JM, et al. Significant orbital and intracranial complications from balloon sinus dilation as a stand-alone and powered dissector-assisted procedure. Laryngoscope 2018; 128:2455–9.

14. Lee JT, DelGaudio J, Orlandi RR. Practice patterns in office-based rhinology: survey of the American Rhinologic Society. Am J Rhinol Allergy 2019;33: 26–35.

15. Sillers MJ, Melroy CT. In-office functional endoscopic sinus surgery for chronic rhinosinusitis utilizing balloon catheter dilation technology. Curr Opin Otolaryngol Head Neck Surg 2013;21:17–22.

16. Silvers SL. Practical techniques in office-based balloon sinus dilation. Oper Tech Otolaryngology-Head Neck Surg 2014;25:206–12.

17. Matjaz R, Jernej P, Mirela KR. Sinus maxillaris mycetoma of odontogenic origin: case report. Braz Dent J 2004;15:248–50.

18. Tomazic PV, Dostal E, Magyar M, et al. Potential correlations of dentogenic factors to the development of clinically verified fungus balls: a retrospective computed tomography-based analysis. Laryngoscope 2016;126:39–43.

19. Torul D, Yuceer E, Sumer M, et al. Maxillary sinus aspergilloma of odontogenic origin: report of 2 cases with cone-beam computed tomographic findings and review of the literature. Imaging Sci Dent 2018;48:139–45.

20. Burnham R, Bridle C. Aspergillosis of the maxillary sinus secondary to a foreign body (amalgam) in the maxillary antrum. Br J Oral Maxillofac Surg 2009;47:313–5.

21. Urs AB, Singh H, Nunia K, et al. Post endodontic Aspergillosis in an immunocompetent individual. J Clin Exp Dent 2015;7:e535–9.

22. Kennedy DW, Zinreich SJ, Shaalan H, et al. Endoscopic middle meatal antrostomy: theory, technique, and patency. Laryngoscope 1987;97:1–9.

23. Kennedy DW, Adappa ND. Endoscopic maxillary antrostomy: not just a simple procedure. Laryngoscope 2011;121:2142–5.

24. Chiu AG, Palmer JN. Maxillary antrostomy. In: Chiu AG, Palmer JN, Adappa ND, editors. Atlas of endoscopic sinus and skull base surgery. Amsterdam: Elsevier, Inc; 2019. p. 41–50.

25. Marino MJ, Luong A, Yao WC, et al. Management of odontogenic cysts by endonasal endoscopic techniques: a systematic review and case series. Am J Rhinol Allergy 2018;32:40–5.

26. Maxfield AZ, Chen TT, Scopel TF, et al. Transnasal endoscopic medial maxillary sinus wall transposition with preservation of structures. Laryngoscope 2016; 126:1504–9.

27. Costa ML, Psaltis AJ, Nayak JV, et al. Long-term outcomes of endoscopic maxillary mega-antrostomy for refractory chronic maxillary sinusitis. Int Forum Allergy Rhinol 2015;5:60–5.

28. Cho DY, Hwang PH. Results of endoscopic maxillary mega-antrostomy in recalcitrant maxillary sinusitis. Am J Rhinol 2008;22:658–62.

29. Leung YY, Lau SL, Tsoi KY, et al. Results of the treatment of keratocystic odontogenic tumours using enucleation and treatment of the residual bony defect with Carnoy's solution. Int J Oral Maxillofac Surg 2016;45:1154–8.

30. Woodworth BA, Parker RO, Schlosser RJ. Modified endoscopic medial maxillectomy for chronic maxillary sinusitis. Am J Rhinol 2006;20:317–9.

31. Woodworth BA, Grayson JW. Modified medial maxillectomy for recalcitrant maxillary sinusitis. In: Chiu AG, Palmer JN, Adappa ND, editors. Atlas of endoscopic sinus and skull base surgery. Amsterdam: Elsevier, Inc; 2019. p. 123–32.

32. Harvey RJ, Sheehan PO, Debnath NI, et al. Transseptal approach for extended endoscopic resections of the maxilla and infratemporal fossa. Am J Rhinol Allergy 2009;23:426–32.

33. Morrissey DK, Wormald PJ, Psaltis AJ. Prelacrimal approach to the maxillary sinus. Int Forum Allergy Rhinol 2016;6:214–8.

34. Zhou B, Han DM, Cui SJ, et al. Intranasal endoscopic prelacrimal recess approach to maxillary sinus. Chin Med J (Engl) 2013;126:1276–80.

35. Suzuki M, Nakamura Y, Yokota M, et al. Modified transnasal endoscopic medial maxillectomy through prelacrimal duct approach. Laryngoscope 2017; 127:2205–9.

36. He S, Bakst RL, Guo T, et al. A combination of modified transnasal endoscopic maxillectomy via transnasal prelacrimal recess approach with or without radiotherapy for selected sinonasal malignancies. Eur Arch Otorhinolaryngol 2015;272:2933–8.

37. Svider PF, Baredes S, Eloy JA. Pitfalls in sinus surgery: an overview of complications. Otolaryngol Clin North Am 2015;48:725–37.

38. Lu VM, Phan K, Oh LJ. Total intravenous versus inhalational anesthesia in endoscopic sinus surgery: a meta-analysis. Laryngoscope 2020;130:575–83.

39. Campbell RG, Solares CA, Mason EC, et al. Endoscopic endonasal landmarks to the greater palatine canal: a radiographic study. J Neurol Surg B Skull Base 2018;79:325–9.

40. Hur K, Ge M, Kim J, et al. Adverse events associated with balloon sinuplasty: a MAUDE database analysis. Otolaryngol Head Neck Surg 2020;162: 137–41.

41. Cohen NA, Antunes MB, Morgenstern KE. Prevention and management of lacrimal duct injury. Otolaryngol Clin North Am 2010;43:781–8.

42. Ali MJ, Nayak JV, Vaezeafshar R, et al. Anatomic relationship of nasolacrimal duct and major lateral wall landmarks: cadaveric study with surgical implications. Int Forum Allergy Rhinol 2014;4:684–8.

43. Chung SK, Cho DY, Dhong HJ. Computed tomogram findings of mucous recirculation between the natural and accessory ostia of the maxillary sinus. Am J Rhinol 2002;16:265–8.

44. DelGaudio JM, Ochsner MC. Office surgery for paranasal sinus recirculation. Int Forum Allergy Rhinol 2015;5:326–8.

Complications of Dentoalveolar Surgery

Patrick J. Louis, DDS, MD

KEYWORDS

- Dentoalveolar complications • Hemorrhage • Displacement

KEY POINTS

- The cause of dentoalveolar complications are discussed.
- Strategies to prevent dentoalveolar complications are stressed.
- Management of dentoalveolar complications can minimize morbidity and mortality.

ALVEOLAR OSTEITIS

Background

Alveolar osteitis (AO) (**Box 1**) is commonly known as a "dry socket" because the socket is many times devoid of a blood clot with exposed bone. The disorder is defined as increased fibrinolytic activity within the early postextraction tooth socket probably secondary to a subclinical infection. It is reported to occur in approximately 2% (1%–3%) of routine extractions and 20% (0.5%–37.5%) of impacted mandibular third molar extractions.[1–7] It usually occurs on the third or fourth day postextraction, although it can occur earlier.[6] The classic triad of AO is: early onset clot lysis, fetor oris, and intense pain. Smoking, oral contraceptives, inexperienced surgeon, poor oral hygiene, increased age, female gender, partial impaction, and periodontal disease have all been reported to increase the risk of AO.[5,8–10]

Prevention

The risk of AO has been reported to be reduced with the use of various agents. Agents that have been used include systemic antibiotics, topical antibiotics, steroids, nonsteroidal anti-inflammatory drugs, clot stabilizers (gelatin sponge, oxidized cellulose, bovine collagen), chlorhexidine mouth rinse, antifibrinolytic agents, antiseptics, and aloe vera.[6,11]

Meta-analyses that investigated the efficacy of prophylactic systemic antibiotic use found a positive effect in reducing the incidence of AO. Tetracycline has been shown to be an effective antibiotic.[12] However, broad- and narrow-spectrum antibiotics have been effective.[13–15]

Multiple topical agents with and without antibiotics, especially tetracycline, have been used with varying degrees of success.[16–20] Topical antibiotics can cause delayed healing, giant cell reaction, nerve injury, and myospherulosis from petroleum-based carrier.[16,21–23] Topical SaliCept (Carrington Laboratories, Inc, Irving, TX) reportedly only had a 1.1% incidence of AO compared with 8.0% in the clindamycin group. SaliCept Patch (Carrington Laboratories, Inc) contains Acemannan Hydrogel, a beta-(1,4)-acetylated mannan, obtained from Aloe Vera L.[24]

Routine use of chlorhexidine rinse 1 week preoperatively and for 1 week postoperatively is recommended in the prevention of AO. This regimen resulted in an 8% incidence (38%–60% reduction) of AO following third molar removal.[5,25,26]

Management

Once a diagnosis is made the wound is irrigated with saline or mouthwash. Dry socket dressing is placed in the socket. Common ingredients include eugenol, benzocaine, and balsam of Peru. Placement of the ointment on a resorbable gelatin or collagen sponge can avoid dressing changes. Another suggested treatment is socket curettage.[2] Treatment with low-level laser therapy reportedly resulted in a more rapid resolution of signs and

Department of Oral and Maxillofacial Surgery, University of Alabama at Birmingham, 1919 7th Avenue South, SDB 419, Birmingham, AL 35294, USA
E-mail address: plouis@uab.edu

Oral Maxillofacial Surg Clin N Am 32 (2020) 649–674
https://doi.org/10.1016/j.coms.2020.07.003
1042-3699/20/© 2020 Elsevier Inc. All rights reserved.

oralmaxsurgery.theclinics.com

Box 1
Alveolar osteitis

Key features	• Early onset clot lysis
	• Fetor oris
	• Intense pain
Prevention	• Perioperative antibiotics
	• Preoperative and postoperative chlorhexidine rinse
	• Topical Acemannan hydrogel
	• Topical chlorhexidine gel
Management	• Irrigation
	• Debridement
	• Sedative dressing place (eugenol, benzocaine, and balsam of Peru)

Box 2
Displacement of teeth, restorations, and instruments

Key features	• Unique anatomy
	• Proximity to other structures
	• Poor surgical technique
	• Failure to use safety precautions
Prevention	• Oropharyngeal screen
	• Proper flap design
	• Adequate exposure
	• Good surgical technique
Management	• Three-dimensional imaging for localization
	• Surgical access
	• Navigation based on location
	• Bronchoscopy if aspirated

symptoms when compared with SaliCept and dry socket dressing.[27]

DISPLACEMENT

Background

Displacement of teeth, implants, dental restorations, small dental instruments, or injection needles is uncommon but difficult to truly estimate (**Box 2**). These objects are displaced into the airway, gastrointestinal tract, buccal space, infratemporal fossa, maxillary sinus, sublingual space, submandibular space, lateral pharyngeal space, and the inferior alveolar canal (IAC).[28] The combination of unique anatomy, poor surgical technique, and failure to use safety precautions can result in displacement.

Prevention

Displacement of root fragments and teeth is sometimes preventable using proper surgical techniques. Proper imaging (plain film and computed tomography [CT] scans) is important in planning the surgical procedure. At the beginning of the procedure an oropharyngeal screen in a conscious patient or a throat pack with umbilical tape during general anesthesia should be used to protect the airway. An adequate flap for visualization and surgical access is an important first step. A broad retractor that rests on the bone, above the level of the tooth or root, can prevent displacement into the buccal or infratemporal space. Displacement of a root into the sinus or through a thin lingual cortex is prevented by proper placement

of the dental elevator between the root and the bone socket and avoiding excessive force. Creating a small window above the level of the apex of the root can allow for excellent access and preserve crestal bone.

Management

The tooth can usually be palpated if it is displaced into the buccal or sublingual space. The clinician should attempt to trap the tooth between their finger and the bone. The tooth can then be pushed toward the occlusal edge of the flap and removed with a large hemostat. A tooth or implant that is displaced into the maxillary sinus is usually removed through a window placed in the canine fossa with a suction tip or aid of an endoscope (**Fig. 1**).[29–31] Teeth or implants that have been displaced into the submandibular space are approached through an osteotomy along the lingual aspect of the third molar tooth socket, leaving it attached to the lingual mucosa.[32] The lingual aspect of the socket is then out-fractured, allowing more direct visual access to the fragment than the traditional sulcular approach. Removal of fragments that have been displaced into the IAC entails obtaining access through a buccal flap. The IAC is exposed with a small to medium size round bur or pieziotome.

Three-dimensional imaging or films at right angles to each other are used for localization.[33] When a tooth or broken needle is displaced into

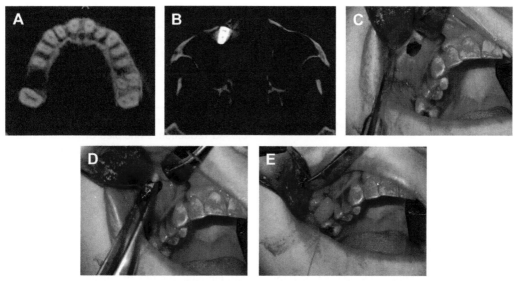

Fig. 1. Displacement of dental implant into the maxillary sinus. (*A*) CT scan showing an oroantral communication during dental implant placement. (*B*) CT scan showing a dental implant in the maxillary sinus. (*C*) Intraoperative view showing a window created into the maxillary sinus. (*D*) Dental implant removed from the maxillary sinus through the sinus window. (*E*) Buccal fat pad flap to close the oroantral communication.

a deep fascial space, the surgeon should consider the use of navigation in the operating room to help in localization.[33] A maxillofacial CT scan is obtained just before surgery. Depending on surgical approach, it may be beneficial to image the patient with a bite-block in place to accurately reflect the position of the mandible at the time of surgery. In cases where the tooth or root fragment has been displaced into the infratemporal fossa a coronal flap may be needed for access. Aspiration in an awake or moderately sedated patient usually results in violent coughing. If this fails to bring the tooth up, then transfer the patient to the hospital for retrieval via bronchoscopy. Chest and abdominal radiographs may be indicated to localize the tooth.

FRACTURE
Background

The reported incidence of iatrogenic mandibular fractures associated with the removal of teeth ranges from 0.0034% to 0.0075%.[34] They can occur during the procedure or within the first 4 weeks (**Box 3**). Iatrogenic mandibular fractures associated with third molar removal may increase with depth of impaction, type of tooth angulation, length of roots, patient age, inexperience of the surgeon, presence of a cyst or tumor around an impacted third molar, systemic disease or medications that may impair bone strength, preoperative infections in the third molar site, and inadequate preoperative examination.[35–40] In a systematic review, men aged greater than 35 years, with teeth in

Box 3	
Fracture associated with dentoalveolar surgery	
Key features	• Mandibular third molar risk factors
	Men >35 y of age
	Depth of impaction
	Amount of bone removal
	Impaired bone healing
	• Maxillary third molar risk factors
	Lone standing
	Widely divergent roots
	Hypereruption
Prevention	• Tooth sectioning
	• Reduce the amount of bone removal
	• Decreased force applied during removal
Management	• Usually treated closed
	• Atrophic fractures may require open repair

positions II/III and B/C, complete bony impaction, and local bone alterations, were found to have a higher frequency of fracture.[41]

Fractures associated with implant placement in the atrophic mandible are most commonly reported in the symphysis region.[42–45] The timing of implant-related mandibular fracture is extremely variable; most occurring either 3 to 6 weeks or 3 months after implant placement, before and after loading.[42,46]

Maxillary tuberosity and alveolar segment fractures can occur during dental extractions and occasionally associated with significant hemorrhage.[47]

Prevention

When removing deeply impacted third molars, it is advisable to perform adequate bone removal, and tooth sectioning, to reduce the amount of bone removal and lessen the force required to remove the tooth.[48–51] A recent literature review reported 74% of fractures occurred postoperatively, and 26% of pathologic mandibular fractures were observed intraoperatively.[46] A soft diet is recommended for 4 weeks postoperatively, especially in patients with full dentition who have risk factors for mandibular fracture.[34,52–54]

In the severely atrophic mandible, the clinician should avoid wide diameter implants and penetration through the inferior border of the mandible, which can significantly weaken the jaw.[45] Good oral hygiene, proper maintenance of implants,

and proper biomechanics of the restoration can prevent late fractures.[42] Nerve repositioning procedures and alveolar osteotomies can also result in fracture of the body of the mandible in atrophic cases (**Fig. 2**).[42,55]

Management

Fractures of the mandible are treated via open or closed reduction. Principles of fracture management must be followed.[56–58] Implants in the line of fracture are left in place when they are osseointegrated, not mobile, not infected, and are not near areas of osteomyelitis.[43]

HEMORRHAGE
Background

The rich network of vessels in the head and neck can increase the risk of persistent hemorrhage in the perioperative period (**Box 4**).[59] The risk of hemorrhage associated with third molar removal is estimated at 0.2% to 1.4%.[60] Causes of bleeding during surgery are caused by local and systemic factors. Local causes of bleeding include normal anatomic structures and pathologic lesions.[61,62] Systemic causes include hereditary and acquired coagulopathies and medications.[63,64]

Life-threatening hemorrhage and airway compromise has been reported during dental implant placement in the mandible.[65,66] Vessels that may be encountered include the lingual, facial, inferior alveolar, sublingual, submental, mental,

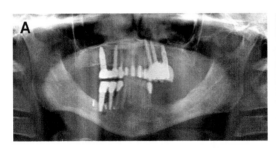
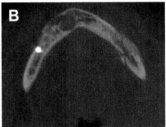
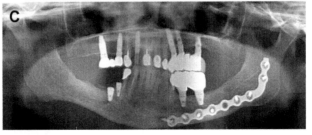

Fig. 2. Mandibular fracture after posterior alveolar osteotomy to increase ridge height. (*A*) Preoperative radiograph showing an atrophic left posterior mandible. (*B*) Postoperative radiograph showing left mandibular fracture after a sandwich osteotomy. (*C*) Postoperative radiograph after repair and healing of the left mandibular fracture.

buccal, and greater palatine arteries (GPA) and veins.[62]

Pathologic lesions that can bleed if encountered during dentoalveolar procedures include arteriovenous malformation (AVM), hemangioma, giant cell tumor (GCT), aneurysmal bone cyst (ABC).[67–69] AVMs occur from a lack of differentiation of arteries, veins, and capillaries during development. This results in direct communication between arteries and veins. AVMs grow throughout life and are characterized according to the main vessel type and flow that comprise it. The character of the bleeding from an AVM is usually brisk because of the high pressure and high flow associated with these lesions. Hemangiomas are present at birth if not clinically apparent. They typically appear during the first 2 years of life. Classically a rapid proliferative phase occurs that outpaces body growth. Approximately 50% of hemangiomas involute by age 5 and about 70%

by age 7.[70–72] ABCs are reactive lesions and are associated with other bony lesions.[73] The histologic examination reveals sinusoidal blood spaces devoid of endothelial lining.[74] GCTs are characterized by a proliferation of fibroblast with various amounts of collagen with multinucleated giant cells dispersed throughout. A recent hypothesis is that these lesions be considered proliferative vascular in origin or angiogenesis-dependent (**Fig. 3**).[75,76]

Systemic disorders associated with an increased risk of bleeding are termed coagulopathies. They are divided into hereditary and acquired causes. The more common hereditary clotting factor deficiencies include hemophilia A, hemophilia B, and von Willebrand disease (VWD). These are x-linked recessive diseases. Hemophilia A and hemophilia B are caused by missing or deficient normal factor VIII and IX, respectively. In the general population the incidence of these disorders is 1:5000 to 10,000 male births for hemophilia A, and 1:20,000 to 34,000 male births for hemophilia B. Mild disease is characterized by 5% to 35% factor level, moderate disease has 1% to 5% factor level, and severe disease has less than 1% factor level. VWD is caused by deficient or defective plasma von Willebrand factor (VWF). It mediates platelet hemostatic function and stabilizing blood coagulation factor VIII. It affects 0.16% to 1% of the population (approximately 1 in 10,000).[77–79] It is classified into three subtypes. Type 1 VWD is a partial quantitative deficiency of essentially normal VWF. Type 2 VWD is characterized by a qualitative deficiency and defective VWF (further subdivided into types 2A, 2B, 2M, and 2N). Type 3 VWD is a virtually complete quantitative deficiency of VWF.[80] Acquired VWD has been described from multiple causes.[81–83]

Thrombocytopenia is defined as a platelet count lower than the 2.5th lower percentile of the normal platelet count distribution. However, the adoption of a cutoff value of 100×10^9/L may be more appropriate to identify a pathologic condition.[84,85] The major mechanisms for a reduced platelet count are decreased production (eg, aplastic anemia, myelodysplastic syndromes, and chemotherapy-induced thrombocytopenia) and increased destruction of platelets (eg, disseminated intravascular coagulation and the thrombotic microangiopathies). Less common mechanisms are platelet sequestration (congestive splenomegaly) and hemodilution (massive blood transfusion).[86,87] Other platelet disorders include adhesion effects, aggregation defects, and granular defects.[88,89]

Medications that prolong bleeding include antiplatelet drugs (cyclooxygenase [COX] inhibitors,

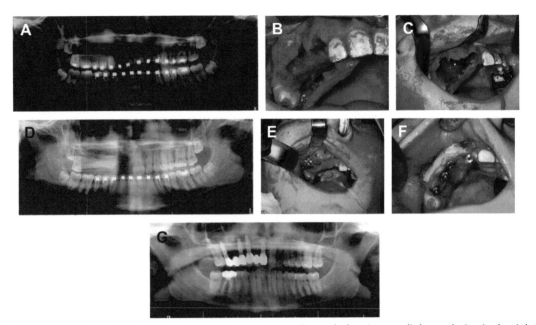

Fig. 3. Giant cell tumor of the right maxilla. (*A*) Preoperative radiograph showing a radiolucent lesion in the right maxilla with root resorption. (*B*) Intraoperative view of right maxillary sinus lesion. (*C*) Intraoperative view after resection of right maxillary tumor. (*D*) Postoperative radiograph after removal of the right maxillary lesion. (*E*) Intraoperative view after staged bone graft. (*F*) Intraoperative view after reconstruction with implants and epithelial graft. (*G*) Postoperative radiograph after reconstruction of the right maxilla with bone graft and implants.

GPIIb/IIIa inhibitors, P2Y12 inhibitors, and phosphodiesterase inhibitors) and anticoagulants (direct thrombin inhibitors, indirect thrombin inhibitors, direct Xa inhibitors, and vitamin K antagonist). Additionally, some herbal remedies can interfere with coagulation.

- COX-1 inhibitors: inhibits COX-1 in such a way that only thromboxane A_2 production is inhibited and not prostaglandin I_2. Aspirin antiplatelet affects are irreversible and last for the life of the platelet (7–10 days). Other COX-1 inhibitor effects are reversible.
- GPIIb/IIIa inhibitors: various modes of action to inhibit GPIIb/IIIa.[90]
- P2Y12 inhibitor: irreversibly binds to the P2Y12 adenosine diphosphate receptors, reducing platelet aggregation and adhesion. The antiplatelet affects are irreversible and last for the life of the platelet (7–10 days).[91]
- Phosphodiesterase inhibitors: aid in degradation of cyclic adenosine monophosphate and cyclic guanosine monophosphate, two substances that play a pivotal role in platelet activation.[92]
- Indirect thrombin inhibitors: binds to antithrombin III and accelerates activity, inhibiting thrombin and factor Xa.

- Direct thrombin inhibitors: directly and reversibly inhibits thrombin by interfering with the conversion of fibrinogen into fibrin.[93]
- Direct factor Xa inhibitors: bind to factor Xa.[93]
- Vitamin K antagonist: inhibits vitamin K–dependent coagulation factors and its effect is dose dependent.

Table 1 summarizes the antiplatelet and anticoagulation medications, their half-life, the recommended time for discontinuation of therapy for more invasive procedures, reversal agents, and the recommended management of uncontrolled bleeding.[90,92,94]

Prevention

Damage to the GPA is avoided by placing full-thickness incisions in the midline or along the palatal gingival crevice. A subperiosteal dissection can proceed to and around the foramen with care. The greater palatine foramen was palatal to the second molar (35.7%), and, interproximal to the second and third molars (35.7%) in women, and palatal to the second molar in men (65%).[95] When harvesting connective tissue grafts, partial-thickness incisions are generally placed in the premolar region and anteriorly to avoid the GPA. The

Table 1
Antiplatelet and anticoagulation medications

Drug	Receptor Binding	Half-Life	Recommended Discontinuation	Reversal	Treatment
Cox inhibitor					
Aspirin	Irreversible	2–6 h	5–7 d	None	Platelet transfusion Desmopressin
P2Y12 inhibitors					
Cangrelor (Inj)	Reversible	6 min	90 min	None	Platelet transfusion Desmopressin
Clopidogrel	Irreversible	6 h	5–7 d		
Prasugrel	Irreversible	7 h	5–9 d		
Ticagrelor	Reversible	7–9 h	4–5 d		
GP IIb/IIIa inhibitors					
Abciximab (Inj)	Irreversibly binds	10–30 min	2–3 d	None	Platelet transfusion Desmopressin Cryoprecipitate
Eptifibatide (Inj)	Reversibly binds	15 min–2.5 h	8–12 h		
Tirofiban (Inj)	Reversibly binds	2 h	8 h		
Phosphodiesterase inhibitors					
Cilostazol		11–13 h	2 d	None	Platelet transfusion Desmopressin
Dipyridamole		10 h	2 d		
Direct thrombin inhibitors					
Argatroban (Inj)		39–51 min	5 h	None	None
Bivalirudin (Inj)		25–34 min	3 h		
Dabigatran		12–17 h	3–4 d	Idarucizumab	Idarucizumab
Indirect thrombin inhibitors					
Dalteparin (Inj)		3–5 h	12–24 h	Protamine	Protamine PCC Andexanet alpha
Enoxaparin (Inj)		4.5–7 h	12–24 h	Andexanet alpha	
Fondaparinux		17–21 h	4 d		
Heparin		1.5 h	6–24 h	Protamine	Protamine
Direct Xa inhibitors					
Apixaban		12 h	3 d	Protamine	Protamine PCC Andexanet alpha
Betrixaban		19–27 h	5 d	Andexanet alpha	
Edoxaban		10–14 h	3 d		
Rivaroxaban		5–9 h	3 d		

(continued on next page)

Table 1
(continued)

Drug	Receptor Binding	Half-Life	Recommended Discontinuation	Reversal	Treatment
Vitamin K antagonist					
Warfarin		36 h	5 d	Vitamin K	PCC Fresh frozen plasma Vitamin K

Antiplatelet and anticoagulation medications; half-life, recommended discontinuation time before surgery, reversal agents, and treatment of correct the antiplatelet or anticoagulant medication.

Abbreviation: Inj, Injectable; PCC, prothrombin complex concentrate.

GPA branches most frequently at the level of first premolar (38%) and at the first and second molar region (43%) in women. In men, branching was commonly observed at the level of first and second premolars region (56%), and at the level of second and third molars region (32%).[95] The sublingual artery is avoided by performing a subperiosteal dissection along the lingual aspect of the mandible. Life-threatening hemorrhage can occur during implant placement secondary to lingual cortical perforation.[65,66] In the inferior neurovascular bundle, the vein was superior to the nerve and there are often multiple veins. The artery was solitary and lingual to the nerve, slightly above the horizontal position. This position seemed to be consistent in all cases.[96] Thus, it is possible to have injury to the vessels without injury to the nerves.

Vascular lesions may seem to be a periapical granuloma or abscess on plain films. Many patients give a history of previous episodes of bleeding from the area. When performing a biopsy of a radiolucent lesion, it is recommended that needle aspiration be performed first. When the aspirate is blood under pressure the lesion is considered to be an AVM until proven otherwise. Bleeding from these lesions is life threatening, thus additional work-up is indicated, including a CT scan with contrast. If the aspirate is blood but low flow, then other lesions should be considered, such as an ABC or GCT.

The two main treatments for VWD are desmopressin (1-deamino-8-Darginine vasopressin) and clotting factor concentrates containing VWF and FVIII (VWF/FVIII concentrate). For surgical procedures where significant bleeding is anticipated the goal is to achieve a factor level between 60% and 100%, depending on the type of hemophilia. The use of epsilon aminocaproic acid can help with clot stabilization and reduce the need for additional factor after tooth extraction.[97] Thrombocytopenia is managed by transfusion with platelets. Platelet counts less than 30,000 to 50,000 are usually transfused when performing procedures that are more invasive.[98,99] Patients with end-stage liver disease must be thoroughly evaluated to determine the risk of bleeding. International normalized ratio (INR) close to a normal range is recommended in these patients because of a significant risk of bleeding.

When discontinuing antiplatelet and anticoagulant therapies, it is important to consult the prescribing physician to determine whether bridging-therapy with enoxaparin or heparin is indicated. This is always indicated in high-risk patients, to shorten the time they are at risk for a thrombotic event. It is considered safe to proceed with minor dentoalveolar procedures, such as dental extractions, when the patient's INR is between 2 and 4.[100–102] Surgical extractions and dentoalveolar procedures with significant risk of bleeding require an INR of less than 2 or discontinuing other antiplatelet and anticoagulant therapy.

Low risk for thrombotic event
1. When indicated, consult the prescribing physician regarding holding anticoagulant therapy.
2. Hold anticoagulant and antiplatelet therapy based on recommendations (see **Table 1**).

High risk for thrombotic event
1. When indicated, consult the prescribing physician regarding holding anticoagulant therapy.
2. Hold anticoagulant and antiplatelet therapy based on recommendations (see **Table 1**).
3. Begin bridging therapy with short-acting anticoagulant (eg, enoxaparin) the day after holding anticoagulant.
4. Hold short-acting anticoagulant on the morning of surgery based on half-life.
5. After surgery, restart short-acting anticoagulant based on current recommendations.
6. Restart long-acting anticoagulant when considered safe, based on type of surgery.

Laboratory monitoring of the newer anticoagulants is not usually recommended. Ecarin clotting time is the most sensitive assay for monitoring dabigatran, but it is not readily available.[103] Thrombin time has been reported to be inaccurate at high concentrations of dabigatran. Because rivaroxaban and apixaban inhibit factor Xa levels, ecarin clotting time or thrombin time are not affected. Activated partial thromboplastin time is the best test for monitoring dabigatran, but sensitivity is reduced at higher concentrations. Although activated partial thromboplastin time also may be prolonged by rivaroxaban, the activated partial thromboplastin time is less reliable than prothrombin time at high concentrations of rivaroxaban.[93,103] The chromogenic anti-FXa assay is used to quantitatively measure the anticoagulant activity of the FXa inhibitors.

Management

When acute hemorrhage is encountered from an extraction site, digital pressure is placed. The socket should be packed tightly with a hemostatic agent, such as a gelatin sponge or oxidized cellulose. The socket is sutured in a figure-of-eight fashion. Pressure with gauze is held for 20 to 30 minutes. With soft tissue bleeding or bone sources that are not as easily packed, other techniques must be used. Digital pressure is the first line of treatment. Electrocautery is used for small vessels, whereas larger vessels are usually ligated.

If the bleeding is not controlled with these maneuvers, then transport the patient to the hospital. Intravenous (IV) access must be established and fluid resuscitation started with lactated Ringer or normal saline. If the airway is compromised secondary to the amount of bleeding or airway swelling, then secure the airway with a laryngeal mask or endotracheal tube. In some cases, a surgical airway must be established. Once in the hospital, consider blood transfusion with O⁻ or type and crossmatched blood. The restrictive transfusion strategy is a threshold for transfusion of red blood cells for a hemoglobin level of 7 g/dL, with a target of 7 to 9 g/dL (70–90 g/L) in adults and most children.[99,104,105] A more liberal transfusion strategy is recommended for preterm infants or children with cyanotic heart disease, severe hypoxemia, active blood loss, or hemodynamic instability with a threshold of 9.5 g/dL and a target of 11 to 12 g/dL.[99,104,105] Laboratory test should include prothrombin time (INR), partial thromboplastin time, and complete blood count with platelets. CT scan with contrast is beneficial in evaluating pathology (neoplasm or hematoma).

When normal structures are the source of the bleeding or when a pathologic lesion is the source of hemorrhage, ligation or embolization is the treatment of choice. The choice is determined by the accessibility to the source of bleeding and potential complexity of surgery. Ligation close to the source of bleeding is more effective than external carotid ligation because of the rich anastomosis of vessels in the head and neck.[106] Selective embolization is recommended for AVMs, bleeding sources that are difficult to access, and/or have failed previous surgery.

When a coagulopathy is suspected to be the cause of the bleeding, this must be corrected. Additional laboratory test that may be helpful include clotting factor assay. This takes valuable time and treatment cannot be delayed while waiting for results. Acute correction of a coagulopathy is performed with the use of fresh frozen plasma (FFP) or prothrombin complex concentrates (PCCs). Plasma transfusion is recommended in patients with active bleeding and an INR greater than 1.6 or before an invasive procedure or surgery if a patient has been anticoagulated.[98] Platelet transfusion is indicated for the management of patients on antiplatelet therapy or patients with thrombocytopenia of less than 20,000 or between 20,000 and 30,000 when there is active bleeding.

PCCs are concentrated pooled plasma products that typically contain three (factors II, IX, and X) or four (factors II, VII, IX, and X) clotting factors.[93] PCCs have been reported to have advantages over FFP.[107] PCCs correct the INR more rapidly than does FFP in patients taking warfarin who develop nontraumatic intracranial hemorrhage.[108] Preparation time for PCCs is shorter than for FFP, which must be thawed before use.[109] PCCs contain a higher concentration of clotting factors than FFP, thus smaller infusion volumes are required.[93,109]

Delayed bleeding after a surgical procedure is just as serious as immediate hemorrhage. When the patient calls or returns to the office with the concern of postoperative bleeding, the clinician must determine the amount and intensity of the bleeding. If the bleeding is slow, then pressure with gauze over the site may be helpful. When bleeding is moderate to severe or has occurred over a prolonged period, then the patient should return to the office or go to the emergency room of a hospital. Of particular concern is an expanding hematoma because of the potential for airway issues. Pressure over the suspected source, airway management, CT scan with contrast, and laboratory data should be part of the initial management. The definitive management may require embolization and/or surgery, and correction of any coagulopathy.

INFECTION
Background

As categorized by the American Society of Health-System Pharmacists, most of the dentoalveolar procedures are classified as clean-contaminated (procedures that violate the gastrointestinal or respiratory tract), and contaminated (procedures in acute inflammation situations). In a systematic review on lower third molar surgery, the incidence of infection in the control groups ranged from 0% to 14.8%[110,111] and from 0% to 6.5% in the antibiotic prophylaxis groups.[110,112,113] The bacteria associated with surgical site infections (SSI) for dentoalveolar procedures are usually opportunistic, from the existing microflora of the oral cavity. The culturable bacterial microbiota of the saliva is dominated by the Streptococcus, Prevotella, and Veillonella genera, which comprise 70% of this microbiota.[114] The most predominant bacteria in the oral cavity include Fusobacteria, Actinobacteria, Proteobacteria, Bacteroidetes, and Spirochaete (**Box 5**).[115,116] When categorizing the microbiota by location in the oral cavity, most sites are

<table>
<tr><td colspan="2">Box 5
Infection</td></tr>
<tr><td>Key features</td><td>• Risk of infection is low
• Predominant bacteria in the oral cavity

Fusobacteria, Actinobacteria, Proteobacteria, Bacteroidetes, and Spirochaeta</td></tr>
<tr><td>Prevention</td><td>• Perioperative antibiotics especially in the immunocompromised</td></tr>
<tr><td>Management</td><td>• Irrigation
• Debridement
• Antibiotics of choice

Penicillins

Clindamycin
• Antibiotics for resistant organisms

B-lactamase inhibitors

Flagyl

Cephalosporins

Fluoroquinolones</td></tr>
</table>

dominated by the *Streptococcus* genus, followed by *Hemophilus* in the buccal mucosa, *Actinomyces* in the supragingival plaque, and *Prevotella* in the subgingival plaque.[117,118]

Prevention

Patient-related risk factors, such as poor nutritional status, smoking, diabetes, and impaired immune system, can increase the risk of SSI and must be taken into consideration. A systematic review of latest evidence on the use of prophylactic antibiotic in oral surgical procedures reported no justification for antibiotics when performing intraalveolar dental extraction.[119] For third molar surgery, there is good evidence to support the use of perioperative antibiotics,[120,121] but three meta-analyses concluded no support for routine prescription for healthy people undergoing third molar removal.[122–124]

For dental implants, there is good evidence that perioperative antibiotic as a single-shot prophylaxis before placement can reduce dental implant failure but not SSI.[125–129] A retrospective study with high risk of bias found antibiotics for 7 days effective in implant survival.[130] However, other studies with low risk of bias reported no statistically significant differences in survival between single-shot prophylaxis and a prolonged postoperative course of antibiotics.[129,131–133] Thus, except in patients with an increased risk of infection, only perioperative antibiotics are recommended for routine dentoalveolar surgeries.

Management

An important aspect of treatment is reduction of the bacterial load by incision and drainage if an abscess has developed, wound debridement to remove necrotic tissue, and wound irrigation. Amoxicillin and clindamycin provide adequate coverage for the usual organisms that are encountered for odontogenic infections after dentoalveolar alveolar procedures. Estimates of penicillin and clindamycin resistance vary but some reports are as high as 20%. B-lactamase inhibitor, or Flagyl are often added to the regimen to expand coverage. Less resistance is seen with cephalosporins and fluoroquinolones and could be considered.[134–136]

Although not the scope of this article, patients that are immunocompromised, or that develop deep space infections, airway compromise, sepsis, other complications of deep space infections or osteomyelitis, usually require admission to the hospital for more aggressive management.

NONHEALING WOUND
Background

Failure of a wound to heal can result from local and systemic disorders.[137–141] Medications that suppress steps of wound healing, radiation therapy, and nutritional deficiencies can have devastating effect on the body's ability to heal. These are initialed by dentoalveolar surgery but are associated with trauma or uncertain cause (**Box 6**).[142]

OSTEORADIONECROSIS
Background

Radiation-induced osteonecrosis (ORN) is defined as an area of exposed devitalized irradiated bone that fails to heal over a period of 3 to 6 months in the absence of local neoplastic disease.[143,144] Radiation results in a hypovascular, hypocellular, and hypoxic tissue bed with poor healing capabilities.[145] The radiation-induced fibroatrophic theory has been proposed.[146] Cellular injury is caused by interactions with H_2O molecules creating secondary particles that interact with cellular DNA.[140] Ionizing radiation induces a variety of DNA lesions, including oxidized base damage, abasic sites, single-strand breaks, and double-strand breaks.

Box 6
Nonhealing wounds

Key features	• Exposed devitalized bone that fails to heal
	• Previous exposure to radiation therapy or bisphosphonates
Prevention	• Comprehensive dental evaluation
	• Optimize dental health
	• Close follow-up
	• Avoid elective dentoalveolar procedures in high-risk patients
	• Drug holidays remain controversial in medication-related osteonecrosis of the jaw prevention
	• Pentoxifylline-tocopherol-clodronate combination (Pentoclo) protocol for radiation-induced osteonecrosis prevention
Management	• Topical antimicrobial rinses
	• Systemic antibiotic therapy
	• Sequestrectomy and/or surgical debridement
	• Resection and reconstruction with free flap for advanced stages
	• Bisphosphonates should be held when possible
	• Hyperbaric oxygen therapy remains controversial

Table 2
Osteoradionecrosis of the jaw staging system

Staging of ORN Based on the Anatomic Extent	
Stage I	Confined to the alveolar bone
Stage II	Extent above the mandibular alveolar canal
Stage III	Extent below the level of the mandibular alveolar canal with a skin fistula and/or pathologic fracture

From Notani K, Yamazaki Y, Kitada H, et al. Management of mandibular osteoradionecrosis corresponding to the severity of osteoradionecrosis and the method of radiotherapy. Head Neck. 2003;25(3):181–6; with permission.

common cause of ORN in the irradiated maxilla or mandible.[149,150] Mandibular surgery, the use of Cobalt radiation, and higher radiation doses over biologically equivalent dose values of 102.6 Gy were significantly associated with the development of ORN.[147] Radiation dose greater than 60 Gy resulted in a 12% risk of developing ORN, whereas doses of less than 60 Gy resulted in no patients developing ORN.[151] Advances in the delivery of radiation therapy, such as intensity-modulated radiation therapy, may reduce the risk to 6% or less.[152,153]

Pentoxifylline-tocopherol-clodronate combination (Pentoclo) may be beneficial in the management and prevention of ORN. Pentoxifylline, a methylxanthine derivative, exerts an anti–tumor necrosis factor-α effect, vasodilates, and inhibits inflammatory reactions. Tocopherol (vitamin E) scavenges the reactive oxygen species generated during oxidative stress. These two drugs work synergistically as potent antifibrotic agents. Clodronate is a bisphosphonate (BP) that inhibits osteoclastic bone destruction and osteolysis.[154] With the cost of hyperbaric oxygen (HBO) therapy and the difficulty in obtaining insurance approval for prophylactic use, many clinicians have adopted the use of pentoxifylline and vitamin E before and after dental extractions until the wound has healed.

Patients with higher-stage tumors, patients who continued to smoke or consume alcohol, and patients who received a radiation dose greater than 60 Gy had a poor response to conservative management of ORN, and often required surgical resection.[155] A recent systematic review did not identify any reliable evidence to either support or refute the efficacy of HBO in the prevention of postextraction ORN in irradiated patients.[156] In cohort and observational studies, the occurrence rate of ORN in patients undergoing prophylactic

Areas that receive higher doses of radiation (Gy = 1 J of absorbed dose per kilogram) are at risk for ORN when undergoing surgical procedures, such as extraction.[147] ORN is has been classified into three stages based on extent of the disease (**Table 2**).[148]

Prevention

Identifying the risk of developing ORN entails obtaining the patient's radiation dosimetry map to determine the amount of radiation exposure to the area that requires treatment. The incidence of ORN in the mandible following radiation treatment ranges from 2.6% to 18%. Dental extraction, before or after radiation, is reported as the most

HBO therapy ranged from 0% to 11% (median, 4.1%), whereas in the non-HBO patients the range was from 0% to 29.9% (median, 7.1%).[156] Marx and coworkers showed in a randomized, prospective study that patients undergoing HBO therapy had a lower incidence of ORN compared with an antibiotic group (5.4% vs 29.9%).[157,158]

Before radiation the following is recommended:

- Comprehensive dental evaluation
- Teeth with a poor or questionable prognosis must be extracted
  - 21 days before or within 4 months of completion of therapy[149]
- Optimize oral health
  - Cleaning, fluoride treatment, restorations, and tori removal
- Meticulous oral hygiene instructions
  - Brush and floss twice daily
  - Use of interproximal brushes
  - Avoid alcohol-containing mouth rinse
  - Use mouth moisturizing rinses
- Custom fluoride trays daily
- Weekly dental evaluation during radiation therapy
- Monthly dental evaluations for the first 6 months following radiation
- Postradiation 4-month recall appointments

Management

The treatment of ORN is based on the clinical stage and management philosophy. Systematic reviews have not shown consistent evidence to support HBO therapy in the management of ORN. Some institutions continue to use HBO therapy, whereas others do not continue to use it. Both treatment protocols are presented in **Tables 3** and **4**.[148,158,159]

MEDICATION-RELATED OSTEONECROSIS OF THE JAW
Background

Medication-related osteonecrosis of the jaw (MRONJ) is defined as exposed bone or bone that can be probed through an intraoral or extraoral fistula in the maxillofacial region, without resolution for greater than 8 weeks in patients treated with an antiresorptive and/or an antiangiogenic agent, who have not received radiation therapy to the jaws or have obvious metastatic disease to the jaws (**Fig. 4**).[160] BPs are used to treat osteopenia, osteoporosis, and metastatic bone disease.[161–168]

BPs are analogues of pyrophosphate that are resistant to chemical or enzymatic breakdown caused by a modification of their structure. They bind to bone hydroxyapatite during its turnover and seem to have a biologic half-life of greater than 10 years.[169] During osteoclastic resorption, BPs are internalized via pinocytosis and inhibition of the enzyme farnesyl pyrophosphate synthase. This leads to reduction of the cell's activity, cell differentiation, and apoptosis, depending on the concentration of the BP.[170–172]

Precursors to osteoclasts, preosteoclasts, express surface receptors called receptor activator of nuclear factor-kappa B (RANK). RANK is activated by RANKL (the RANK ligand), which exists as cell surface molecules on osteoblasts. Activation of RANK by RANKL promotes the maturation of preosteoclasts into osteoclasts. Denosumab is a human monoclonal IgG2-anti-RANKL antibody that inhibits this maturation of osteoclasts by selectively binding to RANKL on the osteoclast and its precursors. By doing so, osteoclast-mediated bone resorption is inhibited.[173,174]

Table 3
Treatment sequence for ORN of the jaw without HBO therapy

Sequence of Treatment Based on Response to Treatment	
Sequence	Treatment
Phase I initial treatment	Topical antimicrobial mouth rinses with chlorhexidine 0.12% Nonsurgical sequestrectomy and/or debridement
Phase II (failure of phase I)	Topical antimicrobial mouth rinses with chlorhexidine 0.12% Initiate systemic antibiotic therapy Nonsurgical sequestrectomy and/or debridement
Phase III (failure of phase II)	Topical antimicrobial mouth rinses with chlorhexidine 0.12% Systemic antibiotic therapy Surgical resection of necrotic bone with or without adjunctive HBO

From Sultan A, Hanna GJ, Margalit DN, et al. The use of hyperbaric oxygen for the prevention and management of osteoradionecrosis of the Jaw: A Dana-Farber/Brigham and Women's Cancer Center multidisciplinary guideline. Oncologist. 11 2017;22(11):348; with permission.

Table 4
Treatment of ORN of the jaw base on stage with HBO therapy

Treatment Based on Stage of Disease	
Stage	**Treatment**
Stage I	Topical antimicrobial mouth rinses with chlorhexidine 0.12% Systemic antibiotic therapy HBO therapy (20 dives before and 10 dives after surgery) Surgical sequestrectomy and/or debridement based on response
Stage II	Topical antimicrobial mouth rinses with chlorhexidine 0.12% Systemic antibiotic therapy HBO therapy (20 dives before and 10 dives after surgery) Surgical debridement Primary closure of the defect with or without a free flap
Stage III	Systemic antibiotic therapy Surgical resection Reconstruction with free flap HBO therapy usually not indicated

From Notani K, Yamazaki Y, Kitada H, et al. Management of mandibular osteoradionecrosis corresponding to the severity of osteoradionecrosis and the method of radiotherapy. Head Neck. 2003;25(3):181–6; with permission.

The mandible was the most common site reported for MRONJ (70.6%), and extraction was the most frequently reported preceding event (48.5%).[175] Alendronate was the most commonly reported antiresorptive drug, reported in 72.6% of the cases, followed by risedronate (5.4%), ibandronate (5.2%), zoledronate (4.3%), and denosumab (2.1%). BPs were administered orally in 86.7% of the patients and intravenously in 7.9%.[142,175]

The risk of developing MRONJ in postmenopausal patients on oral BP is 0.02% to 0.1%.[176–178] This risk increased to 0.21% for patients that were on oral BP therapy for more than 4 years.[176]

Zoledronate IV once yearly for the management of osteoporosis seems to be associated with a low risk for developing osteonecrosis of the jaw over a 3-year period (0.017% and 0.35%).[179,180] The risk of developing MRONJ while on denosumab for patients with osteoporosis was reported to be 0.04% and 0.3%.[178,181]

Factors that have been reported to increase the risk of developing MRONJ include: chemotherapy, corticosteroid therapy, erythropoietin therapy, renal dialysis, hypothyroidism, diabetes mellitus, duration of BP therapy, age of the patient, smoking, and obesity.[142,180–182]

As reported in the American Association of Oral and Maxillofacial Surgeons position paper on MRONJ, patients receiving antiresorptives for the management of skeletal-related events associated with metastatic bone disease may be at higher risk for developing MRONJ.[160] The cumulative incidence of MRONJ among patients with cancer exposed to zoledronate ranged from 0.7% to 6.7%.[183,184] Studies with Level 1 evidence revealed the risk of MRONJ in subjects exposed to zoledronate was approximately 1%.[183,185–18] In reviewing studies of patients with cancer exposed to denosumab, the risk of MRONJ ranges from 0.7% to 1.9%.[185,187] The reported risk for osteonecrosis of the jaw among patients with cancer exposed to bevacizumab, an antiangiogenic agent, was 0.2% (**Table 5**).[188]

Prevention

It remains controversial whether the secession of BPs, denosumab, and angiogenesis inhibitors is effective in the prevention or reduction of MRONJ.[189,190] There is no evidence that the secession of oral BPs prevents or reduces the risk of MRONJ after invasive surgery.[191] However, because of the morbidity associated with MRONJ, many clinicians continue to use drug holidays and delaying treatment in high-risk patients.

For individuals on oral BP therapy, elective dentoalveolar surgery is not contraindicated. Patients should be adequately informed about the risk of compromised bone healing. Alteration in surgical planning is not necessary in patients on oral BPs for less than 4 years with no other risk factors. For patients undergoing oral surgery that have risk factors for developing MRONJ, the International Task Force on Osteonecrosis of the Jaw recommends discontinuation of antiresorptive therapy if bone health is not disturbed.[192] Treatment may be resumed after bone healing is completed. This decision should be made after consulting the treating physician and only if systemic conditions permit. Before initiating BP therapy the following is recommended:

- Comprehensive dental and head and neck evaluation
- Teeth with a poor or questionable prognosis should be extracted
  - Before initiating IV therapy or before 3 years of oral therapy

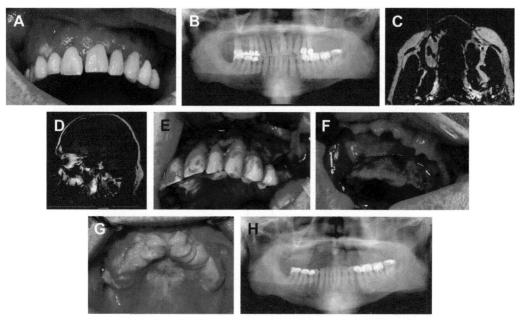

Fig. 4. Medication osteonecrosis of the jaw in patient on IV zoledronate for the management of skeletal-related events associated with metastatic bone disease. (*A*) Preoperative intraoral view of the maxilla with loose teeth and sinus tracts. (*B*) Preoperative radiograph with radiolucency along the left maxillary teeth. (*C*) Preoperative axial view MRI showing increased signal in the left and right maxilla. (*D*) Preoperative sagittal view MRI showing increased signal in the maxilla. (*E*) Intraoperative view showing necrotic bone of the maxilla. (*F*) Intraoperative view after maxillectomy. (*G*) Postoperative view after healing of the maxilla. (*H*) Postoperative radiograph after subtotal maxillectomy.

- Dental treatment to optimize oral health
  - Dental cleaning and fluoride treatment
  - Dental restorations
  - Removal of large to moderate size tori
- Meticulous oral hygiene instructions
  - Brush and floss twice daily
  - Use of interproximal brushes
- Custom dental trays are fabricated for daily fluoride treatments
- 4-month recall appointments

Management

The management of MRONJ is based on the extent of the disease. A staging system for MRONJ has been proposed by Ruggiero and colleagues (**Table 6**).[160] In patients with MRONJ, treatment is directed toward pain management, reducing the risk of infection and extension of bone exposure and necrosis. Because all of the patient's bone has been exposed to BP, surgical resection may not be effective. Mobile necrotic bone segments should be removed without exposing uninvolved bone. When possible, in consultation with the prescribing physician, BP therapy should be stopped or modified. Discontinuation of oral BP therapy in patients with MRONJ has been associated with gradual improvement in clinical disease (**Table 7**).[193]

OROANTRAL COMMUNICATION
Background

Predisposition to developing an oroantral communication (OAC) includes increased pneumatization of the sinus, proximity of the roots to the sinus, widely divergent roots, periapical pathology,

Table 5
MRONJ based on application of the medication and associated risk factors

Risk of MRONJ Based on Medication and Indication	
Oral bisphosphonates	0.02%–0.1%
Oral bisphosphonates >4 y	0.21%
IV bisphosphonates for osteoporosis	0.017%–0.35%
Denosumab for osteoporosis	0.04%–0.3%
IV bisphosphonates for cancer	0.7%–6.7%
Denosumab for cancer	0.7%–1.9%
Bevacizumab for cancer	0.2%

Risk of MRONJ based on the use of bisphosphonates, monoclonal IgG2-anti-RANKL antibody, and antiangiogenic agent in the management of osteoporosis or skeletal-related events associated with metastatic bone disease.

Table 6
MRONJ staging

MRONJ Staging System Based on Extent of the Disease	
MRONJ Staging	**Description**
Stage 0	No clinical evidence of necrotic bone, but nonspecific clinical findings, radiographic changes, and symptoms
Stage 1	Exposed and necrotic bone, or fistulae that probes to bone, in patients who are asymptomatic and have no evidence of infection
Stage 2	Exposed and necrotic bone, or fistulae that probes to bone, associated with infection as evidenced by pain and erythema in the region of the exposed bone with or without purulent drainage
Stage 3	Exposed and necrotic bone or a fistula that probes to bone in patients with pain, infection, and one or more of the following: exposed and necrotic bone extending beyond the region of alveolar bone (ie, inferior border and ramus in the mandible, maxillary sinus, and zygoma in the maxilla) resulting in pathologic fracture, extraoral fistula, oral antral/oral nasal communication, or osteolysis extending to the inferior border of the mandible of sinus floor

From Ruggiero SL, Dodson TB, Fantasia J, et al. American Association of Oral and Maxillofacial Surgeons position paper on medication-related osteonecrosis of the jaw–2014 update. J Oral Maxillofac Surg. Oct 2014;72(10):1949; with permission.

Table 7
Treatment for MRONJ based on stage

Management of MRONJ Based on Extent of Disease	
Stage	**Treatment**
Stage 0	Systemic management that may include analgesics and antibiotics Patient education and review of indications for continued bisphosphonate therapy Optimize oral health
Stage 1	Antibacterial mouth rinse Clinical follow-up on a quarterly basis Patient education and review of indications for continued bisphosphonate therapy
Stage 2	Antibacterial mouth rinse Oral antibiotics Analgesics as needed Surgical debridement for soft tissue irritation and infection control
Stage 3	Antibacterial mouth rinse Antibiotic therapy Analgesics as needed Surgical debridement/resection for infection and pain management

From Ruggiero SL, Dodson TB, Fantasia J, et al. American Association of Oral and Maxillofacial Surgeons position paper on medication-related osteonecrosis of the jaw–2014 update. J Oral Maxillofac Surg. Oct 2014;72(10):1949; with permission.

is reported as the most common cause of OAC (73.3%) followed by maxillofacial pathology removal.[198,199] Performance of an incision (odds ratio, 5.16), mesioangular tooth angulation and type 3 RS classification, and superimposition of the roots with the sinus floor are significant risk factors.[200]

Prevention

The thickness of the bone between the maxillary sinus and the molar and premolar roots has been reported to have a wide range (1–7 mm).[201] When the bone is thin, a surgical extraction, removing each root separately may be helpful in these situations. An OAC is sometimes unavoidable when excising a pathologic lesion. When a hard tissue tuberosity reduction is indicated and there is a small amount of crestal bone present, a segmental osteotomy should be considered to reduce the bone height.

excessive force, posterior maxillary pathology, and maxillary sinusitis (**Box 7**, **Fig. 5**). The relative incidence of developing an OAC during tooth extraction is reported to be around 5%.[194,195] When removing maxillary third molars the incidence is reported between 11% and 13%.[196,197] Intraoperative fracture of the root, higher degree of impaction, and higher age of the patient are associated with a greater risk. Dental extraction

Box 7
Oroantral communication

Key Features

- Pneumatization of the sinus
- Proximity of the procedure to the sinus

Prevention

- Radiographic imaging to determine thickness of bone below the sins floor
- Tailoring the surgical procedure to minimize sinus perforation

Management

- Topical antimicrobial rinses
- Systemic antibiotic therapy
- Systemic decongestants
- Remove diseased sinus mucosa
- Excision of the sinus tract
- 2-layered closure

Management

If an OAC occurs at the time of dental extraction, then a simple closure is usually sufficient. Size of the defect has been reported to be a factor in determining whether the clinician should achieve primary closure at the time of the initial development of an OAC. Although spontaneous healing of defects of less than 5 mm has been reported, randomized trials evaluating this topic do not exist in the literature.[202] Thus, OAC should be closed immediately or within 24 to 48 hours, to prevent the development of an infection.[203] Chronic defects require the exploration of the sinus through a window in the canine fossa; removal of only diseased mucosa, usually with a suction tip; removal of foreign bodies; excision of the fistulous tract; and a two-layered closure. In patients with a patent ostium, a nasal antrostomy is not required to establish drainage for the sinus.[204] If the ostium for the maxillary sinus is blocked, then consider functional endoscopic sinus surgery. Teeth without bone along the root surface that are adjacent to the OAC must be extracted; otherwise this results in failure to achieve closure.

The buccal fat pad flap has a reported success rate of 93%.[205,206] It is used alone as a single-layer closure.[207] It has been reported to undergo complete epithelialization in 6 to 8 weeks and is slowly replaced by fibrous tissue.[208,209] Using the buccal flap in combination with the buccal fat pad flap may offer the advantage of improved predictability in case of large defects or when there is a hole or tear in the fat pad flap.[206,210]

Full-thickness mucoperiosteal palatal flaps are used for closure of OAC.[211] It has a reported success rate of 76% when used as a random palatal flap.[212] Modification of the palatal flap used for closure of the cleft palate has been advocated for large OAC.[213] The submucosal palatal flap has been advocated to avoid denuded areas of the palate to minimize postoperative morbidity.[214]

The patient is placed on antibiotics, nasal decongestants, and saline nasal spray postoperatively. Sinus precaution instructions including no nose blowing and sneezing with the mouth open are recommended for the first 2 weeks.

SWELLING AND TRISMUS
Background

Concerns associated with postoperative edema include wound dehiscence; increased pain; decreased function; and delay in return to daily activities, such as work or social activities (**Box 8**). When performing third molar surgery, older age (greater than 30 years), deeply impacted teeth, and long operation times (greater than 10 minutes) are associated with significantly higher

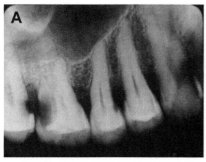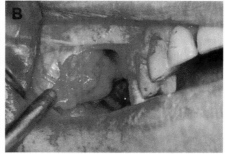

Fig. 5. Oroantral communication caused by extraction of maxillary first molar with proximity to the maxillary sinus. (*A*) Preoperative periapical radiograph showing tooth #3 with roots near the sinus. (*B*) Intraoperative view showing mobilization of the buccal fat pad to close and OAC.

Box 8
Swelling and Trismus

Key Features
- Edema with increase risk of complications
- Limited mouth opening

Prevention
- Use of ice and anti-inflammatory drugs
- Bite block for lower extractions
- Controlled force during extractions

Management
- Anti-inflammatory medications
- Physical therapy

---

swelling.[215] Deeply impact teeth and longer operation times are also associated with higher postoperative pain scores.

Trismus is defined as limited opening of the jaw secondary to spasm of the closing muscles of the mandible. The overriding cause is inflammation of the closing muscles of the mandible or the temporomandibular joint. Causes of trismus associated with dentoalveolar surgery include local anesthetic injection, deep space infection, hematoma or bleeding in the masticatory muscles, muscle reflection for surgical access, or temporomandibular joint trauma secondary to forceful dental extraction and prolonged opening. The incidence of trismus after impacted mandibular third molars of more than 10 mm at postoperative day 1 was 18.3% and was significantly associated with the depth of impaction.[215]

Prevention

Preventive measures currently used include the use of ice and corticosteroids. Patients receiving corticosteroids have significantly less edema and trismus during early and late postoperative periods.[216] Additionally, steroids have been reported to decrease postoperative nausea vomiting.[217,218] Additional measures to reduce the risk of trismus include preoperative antimicrobial mouth rinse, perioperative nonsteroidal anti-inflammatory drugs, proper injection techniques for local anesthesia administration, avoiding excessive force on the mandible, limiting surgical access when possible, use a bite block for mandibular extractions, and avoiding excessive mouth opening.

Management

The management of postoperative swelling and trismus is based on degree and cause. Intubation secondary to postoperative edema alone should be rare. Corticosteroid administration may aid in reduction of swelling and trismus.[219]

In the absence of fracture, the treatment should include physical therapy (jaw stretching exercise, ice/heat, and ultrasound), soft diet, and medications (nonsteroidal anti-inflammatory drugs, corticosteroids, muscle relaxants). Antibiotics are indicated only when infection is suspected as the cause of trismus.

DISCLOSURE

The authors have nothing to disclose.

REFERENCES

1. Field EA, Speechley JA, Rotter E, et al. Dry socket incidence compared after a 12 year interval. Br J Oral Maxillofac Surg 1985;23(6):419–27.
2. Turner PS. A clinical study of "dry socket". Int J Oral Surg 1982;11(4):226–31.
3. Osborn TP, Frederickson G Jr, Small IA, et al. A prospective study of complications related to mandibular third molar surgery. J Oral Maxillofac Surg 1985;43(10):767–9.
4. Kolokythas A, Olech E, Miloro M. Alveolar osteitis: a comprehensive review of concepts and controversies. Int J Dent 2010;2010:249073.
5. Larsen PE. Alveolar osteitis after surgical removal of impacted mandibular third molars. Identification of the patient at risk. Oral Surg Oral Med Oral Pathol 1992;73(4):393–7.
6. Blum IR. Contemporary views on dry socket (alveolar osteitis): a clinical appraisal of standardization, aetiopathogenesis and management: a critical review. Int J Oral Maxillofac Surg 2002;31(3):309–17.
7. Heasman PA, Jacobs DJ. A clinical investigation into the incidence of dry socket. Br J Oral Maxillofac Surg 1984;22(2):115–22.
8. Nitzan DW. On the genesis of "dry socket". J Oral Maxillofac Surg 1983;41(11):706–10.
9. Rood JP, Murgatroyd J. Metronidazole in the prevention of 'dry socket'. Br J Oral Surg 1979;17(1):62–70.
10. Catellani JE, Harvey S, Erickson SH, et al. Effect of oral contraceptive cycle on dry socket (localized alveolar osteitis). J Am Dent Assoc 1980;101(5):777–80.
11. Bergdahl M, Hedstrom L. Metronidazole for the prevention of dry socket after removal of partially impacted mandibular third molar: a randomised controlled trial. Br J Oral Maxillofac Surg 2004;42(6):555–8.
12. Hedstrom L, Sjogren P. Effect estimates and methodological quality of randomized controlled trials about prevention of alveolar osteitis following tooth

extraction: a systematic review. Oral Surg Oral Med Oral Pathol Oral Radiol Endod 2007;103(1):8–15.

13. Ren YF, Malmstrom HS. Effectiveness of antibiotic prophylaxis in third molar surgery: a meta-analysis of randomized controlled clinical trials. J Oral Maxillofac Surg 2007;65(10):1909–21.

14. Lodi G, Figini L, Sardella A, et al. Antibiotics to prevent complications following tooth extractions. Cochrane Database Syst Rev 2012;(11):CD003811.

15. Ataoglu H, Oz GY, Candirli C, et al. Routine antibiotic prophylaxis is not necessary during operations to remove third molars. Br J Oral Maxillofac Surg 2008;46(2):133–5.

16. Swanson AE. A double-blind study on the effectiveness of tetracycline in reducing the incidence of fibrinolytic alveolitis. J Oral Maxillofac Surg 1989; 47(2):165–7.

17. Davis WM Jr, Buchs AU, Davis WM. The use of granular gelatin-tetracycline compound after third molar removal. J Oral Surg 1981;39(6):466–7.

18. Sorensen DC, Preisch JW. The effect of tetracycline on the incidence of postextraction alveolar osteitis. J Oral Maxillofac Surg 1987;45(12):1029–33.

19. Akota I, Alvsaker B, Bjornland T. The effect of locally applied gauze drain impregnated with chlortetracycline ointment in mandibular third-molar surgery. Acta Odontol Scand 1998;56(1):25–9.

20. Fridrich KL, Olson RA. Alveolar osteitis following surgical removal of mandibular third molars. Anesth Prog 1990;37(1):32–41.

21. Schow SR. Evaluation of postoperative localized osteitis in mandibular third molar surgery. Oral Surg Oral Med Oral Pathol 1974;38(3):352–8.

22. Zuniga JR, Leist JC. Topical tetracycline-induced neuritis: a case report. J Oral Maxillofac Surg 1995;53(2):196–9.

23. Lynch DP, Newland JR, McClendon JL. Myospherulosis of the oral hard and soft tissues. J Oral Maxillofac Surg 1984;42(6):349–55.

24. Poor MR, Hall JE, Poor AS. Reduction in the incidence of alveolar osteitis in patients treated with the SaliCept patch, containing Acemannan hydrogel. J Oral Maxillofac Surg 2002;60(4):374–9 [discussion: 379].

25. Hermesch CB, Hilton TJ, Biesbrock AR, et al. Perioperative use of 0.12% chlorhexidine gluconate for the prevention of alveolar osteitis: efficacy and risk factor analysis. Oral Surg Oral Med Oral Pathol Oral Radiol Endod 1998;85(4):381–7.

26. Teshome A. The efficacy of chlorhexidine gel in the prevention of alveolar osteitis after mandibular third molar extraction: a systematic review and meta-analysis. BMC Oral Health 2017;17(1):82.

27. Kaya GS, Yapici G, Savas Z, et al. Comparison of alvogyl, SaliCept patch, and low-level laser therapy in the management of alveolar osteitis. J Oral Maxillofac Surg 2011;69(6):1571–7.

28. Esen E, Aydogan LB, Akcali MC. Accidental displacement of an impacted mandibular third molar into the lateral pharyngeal space. J Oral Maxillofac Surg 2000;58(1):96–7.

29. Gay-Escoda C, Berini-Aytes L, Pinera-Penalva M. Accidental displacement of a lower third molar. Report of a case in the lateral cervical position. Oral Surg Oral Med Oral Pathol 1993;76(2):159–60.

30. Iwai T, Matsui Y, Hirota M, et al. Endoscopic removal of a maxillary third molar displaced into the maxillary sinus via the socket. J Craniofac Surg 2012;23(4):e295–6.

31. Iwai T, Chikumaru H, Shibasaki M, et al. Safe method of extraction to prevent a deeply-impacted maxillary third molar being displaced into the maxillary sinus. Br J Oral Maxillofac Surg 2012;51(5):e75–6.

32. Huang IY, Wu CW, Worthington P. The displaced lower third molar: a literature review and suggestions for management. J Oral Maxillofac Surg 2007;65(6):1186–90.

33. Campbell A, Costello BJ. Retrieval of a displaced third molar using navigation and active image guidance. J Oral Maxillofac Surg 2010;68(2):480–5.

34. Libersa P, Roze D, Cachart T, et al. Immediate and late mandibular fractures after third molar removal. J Oral Maxillofac Surg 2002;60(2):163–5 [discussion: 165–6].

35. Sakr K, Farag IA, Zeitoun IM. Review of 509 mandibular fractures treated at the University Hospital, Alexandria, Egypt. Br J Oral Maxillofac Surg 2006;44(2):107–11.

36. Yamaoka M, Furusawa K, Iguchi K, et al. The assessment of fracture of the mandibular condyle by use of computerized tomography. Incidence of sagittal split fracture. Br J Oral Maxillofac Surg 1994;32(2):77–9.

37. Thorn JJ, Mogeltoft M, Hansen PK. Incidence and aetiological pattern of jaw fractures in Greenland. Int J Oral Maxillofac Surg 1986;15(4):372–9.

38. Cankaya AB, Erdem MA, Cakarer S, et al. Iatrogenic mandibular fracture associated with third molar removal. Int J Med Sci 2011;8(7):547–53.

39. Dunstan SP, Sugar AW. Fractures after removal of wisdom teeth. Br J Oral Maxillofac Surg 1997; 35(6):396–7.

40. Krimmel M, Reinert S. Mandibular fracture after third molar removal. J Oral Maxillofac Surg 2000; 58(10):1110–2.

41. Pires WR, Bonardi JP, Faverani LP, et al. Late mandibular fracture occurring in the postoperative period after third molar removal: systematic review and analysis of 124 cases. Int J Oral Maxillofac Surg 2017;46(1):46–53.

42. Chrcanovic BR, Custodio AL. Mandibular fractures associated with endosteal implants. Oral Maxillofac Surg 2009;13(4):231–8.

43. Mason ME, Triplett RG, Van Sickels JE, et al. Mandibular fractures through endosseous cylinder implants: report of cases and review. J Oral Maxillofac Surg 1990;48(3):311–7.

44. Raghoebar GM, Stellingsma K, Batenburg RH, et al. Etiology and management of mandibular fractures associated with endosteal implants in the atrophic mandible. Oral Surg Oral Med Oral Pathol Oral Radiol Endod 2000;89(5):553–9.

45. Oh WS, Roumanas ED, Beumer J 3rd. Mandibular fracture in conjunction with bicortical penetration, using wide-diameter endosseous dental implants. J Prosthodont 2010;19(8):625–9.

46. Boffano P, Roccia F, Gallesio C, et al. Pathological mandibular fractures: a review of the literature of the last two decades. Dent Traumatol 2013;29(3): 185–96.

47. Bertram AR, Rao AC, Akbiyik KM, et al. Maxillary tuberosity fracture: a life-threatening haemorrhage following simple exodontia. Aust Dent J 2011; 56(2):212–5.

48. Coletti D, Ord RA. Treatment rationale for pathological fractures of the mandible: a series of 44 fractures. Int J Oral Maxillofac Surg 2008;37(3):215–22.

49. Grau-Manclus V, Gargallo-Albiol J, Almendros-Marques N, et al. Mandibular fractures related to the surgical extraction of impacted lower third molars: a report of 11 cases. J Oral Maxillofac Surg 2011;69(5):1286–90.

50. Bodner L, Brennan PA, McLeod NM. Characteristics of iatrogenic mandibular fractures associated with tooth removal: review and analysis of 189 cases. Br J Oral Maxillofac Surg 2011;49(7): 567–72.

51. Al-Belasy FA, Tozoglu S, Ertas U. Mastication and late mandibular fracture after surgery of impacted third molars associated with no gross pathology. J Oral Maxillofac Surg 2009;67(4):856–61.

52. Perry PA, Goldberg MH. Late mandibular fracture after third molar surgery: a survey of Connecticut oral and maxillofacial surgeons. J Oral Maxillofac Surg 2000;58(8):858–61.

53. Komerik N, Karaduman AI. Mandibular fracture 2 weeks after third molar extraction. Dent Traumatol 2006;22(1):53–5.

54. Kao YH, Huang IY, Chen CM, et al. Late mandibular fracture after lower third molar extraction in a patient with Stafne bone cavity: a case report. J Oral Maxillofac Surg 2010;68(7):1698–700.

55. Karlis V, Bae RD, Glickman RS. Mandibular fracture as a complication of inferior alveolar nerve transposition and placement of endosseous implants: a case report. Implant Dent 2003;12(3):211–6.

56. Moreno JC, Fernandez A, Ortiz JA, et al. Complication rates associated with different treatments for mandibular fractures. J Oral Maxillofac Surg 2000;58(3):273–80 [discussion: 280–1].

57. Ellis E 3rd, Walker LR. Treatment of mandibular angle fractures using one noncompression miniplate. J Oral Maxillofac Surg 1996;54(7):864–71 [discussion: 871–2].

58. Ellis E 3rd. Treatment methods for fractures of the mandibular angle. J Craniomaxillofac Trauma 1996;2(1):28–36.

59. Wasson M, Ghodke B, Dillon JK. Exsanguinating hemorrhage following third molar extraction: report of a case and discussion of materials and methods in selective embolization. J Oral Maxillofac Surg 2012;70(10):2271–5.

60. Moghadam HG, Caminiti MF. Life-threatening hemorrhage after extraction of third molars: case report and management protocol. J Can Dent Assoc 2002;68(11):670–4.

61. Lamberg MA, Tasanen A, Jaaskelainen J. Fatality from central hemangioma of the mandible. J Oral Surg 1979;37(8):578–84.

62. Flanagan D. Important arterial supply of the mandible, control of an arterial hemorrhage, and report of a hemorrhagic incident. J Oral Implantol 2003;29(4):165–73.

63. Orlian AI, Karmel R. Postoperative bleeding in an undiagnosed hemophilia A patient: report of case. J Am Dent Assoc 1989;118(5):583–4.

64. Hong C, Napenas JJ, Brennan M, et al. Risk of postoperative bleeding after dental procedures in patients on warfarin: a retrospective study. Oral Surg Oral Med Oral Pathol Oral Radiol 2012; 114(4):464–8.

65. Givol N, Chaushu G, Halamish-Shani T, et al. Emergency tracheostomy following life-threatening hemorrhage in the floor of the mouth during immediate implant placement in the mandibular canine region. J Periodontol 2000;71(12):1893–5.

66. Mason ME, Triplett RG, Alfonso WF. Life-threatening hemorrhage from placement of a dental implant. J Oral Maxillofac Surg 1990;48(2):201–4.

67. Ennis JT, Bateson EM, Moule NJ. Uncommon arterio-venous fistulae. Clin Radiol 1972;23(3): 392–8.

68. Hassard AD, Byrne BD. Arteriovenous malformations and vascular anatomy of the upper lip and soft palate. Laryngoscope 1985;95(7 Pt 1): 829–32.

69. Darlow LD, Murphy JB, Berrios RJ, et al. Arteriovenous malformation of the maxillary sinus: an unusual clinical presentation. Oral Surg Oral Med Oral Pathol 1988;66(1):21–3.

70. Mulliken JB, Glowacki J. Classification of pediatric vascular lesions. Plast Reconstr Surg 1982;70(1): 120–1.

71. Mulliken JB, Glowacki J. Hemangiomas and vascular malformations in infants and children: a classification based on endothelial characteristics. Plast Reconstr Surg 1982;69(3):412–22.

72. Buckmiller LM. Update on hemangiomas and vascular malformations. Curr Opin Otolaryngol Head Neck Surg 2004;12(6):476–87.

73. Padwa BL, Denhart BC, Kaban LB. Aneurysmal bone cyst-"plus": a report of three cases. J Oral Maxillofac Surg 1997;55(10):1144–52.

74. Vollmer E, Roessner A, Lipecki KH, et al. Biologic characterization of human bone tumors. VI. The aneurysmal bone cyst: an enzyme histochemical, electron microscopical, and immunohistological study. Virchows Arch B Cell Pathol Incl Mol Pathol 1987;53(1):58–65.

75. O'Malley M, Pogrel MA, Stewart JC, et al. Central giant cell granulomas of the jaws: phenotype and proliferation-associated markers. J Oral Pathol Med 1997;26(4):159–63.

76. Kaban LB, Dodson TB. Management of giant cell lesions. Int J Oral Maxillofac Surg 2006;35(11): 1074–5 [author reply: 1076].

77. Rodeghiero F, Castaman G, Dini E. Epidemiological investigation of the prevalence of von Willebrand's disease. Blood 1987;69(2):454–9.

78. Werner EJ, Broxson EH, Tucker EL, et al. Prevalence of von Willebrand disease in children: a multiethnic study. J Pediatr 1993;123(6):893–8.

79. Bloom AL. von Willebrand factor: clinical features of inherited and acquired disorders. Mayo Clin Proc 1991;66(7):743–51.

80. Sadler JE, Budde U, Eikenboom JC, et al. Update on the pathophysiology and classification of von Willebrand disease: a report of the Subcommittee on von Willebrand Factor. J Thromb Haemost 2006;4(10):2103–14.

81. Sucker C, Michiels JJ, Zotz RB. Causes, etiology and diagnosis of acquired von Willebrand disease: a prospective diagnostic workup to establish the most effective therapeutic strategies. Acta Haematol 2009;121(2–3):177–82.

82. Federici AB. Acquired von Willebrand syndrome: an underdiagnosed and misdiagnosed bleeding complication in patients with lymphoproliferative and myeloproliferative disorders. Semin Hematol 2006;43(1 Suppl 1):S48–58.

83. James PD, Goodeve AC. von Willebrand disease. Genet Med 2011;13(5):365–76.

84. Cheng CK, Chan J, Cembrowski GS, et al. Complete blood count reference interval diagrams derived from NHANES III: stratification by age, sex, and race. Lab Hematol 2004;10(1):42–53.

85. Rodeghiero F, Stasi R, Gernsheimer T, et al. Standardization of terminology, definitions and outcome criteria in immune thrombocytopenic purpura of adults and children: report from an international working group. Blood 2009;113(11):2386–93.

86. Stasi R. How to approach thrombocytopenia. Hematology Am Soc Hematol Educ Program 2012; 2012:191–7.

87. Aster RH. Pooling of platelets in the spleen: role in the pathogenesis of "hypersplenic" thrombocytopenia. J Clin Invest 1966;45(5):645–57.

88. Clemetson KJ. Platelet glycoproteins and their role in diseases. Transfus Clin Biol 2001;8(3):155–62.

89. Cattaneo M. Inherited platelet-based bleeding disorders. J Thromb Haemost 2003;1(7):1628–36.

90. Dornbos D, Nimjee SM. Reversal of systemic anticoagulants and antiplatelet therapeutics. Neurosurg Clin N Am 2018;29(4):537–45.

91. Committee CS. A randomised, blinded, trial of clopidogrel versus aspirin in patients at risk of ischaemic events (CAPRIE). CAPRIE Steering Committee. Lancet 1996;348(9038):1329–39.

92. Hart BM, Ferrell SM, Motejunas MW, et al. New anticoagulants, reversal agents, and clinical considerations for perioperative practice. Best Pract Res Clin Anaesthesiol 2018;32(2):165–78.

93. Nitzki-George D, Wozniak I, Caprini JA. Current state of knowledge on oral anticoagulant reversal using procoagulant factors. Ann Pharmacother 2013;47(6):841–55.

94. Narouze S, Benzon HT, Provenzano D, et al. Interventional spine and pain procedures in patients on antiplatelet and anticoagulant medications (second edition): Guidelines From the American Society of Regional Anesthesia and Pain Medicine, the European Society of Regional Anaesthesia and Pain Therapy, the American Academy of Pain Medicine, the International Neuromodulation Society, the North American Neuromodulation Society, and the World Institute of Pain. Reg Anesth Pain Med 2018;43(3):225–62.

95. Klosek SK, Rungruang T. Anatomical study of the greater palatine artery and related structures of the palatal vault: considerations for palate as the subepithelial connective tissue graft donor site. Surg Radiol Anat 2009;31(4):245–50.

96. Pogrel MA, Dorfman D, Fallah H. The anatomic structure of the inferior alveolar neurovascular bundle in the third molar region. J Oral Maxillofac Surg 2009;67(11):2452–4.

97. Needleman HL, Kaban LB, Kevy SV. The use of epsilon-aminocaproic acid for the management of hemophilia in dental and oral surgery patients. J Am Dent Assoc 1976;93(3):586–90.

98. Holland LL, Brooks JP. Toward rational fresh frozen plasma transfusion: the effect of plasma transfusion on coagulation test results. Am J Clin Pathol 2006;126(1):133–9.

99. Sharma S, Sharma P, Tyler LN. Transfusion of blood and blood products: indications and complications. Am Fam Physician 2011;83(6):719–24.

100. Beirne OR. Evidence to continue oral anticoagulant therapy for ambulatory oral surgery. J Oral Maxillofac Surg 2005;63(4):540–5.

101. Evans IL, Sayers MS, Gibbons AJ, et al. Can warfarin be continued during dental extraction? Results of a randomized controlled trial. Br J Oral Maxillofac Surg 2002;40(3):248–52.

102. Dodson TB. Strategies for managing anticoagulated patients requiring dental extractions: an exercise in evidence-based clinical practice. J Mass Dent Soc 2002;50(4):44–50.

103. Favaloro EJ, Lippi G, Koutts J. Laboratory testing of anticoagulants: the present and the future. Pathology 2011;43(7):682–92.

104. Hebert PC, Wells G, Blajchman MA, et al. A multicenter, randomized, controlled clinical trial of transfusion requirements in critical care. Transfusion Requirements in Critical Care Investigators, Canadian Critical Care Trials Group. N Engl J Med 1999;340(6):409–17.

105. Carless PA, Henry DA, Carson JL, et al. Transfusion thresholds and other strategies for guiding allogeneic red blood cell transfusion. Cochrane Database Syst Rev 2010;(10):CD002042.

106. Yin NT. Effect of multiple ligations of the external carotid artery and its branches on blood flow in the internal maxillary artery in dogs. J Oral Maxillofac Surg 1994;52(8):849–54.

107. Bershad EM, Suarez JI. Prothrombin complex concentrates for oral anticoagulant therapy-related intracranial hemorrhage: a review of the literature. Neurocrit Care 2010;12(3):403–13.

108. Fredriksson K, Norrving B, Stromblad LG. Emergency reversal of anticoagulation after intracerebral hemorrhage. Stroke 1992;23(7):972–7.

109. Lemon SJ Jr, Crannage AJ. Pharmacologic anticoagulation reversal in the emergency department. Adv Emerg Nurs J 2011;33(3):212–23 [quiz: 224–5].

110. Bortoluzzi MC, Capella DL, Barbieri T, et al. A single dose of amoxicillin and dexamethasone for prevention of postoperative complications in third molar surgery: a randomized, double-blind, placebo controlled clinical trial. J Clin Med Res 2013;5(1):26–33.

111. Monaco G, Tavernese L, Agostini R, et al. Evaluation of antibiotic prophylaxis in reducing postoperative infection after mandibular third molar extraction in young patients. J Oral Maxillofac Surg 2009;67(7):1467–72.

112. Pasupathy S, Alexander M. Antibiotic prophylaxis in third molar surgery. J Craniofac Surg 2011;22(2):551–3.

113. Marcussen KB, Laulund AS, Jørgensen HL, et al. A systematic review on effect of single-dose preoperative antibiotics at surgical osteotomy extraction of lower third molars. J Oral Maxillofac Surg 2016;74(4):693–703.

114. Nasidze I, Li J, Quinque D, et al. Global diversity in the human salivary microbiome. Genome Res 2009;19(4):636–43.

115. Nadell CD, Xavier JB, Foster KR. The sociobiolog of biofilms. FEMS Microbiol Rev 2009;33(1) 206–24.

116. Rogers GB, Hoffman LR, Carroll MP, et al. Interpreting infective microbiota: the importance of a ecological perspective. Trends Microbiol 2013 21(6):271–6.

117. Cho I, Blaser MJ. The human microbiome: at th interface of health and disease. Nat Rev Gene 2012;13(4):260–70.

118. Le Bars P, Matamoros S, Montassier E, et al. The oral cavity microbiota: between health, oral disease, and cancers of the aerodigestive tract. Ca J Microbiol 2017;63(6):475–92.

119. Sidana S, Mistry Y, Gandevivala A, et al. Evaluation of the need for antibiotic prophylaxis during routine intra-alveolar dental extractions in healthy patients a randomized double-blind controlled trial. J Evi Based Dent Pract 2017;17(3):184–9.

120. López-Cedrún JL, Pijoan JI, Fernández S, et al. E ficacy of amoxicillin treatment in preventing pos operative complications in patients undergoin third molar surgery: a prospective, randomizec double-blind controlled study. J Oral Maxillofa Surg 2011;69(6):e5–14.

121. Lang MS, Gonzalez ML, Dodson TB. Do antibiotic decrease the risk of inflammatory complications af ter third molar removal in community practices J Oral Maxillofac Surg 2017;75(2):249–55.

122. Marghalani A. Antibiotic prophylaxis reduces infec tious complications but increases adverse effect after third-molar extraction in healthy patients J Am Dent Assoc 2014;145(5):476–8.

123. Isiordia-Espinoza MA, Aragon-Martinez OH, Mart nez-Morales JF, et al. Risk of wound infection an safety profile of amoxicillin in healthy patient which required third molar surgery: a systemati review and meta-analysis. Br J Oral Maxillofa Surg 2015;53(9):796–804.

124. Cho H, Lynham AJ, Hsu E. Postoperative interver tions to reduce inflammatory complications afte third molar surgery: review of the current evidence Aust Dent J 2017;62(4):412–9.

125. Ata-Ali J, Ata-Ali F. Do antibiotics decrease implar failure and postoperative infections? A systemati review and meta-analysis. Int J Oral Maxillofa Surg 2014;43(1):68–74.

126. Esposito M, Grusovin MG, Worthington HV. Inter ventions for replacing missing teeth: antibiotics a dental implant placement to prevent complications Cochrane Database Syst Rev 2013;(7):CD004152

127. Chrcanovic BR, Albrektsson T, Wennerberg A. Pro phylactic antibiotic regimen and dental implant fail ure: a meta-analysis. J Oral Rehabil 2014;41(12 941–56.

128. Lund B, Hultin M, Tranaeus S, et al. Comple systematic review: perioperative antibiotics i

conjunction with dental implant placement. Clin Oral Implants Res 2015;26(Suppl 11):1–14.

129. Sharaf B, Jandali-Rifai M, Susarla SM, et al. Do perioperative antibiotics decrease implant failure? J Oral Maxillofac Surg 2011;69(9):2345–50.

130. Krasny M, Krasny K, Zadurska M, et al. Evaluation of treatment outcomes and clinical indications for antibiotic prophylaxis in patients undergoing implantation procedures. Adv Med Sci 2016;61(1): 113–6.

131. El-Kholey KE. Efficacy of two antibiotic regimens in the reduction of early dental implant failure: a pilot study. Int J Oral Maxillofac Surg 2014;43(4):487–90.

132. Park J, Tennant M, Walsh LJ, et al. Is there a consensus on antibiotic usage for dental implant placement in healthy patients? Aust Dent J 2018; 63(1):25–33.

133. Arduino PG, Tirone F, Schiorlin E, et al. Single preoperative dose of prophylactic amoxicillin versus a 2-day postoperative course in dental implant surgery: a two-centre randomised controlled trial. Eur J Oral Implantol 2015;8(2): 143–9.

134. Brook I. Microbiology and management of peritonsillar, retropharyngeal, and parapharyngeal abscesses. J Oral Maxillofac Surg 2004;62(12): 1545–50.

135. Stefanopoulos PK, Kolokotronis AE. The clinical significance of anaerobic bacteria in acute orofacial odontogenic infections. Oral Surg Oral Med Oral Pathol Oral Radiol Endod 2004;98(4): 398–408.

136. Fating NS, Saikrishna D, Vijay Kumar GS, et al. Detection of bacterial flora in orofacial space infections and their antibiotic sensitivity profile. J Maxillofac Oral Surg 2014;13(4):525–32.

137. Akintoye SO, Hersh EV. Risks for jaw osteonecrosis drastically increases after 2 years of bisphosphonate therapy. J Evid Based Dent Pract 2012;12(3 Suppl):251–3.

138. Allen MR, Burr DB. The pathogenesis of bisphosphonate-related osteonecrosis of the jaw: so many hypotheses, so few data. J Oral Maxillofac Surg 2009;67(5 Suppl):61–70.

139. Lambade PN, Lambade D, Goel M. Osteoradionecrosis of the mandible: a review. Oral Maxillofac Surg 2012;17(4):243–9.

140. Carlson ER. The radiobiology, treatment, and prevention of osteoradionecrosis of the mandible. Recent Results Cancer Res 1994;134:191–9.

141. Sisson R, Lang S, Serkes K, et al. Comparison of wound healing in various nutritional deficiency states. Surgery 1958;44(4):613–8.

142. Mücke T, Krestan CR, Mitchell DA, et al. Bisphosphonate and medication-related osteonecrosis of the jaw: a review. Semin Musculoskelet Radiol 2016;20(3):305–14.

143. Beumer J, Harrison R, Sanders B, et al. Osteoradionecrosis: predisposing factors and outcomes of therapy. Head Neck Surg 1984;6(4):819–27.

144. Epstein JB, Rea G, Wong FL, et al. Osteonecrosis: study of the relationship of dental extractions in patients receiving radiotherapy. Head Neck Surg 1987;10(1):48–54.

145. Marx RE. Osteoradionecrosis: a new concept of its pathophysiology. J Oral Maxillofac Surg 1983; 41(5):283–8.

146. Delanian S, Lefaix JL. The radiation-induced fibroatrophic process: therapeutic perspective via the antioxidant pathway. Radiother Oncol 2004;73(2): 119–31.

147. Lee IJ, Koom WS, Lee CG, et al. Risk factors and dose-effect relationship for mandibular osteoradionecrosis in oral and oropharyngeal cancer patients. Int J Radiat Oncol Biol Phys 2009;75(4): 1084–91.

148. Notani K, Yamazaki Y, Kitada H, et al. Management of mandibular osteoradionecrosis corresponding to the severity of osteoradionecrosis and the method of radiotherapy. Head Neck 2003;25(3):181–6.

149. Marx RE, Johnson RP. Studies in the radiobiology of osteoradionecrosis and their clinical significance. Oral Surg Oral Med Oral Pathol 1987; 64(4):379–90.

150. Thorn JJ, Hansen HS, Specht L, et al. Osteoradionecrosis of the jaws: clinical characteristics and relation to the field of irradiation. J Oral Maxillofac Surg 2000;58(10):1088–93 [discussion: 1093–5].

151. Nabil S, Samman N. Incidence and prevention of osteoradionecrosis after dental extraction in irradiated patients: a systematic review. Int J Oral Maxillofac Surg 2011;40(3):229–43.

152. Studer G, Gratz KW, Glanzmann C. Osteoradionecrosis of the mandibula in patients treated with different fractionations. Strahlenther Onkol 2004; 180(4):233–40.

153. Vissink A, Jansma J, Spijkervet FK, et al. Oral sequelae of head and neck radiotherapy. Crit Rev Oral Biol Med 2003;14(3):199–212.

154. Delanian S, Chatel C, Porcher R, et al. Complete restoration of refractory mandibular osteoradionecrosis by prolonged treatment with a pentoxifylline-tocopherol-clodronate combination (PENTOCLO): a phase II trial. Int J Radiat Oncol Biol Phys 2011; 80(3):832–9.

155. Oh HK, Chambers MS, Martin JW, et al. Osteoradionecrosis of the mandible: treatment outcomes and factors influencing the progress of osteoradionecrosis. J Oral Maxillofac Surg 2009;67(7): 1378–86.

156. Chuang SK. Limited evidence to demonstrate that the use of hyperbaric oxygen (HBO) therapy reduces the incidence of osteoradionecrosis in

irradiated patients requiring tooth extraction. J Evid Based Dent Pract 2012;12(3 Suppl): 248–50.

157. Marx RE, Johnson RP, Kline SN. Prevention of osteoradionecrosis: a randomized prospective clinical trial of hyperbaric oxygen versus penicillin. J Am Dent Assoc 1985;111(1):49–54.

158. Sultan A, Hanna GJ, Margalit DN, et al. The use of hyperbaric oxygen for the prevention and management of osteoradionecrosis of the jaw: a Dana-Farber/Brigham and Women's Cancer Center multidisciplinary guideline. Oncologist 2017;22(11): 1413.

159. Gal TJ, Yueh B, Futran ND. Influence of prior hyperbaric oxygen therapy in complications following microvascular reconstruction for advanced osteoradionecrosis. Arch Otolaryngol Head Neck Surg 2003;129(1):72–6.

160. Ruggiero SL, Dodson TB, Fantasia J, et al. American Association of Oral and Maxillofacial Surgeons position paper on medication-related osteonecrosis of the jaw: 2014 update. J Oral Maxillofac Surg 2014;72(10):1938–56.

161. Nussbaum SR, Younger J, Vandepol CJ, et al. Single-dose intravenous therapy with pamidronate for the treatment of hypercalcemia of malignancy: comparison of 30-, 60-, and 90-mg dosages. Am J Med 1993;95(3):297–304.

162. Major P, Lortholary A, Hon J, et al. Zoledronic acid is superior to pamidronate in the treatment of hypercalcemia of malignancy: a pooled analysis of two randomized, controlled clinical trials. J Clin Oncol 2001;19(2):558–67.

163. Delmas PD, Meunier PJ. The management of Paget's disease of bone. N Engl J Med 1997;336(8): 558–66.

164. Delmas PD. The use of bisphosphonates in the treatment of osteoporosis. Curr Opin Rheumatol 2005;17(4):462–6.

165. Berenson JR. Treatment of hypercalcemia of malignancy with bisphosphonates. Semin Oncol 2002; 29(6 Suppl 21):12–8.

166. Berenson JR. Advances in the biology and treatment of myeloma bone disease. Semin Oncol 2002;29(6 Suppl 17):11–6.

167. Berenson JR, Hillner BE, Kyle RA, et al. American Society of Clinical Oncology clinical practice guidelines: the role of bisphosphonates in multiple myeloma. J Clin Oncol 2002;20(17):3719–36.

168. Bone HG, Hosking D, Devogelaer JP, et al. Ten years' experience with alendronate for osteoporosis in postmenopausal women. N Engl J Med 2004;350(12):1189–99.

169. Khan SA, Kanis JA, Vasikaran S, et al. Elimination and biochemical responses to intravenous alendronate in postmenopausal osteoporosis. J Bone Miner Res 1997;12(10):1700–7.

170. Murakami H, Takahashi N, Sasaki T, et al. A possible mechanism of the specific action of bisphosphonates on osteoclasts: tiludronate preferentially affects polarized osteoclasts having ruffled borders. Bone 1995;17(2):137–44.

171. Hall A. Rho GTPases and the actin cytoskeleton. Science 1998;279(5350):509–14.

172. Sato M, Grasser W, Endo N, et al. Bisphosphonate action. Alendronate localization in rat bone and effects on osteoclast ultrastructure. J Clin Invest 1991;88(6):2095–105.

173. Saad F, Brown JE, Van Poznak C, et al. Incidence, risk factors, and outcomes of osteonecrosis of the jaw: integrated analysis from three blinded active-controlled phase III trials in cancer patients with bone metastases. Ann Oncol 2012;23(5):1341–7.

174. Castellano D, Sepulveda JM, García-Escobar I, et al. The role of RANK-ligand inhibition in cancer: the story of denosumab. Oncologist 2011;16(2): 136–45.

175. Aljohani S, Fliefel R, Ihbe J, et al. What is the effect of anti-resorptive drugs (ARDs) on the development of medication-related osteonecrosis of the jaw (MRONJ) in osteoporosis patients: a systematic review. J Craniomaxillofac Surg 2017;45(9): 1493–502.

176. Lo JC, O'Ryan FS, Gordon NP, et al. Prevalence of osteonecrosis of the jaw in patients with oral bisphosphonate exposure. J Oral Maxillofac Surg 2010;68(2):243–53.

177. Tanna N, Steel C, Stagnell S, et al. Awareness of medication related osteonecrosis of the jaws (MRONJ) amongst general dental practitioners. Br Dent J 2017;222(2):121–5.

178. Oral health management of patients at risk of medication-related osteonecrosis of the jaw. Br Dent J 2017;222(12):930.

179. Black DM, Delmas PD, Eastell R, et al. Once-yearly zoledronic acid for treatment of postmenopausal osteoporosis. N Engl J Med 2007;356(18): 1809–22.

180. Anagnostis P, Stevenson JC. Bisphosphonate drug holidays: when, why and for how long? Climacteric 2015;18(Suppl 2):32–8.

181. Papapoulos S, Chapurlat R, Libanati C, et al. Five years of denosumab exposure in women with postmenopausal osteoporosis: results from the first two years of the FREEDOM extension. J Bone Miner Res 2012;27(3):694–701.

182. Wessel JH, Dodson TB, Zavras AI. Zoledronate, smoking, and obesity are strong risk factors for osteonecrosis of the jaw: a case-control study. J Oral Maxillofac Surg 2008;66(4):625–31.

183. Coleman R, Woodward E, Brown J, et al. Safety of zoledronic acid and incidence of osteonecrosis of the jaw (ONJ) during adjuvant therapy in a randomised phase III trial (AZURE: BIG 01-04) for

women with stage II/III breast cancer. Breast Cancer Res Treat 2011;127(2):429–38.

184. Vahtsevanos K, Kyrgidis A, Verrou E, et al. Longitudinal cohort study of risk factors in cancer patients of bisphosphonate-related osteonecrosis of the jaw. J Clin Oncol 2009;27(32):5356–62.

185. Qi WX, Tang LN, He AN, et al. Risk of osteonecrosis of the jaw in cancer patients receiving denosumab: a meta-analysis of seven randomized controlled trials. Int J Clin Oncol 2014;19(2):403–10.

186. Mauri D, Valachis A, Polyzos IP, et al. Osteonecrosis of the jaw and use of bisphosphonates in adjuvant breast cancer treatment: a meta-analysis. Breast Cancer Res Treat 2009;116(3):433–9.

187. Scagliotti GV, Hirsh V, Siena S, et al. Overall survival improvement in patients with lung cancer and bone metastases treated with denosumab versus zoledronic acid: subgroup analysis from a randomized phase 3 study. J Thorac Oncol 2012; 7(12):1823–9.

188. Guarneri V, Miles D, Robert N, et al. Bevacizumab and osteonecrosis of the jaw: incidence and association with bisphosphonate therapy in three large prospective trials in advanced breast cancer. Breast Cancer Res Treat 2010;122(1):181–8.

189. Dimopoulos MA, Kastritis E, Bamia C, et al. Reduction of osteonecrosis of the jaw (ONJ) after implementation of preventive measures in patients with multiple myeloma treated with zoledronic acid. Ann Oncol 2009;20(1):117–20.

190. Ripamonti CI, Maniezzo M, Campa T, et al. Decreased occurrence of osteonecrosis of the jaw after implementation of dental preventive measures in solid tumour patients with bone metastases treated with bisphosphonates. The experience of the National Cancer Institute of Milan. Ann Oncol 2009;20(1):137–45.

191. Kuroshima S, Sasaki M, Sawase T. Medication-related osteonecrosis of the jaw: A literature review. J Oral Biosci 2019;61(2):99–104.

192. Khan AA, Morrison A, Hanley DA, et al. Diagnosis and management of osteonecrosis of the jaw: a systematic review and international consensus. J Bone Miner Res 2015;30(1):3–23.

193. Marx RE, Cillo JE Jr, Ulloa JJ. Oral bisphosphonate-induced osteonecrosis: risk factors, prediction of risk using serum CTX testing, prevention, and treatment. J Oral Maxillofac Surg 2007;65(12):2397–410.

194. del Rey-Santamaria M, Valmaseda Castellon E, Berini Aytes L, et al. Incidence of oral sinus communications in 389 upper third molar extraction. Med Oral Patol Oral Cir Bucal 2006;11(4):E334–8.

195. Bodner L, Gatot A, Bar-Ziv J. Technical note: oroantral fistula: improved imaging with a dental computed tomography software program. Br J Radiol 1995;68(815):1249–50.

196. Wachter R, Stoll P. [Complications of surgical wisdom tooth removal of the maxilla. A clinical and roentgenologic study of 1,013 patients with statistical evaluation]. Fortschr Kiefer Gesichtschir 1995; 40:128–33.

197. Rothamel D, Wahl G, d'Hoedt B, et al. Incidence and predictive factors for perforation of the maxillary antrum in operations to remove upper wisdom teeth: prospective multicentre study. Br J Oral Maxillofac Surg 2007;45(5):387–91.

198. Jain MK, Ramesh C, Sankar K, et al. Pedicled buccal fat pad in the management of oroantral fistula: a clinical study of 15 cases. Int J Oral Maxillofac Surg 2012;41(8):1025–9.

199. Yilmaz T, Suslu AE, Gursel B. Treatment of oroantral fistula: experience with 27 cases. Am J Otolaryngol 2003;24(4):221–3.

200. Hasegawa T, Tachibana A, Takeda D, et al. Risk factors associated with oroantral perforation during surgical removal of maxillary third molar teeth. Oral Maxillofac Surg 2016;20(4): 369–75.

201. Skoglund LA, Pedersen SS, Holst E. Surgical management of 85 perforations to the maxillary sinus. Int J Oral Surg 1983;12(1):1–5.

202. von Wowern N. Correlation between the development of an oroantral fistula and the size of the corresponding bony defect. J Oral Surg 1973;31(2): 98–102.

203. Schulz D, Buhrmann K. [Pathological changes in the maxillary sinus: important secondary findings in orthodontic x-ray diagnosis]. Fortschr Kieferorthop 1987;48(4):298–312.

204. Huang YC, Chen WH. Caldwell-Luc operation without inferior meatal antrostomy: a retrospective study of 50 cases. J Oral Maxillofac Surg 2012; 70(9):2080–4.

205. Killey HC, Kay LW. Observations based on the surgical closure of 362 oro-antral fistulas. Int Surg 1972;57(7):545–9.

206. Candamourty R, Jain MK, Sankar K, et al. Double-layered closure of oroantral fistula using buccal fat pad and buccal advancement flap. J Nat Sci Biol Med 2012;3(2):203–5.

207. Poeschl PW, Baumann A, Russmueller G, et al. Closure of oroantral communications with Bichat's buccal fat pad. J Oral Maxillofac Surg 2009;67(7): 1460–6.

208. Fan L, Chen G, Zhao S, et al. Clinical application and histological observation of pedicled buccal fat pad grafting. Chin Med J (Engl) 2002;115(10): 1556–9.

209. Rapidis AD, Alexandridis CA, Eleftheriadis E, et al. The use of the buccal fat pad for reconstruction of oral defects: review of the literature and report of 15 cases. J Oral Maxillofac Surg 2000;58(2): 158–63.

210. Samman N, Cheung LK, Tideman H. The buccal fat pad in oral reconstruction. Int J Oral Maxillofac Surg 1993;22(1):2–6.

211. Ehrl PA. Oroantral communication. Epicritical study of 175 patients, with special concern to secondary operative closure. Int J Oral Surg 1980;9(5):351–8.

212. Lee JJ, Kok SH, Chang HH, et al. Repair of oroantral communications in the third molar region by random palatal flap. Int J Oral Maxillofac Surg 2002;31(6):677–80.

213. James RB. Surgical closure of large oroantral fistulas using a palatal island flap. J Oral Surg 1980;38(8):591–5.

214. Yamazaki Y, Yamaoka M, Hirayama M, et al. The submucosal island flap in the closure of oro-antral fistula. Br J Oral Maxillofac Surg 1985;23(4): 259–63.

215. Kim JC, Choi SS, Wang SJ, et al. Minor complications after mandibular third molar surgery: type, incidence, and possible prevention. Oral Surg Oral Med Oral Pathol Oral Radiol Endod 2006; 102(2):e4–11.

216. Markiewicz MR, Brady MF, Ding EL, et al. Corticosteroids reduce postoperative morbidity after third molar surgery: a systematic review and meta-analysis. J Oral Maxillofac Surg 2008;66(9):1881–94.

217. Tolver MA, Strandfelt P, Bryld EB, et al. Randomized clinical trial of dexamethasone versus placebo in laparoscopic inguinal hernia repair. Br J Surg 2012;99(10):1374–80.

218. Mataruski MR, Keis NA, Smouse DJ, et al. Effect of steroids on postoperative nausea and vomiting. Nurse Anesth 1990;1(4):183–8.

219. Osunde OD, Adebola RA, Omeje UK. Management of inflammatory complications in third molar surgery: a review of the literature. Afr Health Sci 2011;11(3):530–7.

The Trigeminal Nerve Injury

Arshad Kaleem, DMD, MD[a], Paul Amailuk, BDS, FRACDS (OMS)[b], Hisham Hatoum, DMD, MD[a], Ramzey Tursun, DDS[a],*

KEYWORDS

• Lingual nerve injury • Inferior alveolar nerve injury • Trigeminal nerve injury • Microneurosurgery

KEY POINTS

• The fifth cranial nerve is the largest cranial nerve and the largest peripheral sensory nerve in the human body.
• As oral and maxillofacial surgery broadens in scope, the surgeon will increasingly be required to diagnose and grade trigeminal nerve injury accurately and in the case of some surgeons surgically repair these injuries.
• Injury to the branches of the trigeminal nerve is commonly associated with "negative" clinical symptoms of decrease in sensation (hypoesthesia, anesthesia), but may also be accompanied by distressing "positive" symptoms of prolonged or permanent painful or inappropriate sensation (dysesthesia) and hypersensitivity (hyperesthesia).
• The areas most often affected (upper and lower lips, maxilla, mandible, tongue, and chin) are important in eating and touch and communication.

INTRODUCTION

The fifth cranial nerve is the largest cranial nerve and the largest peripheral sensory nerve in the human body. The importance of this primary somatosensory cortex in daily function is well illustrated by the trigeminal nerve representing close to half of the sensory area in the postcentral gyrus. Patients with impaired function of the trigeminal nerve can present with significant functional deficits and a decreased quality of life.[1]

The trigeminal nerve is the primary sensory neuron supplying the head and neck, and its branches are never far from the operating field of the oral and maxillofacial surgeon. As the specialty broadens in scope, the oral and maxillofacial surgeon will increasingly be required to diagnose and grade trigeminal nerve injury accurately and in the case of some surgeons surgically repair these injuries. In addition, litigation for iatrogenic damage to the trigeminal nerve is of increasing concern to oral and maxillofacial surgeons.

Injury to the branches of the trigeminal nerve is commonly associated with "negative" clinical symptoms of decrease in sensation (hypoesthesia, anesthesia), but may also be accompanied by distressing "positive" symptoms of prolonged or permanent painful or inappropriate sensation (dysesthesia) and hypersensitivity (hyperesthesia). The areas most often affected (upper and lower lips, maxilla, mandible, tongue, and chin) are important in eating, touch, and communication.

ETIOLOGY

Injuries to the trigeminal nerve are caused by:

1. Trauma (avulsive motor vehicle trauma, missile injuries, interpersonal violence, military combat [these patients often suffer continuity loss of one or more peripheral branches])

[a] Division of Oral & Maxillofacial Surgery, Department of Surgery, University of Miami, Deering Medical Plaza, 9380 Southwest 150th Street, Suite 170, Miami, FL 33176, USA; [b] Department of oral and maxillofacial surgery, Gold Coast University Hospital, 1 hospital Boulevard, Queensland 4215, Australia
* Corresponding author.
E-mail address: r.tursun@med.miami.edu

Oral Maxillofacial Surg Clin N Am 32 (2020) 675–687
https://doi.org/10.1016/j.coms.2020.07.005
1042-3699/20/© 2020 Elsevier Inc. All rights reserved.

2. Ablative tumor operations in the oral and maxillofacial region (**Fig. 1**)
3. Dentoalveolar surgical procedures[2]
   - Removal of teeth (excluding third molars) and cysts
   - Nerve blocks
   - Third molar removal
   - Endodontic treatment (**Fig. 2**)
   - Implant placement (**Fig. 3**)

In general, third molar removal had the highest incidence of injury (40.8%), followed by endodontic therapy (35.3%), other surgical procedures (20.7%), and lastly implant placement (3.2%).

The data on injury to the first and second division of the trigeminal nerve are sparse. Tay and Zuniga in 2005[3] reported that the third molar was the most common cause of referral for trigeminal nerve injury. Where third division injuries are concerned, lingual nerve (LN) and inferior alveolar nerve (IAN) injuries are the most common. Renton and Yilmaz[4] found that where IAN injury is concerned third molar surgery is the most common cause (60%), followed by local anesthetic injections (19%), implants (18%), and endodontic surgery (18%). Where LN injury is concerned, the same authors found that in their population, third molar removal was the leading cause (73%) followed by local anesthesia injections (17%).

Current literature accepts that the risk of injury to either the IAN or LN occurs in 0.4% to 22% of cases following third molar surgery.[5] More recently Nguyen and colleagues[6] found the incidence of IAN injury as 0.68% and LN injury as 0.15% in their study looking at 11,599 lower third molar extractions in 6803 patients.

Pogrel[7] found that although the true incidence of injury to the IAN from injection was unknown, he estimated that permanent damage might occur in 1 in 25,000 IAN blocks. He found most patients entirely recovered with 85% recovering fully within 8 to 10 weeks, 5% taking longer, and 10% sustaining permanent deficits.

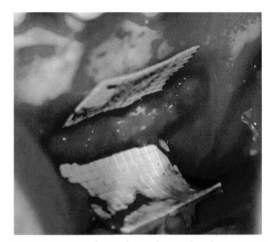

Fig. 2. Gutta-percha within inferior alveolar nerve as result of endodontic injury.

Lost or altered sensation resulting from peripheral trigeminal nerve injuries interferes with standard oral and facial functions and can result in a significantly reduced quality of life for patients.[1] This can mean the difference between an acceptable return to function in the reconstructed tumor patient, detract from an otherwise successful trauma repair, and present as unacceptable morbidity in the elective wisdom tooth or implant patient. Thus, avoiding injury where possible, and offering a reconstruction of the trigeminal nerve where indicated, should be an integral part of the surgical service provided to patients. This is of particular importance in a clinical environment where more professionals are placing implants

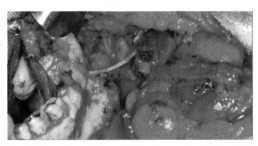

Fig. 1. Resection of mandibular tumor including inferior alveolar nerve.

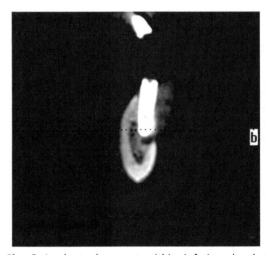

Fig. 3. Implant placement within inferior alveolar canal.

and there is increased awareness of injuries by patients, and increased reporting of incidents by professionals.

PREOPERATIVE EVALUATION
Patient History

A baseline complete neurosensory examination consisting of a thorough history and physical should be conducted with care taken to document the patient's sensory deficit or pain accurately. Is the patient experiencing "positive" symptoms, such as painful or unpleasant sensation (dysesthesia)? Alternatively, are the symptoms more in the "negative" category with absent, decreased, or altered sensation (paresthesia, hypoesthesia, anesthesia)? Is the pain constant (suggesting a long-term injury or neuroma formation)? Is the pain intermittent? If so, are there instigating factors? Is it spontaneous and how long does each episode last? Next, a visual analog scale should be used to quantify the pain on a scale of 1 to 10. Determine further whether there are any relieving or exacerbating factors. Have any medications or treatments been tried and have any succeeded? Lastly, establish from the patient what the effect of the injury is on their quality of life and activities of daily living.

Thus, the patient can be placed in one of three groups based on whether they perceive a neurosensory or functional deficit from the injury, and secondly, whether they are concerned about it or motivated to seek some intervention.

A. Not aware: does not care
B. Aware: does not care
C. Aware: cares

The "aware and cares" patient is the one for whom medical or surgical intervention is an absolute requirement.

Physical Examination

The physical examination should take place in a quiet room with the patient relaxed, seated comfortably, and with their eyes closed when tests are administered. Clinical photography is instrumental in mapping the affected areas and recording any trophic changes, or traumatic injuries and any obviously visible pathology. It is good practice to begin the examination with the "normal" side to establish a baseline. Any difference in sensory testing is then graded using Zuniga's clinical Neurosensory Test (NST).[8] If the patient has reduced or no sensation, then levels of function are tested in a stepwise approach (Fig. 4).

Armamentarium

- Cotton swab
- Boley gauge, or college pliers and a millimeter rule or Axotouch (two-point discriminator [AxoGen, Alachua, FL]) (Fig. 5)
- Semmes-Weinstein filaments
- Dental needle
- Ethyl chloride spray

Level A testing (light touch and direction discrimination)

Fibers evaluated: Larger diameter A-alpha and A-beta (5–12 μm diameter).
Method: The cotton fibers are drawn into a wisp, and 10 strokes are applied with the patient being asked to determine the direction of the strokes. Begin on the normal side and then repeat on the altered side. Record how many attempts are correctly identified (9/10 is a normal score).
Two-point discrimination is then performed using an Axotouch two-point discriminator, Boley gauge, or college pliers and millimeter ruler. The patient is asked the smallest distance at which they can discriminate two separate points (normal IAN distribution is 4 mm; normal LN is 3 mm).[8] Compare the normal side with the altered side. Only if there are abnormal results does one proceed to level B testing.
Allodynia (abnormal pain response to a nonnoxious stimulus) is experienced as pain that ceases with the removal of the stimulus.

Level B testing (static and light touch)

- Fibers evaluated: Smaller A-beta fibers (4–8 μm diameter).
- Method: Lightly touch the skin without indentation using the wooden end of a cotton swab. If there is no response increase the pressure until the skin is slightly indented. Start on the normal side and compare with the altered side. Record whether light or heavy pressure is required. More accuracy is obtained by using Semmes-Weinstein filaments in a stepwise fashion, recording which filament is felt when it is deformed (increasing pressure is required to deform the larger filaments). If the sensation is not present even at higher pressures, then proceed to level C testing.
- Hyperpathia (exaggerated response to a potentially noxious stimulus) is present if the patient has delayed-onset pain, or increasing intensity on repeated stimuli.

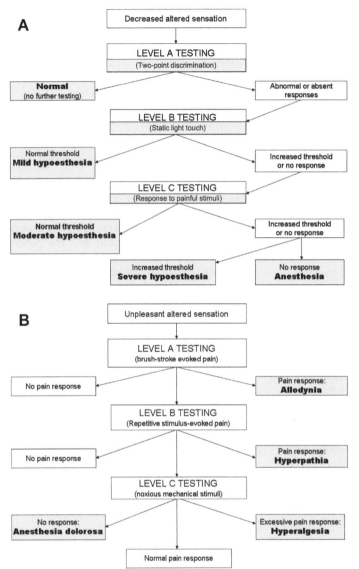

Fig. 4. (*A, B*) NST used to grade trigeminal nerve injury. (*From* Bagheri SC, Meyer R. Microsurgical reconstruction of the trigeminal nerve. Oral Maxillofacial Surg Clin N Am 2013;25(2):289; with permission.)

Level C testing (noxious stimulus)

- Fibers evaluated: Partial myelinated A-delta fibers and nonmyelinated C fibers.
- Method: Lightly touch the skin with a dental needle. If there is no response increase the pressure until light indentation of the skin. The temperature perception of hot and cold stimuli can also be tested with ethyl chloride on a cotton tip or warm gutta-percha.
- Hyperalgesia (abnormally increased sensitivity to pain) is present if the patient has pain out of all proportion in comparison with the normal side.

Diagnostic nerve blocks can be performed at the end of the examination. They are useful in patient who present with constant pain, or dysesthesia. A lack of response to the local anesthetic may indicate a central mechanism to the pain or collateral macrosprouting from adjacent nerves.

No clinical examination, however, is perfect. The NST has been shown to exhibit high positive predictive values (95%) and negative predictive values (100%) for LN injuries and moderate positive predictive values (77%) and negative predictive values (60%) for IAN injuries. This negative predictive value of 60% indicates that the NST may be less efficient at ruling out IAN injury. A

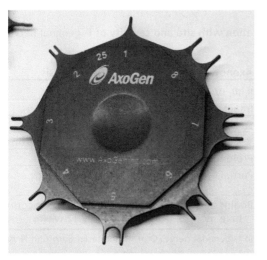

Fig. 5. Axotouch, 2-point discriminator (AxoGen, Alachua, FL). (Copyright© 2020 AxoGen. All rights reserved. Used with AxoGen's permission.)

higher sensory impairment scores, the NST tends to underestimate the degree of nerve injury for IAN and LN. Conversely, at lower sensory impairment scores, the NST tends to minimize the degree of damage.[9] Besides, patients with different degrees of nerve injury may have similar NST scores, and there may be variation with age, duration, and cause of injury. Lastly, there may be added inaccuracy in examinations done less than 1-month postinjury.

Although clinically useful in providing diagnosis and prognosis, as noted by Zuniga and colleagues,[9] the NST has the following shortcomings:

- There may be delays in treatment of higher class injuries that would have benefitted from earlier intervention.
- There may be inaccuracies in delineating the anatomy and exact location of injuries.
- There may be underestimation or overestimation of injuries, especially with variation in patient age, duration of injury, and cause of injury.

The Medical Research Council Scale (MRCS)[10] for sensory recovery is currently the reference standard to identify functional sensory recovery after surgical repair (**Table 1**). The MRCS was originally developed in the United Kingdom to evaluate sensory injuries in the upper extremity, but has since been adapted for use in the head and neck region. The patient is scored according to their NST result with grades from S0 (no sensation) to S4 (normal sensation). S3 is defined as "useful sensory function" and S4 "complete sensory function."

Classification of Nerve Injury Related to Clinical Evaluation and Diagnosis

The date of the nerve injury incident and the progress of symptoms are the features of clinical assessment used in the time-honored Seddon[11] and Sunderland[12] classifications, and the more recent Zuniga and Essick[8] approach to the evaluation of these injuries.

Seddon's classification is more than 75 years old is but is still the most commonly used. He classified nerve damage into three categories:

1. Neuropraxia: Local conduction block with a decrease in conduction; that is, retraction during surgery or postoperative edema.
2. Axonotmesis: The destruction of the axonal conduction and degeneration of the distal segments without disruption of the supporting

Table 1
Medical Research Council Scale for grading sensory function of peripheral nerves as applied to the trigeminal nerve

Grade	Description
S0	No sensation
S1	Deep cutaneous pain in an autonomous zone
S2	Some superficial pain and touch sensation
S2+	Pain and touch sensation with hyperesthesia
S3	Pain and touch sensation without hyperesthesia; static 2-point discrimination >15 mm
S3+	Same as S3 with good stimulus localization and static 2-point discrimination 7–15 mm
S4	Normal sensation

Grades S3, S3+, and S4 are considered functional sensory recovery.
Adapted from Novak CB, Kelly L, Mackinnon SE. Sensory recovery after median nerve grafting. J Hand Surg Am. 1992;17(1):63; with permission.

Table 2
Correlation of Seddon and Sunderland injury classification with site and severity of trigeminal nerve injury

Seddon	Neuropraxia	Axonotmesis	Neurotmesis
Sunderland	I	II, III, IV	V
Nerve sheath	Intact	Intact	Interrupted
Axons	Intact	Some interrupted	All interrupted
Wallerian degeneration	None	Yes, some distal axons	Yes, all distal axons
Conduction failure	Transitory	Prolonged	Permanent
Potential for spontaneous recovery	Complete	Partial	Little or none
Time to spontaneous recovery	Within 4 wk	Begins at 5–12 wk, may take months	None, if not begun by 12 wk

From Bagheri SC, Meyer R. Microsurgical reconstruction of the trigeminal nerve. Oral Maxillofacial Surg Clin N Am 2013;25(2):90; with permission.

structures; that is, a more vigorous localized crushing force.

3 .Neurotmesis: Total interruption of axonal conduction and supporting neural structures.

Sunderland divided these injuries into five types of increasing severity:

1 .Conduction block
2 .Transection of the axon with intact endoneurium
3 .Transection nerve fiber axons and sheath inside intact perineurium
4 .Transection of the fascicles with nerve trunk continuity maintained only by epineural tissues
5 .Transection of the entire nerve trunk

Meyer and Bagheri[10] compared Seddon and Sunderland's classifications of peripheral nerve injuries, concluding that Seddon's classification was most helpful to clinicians in making timely decisions regarding surgical intervention. Jones[13] also found that a neuropraxia often results in a return to sensation within the first 4 weeks, implying an excellent prognosis. Late-onset of the return to function indicates a more severe injury, such as axonotmesis, and no return of sensation within 3 months means neurotmesis is likely. These findings were grouped by Meyer and Bagheri into a table that correlated clinical signs with anatomic injury (**Table 2**).

Magnetic Resonance Neurography

Although they are standards of care at present, the NST and MRCS rely on patient response to stimulus and operator experience and may be inaccurate in distinguishing levels of injury earlier than 1 month postinjury. The shortcomings of the NST were described previously in this article.

Magnetic resonance neurography (MRN) is an imaging technique that increases visualization of peripheral nerves by suppressing the signal from adjacent tissue (primarily fat-containing structures, such as bone and muscle). The nerve signal remains unsuppressed because the nerve contains little fat.[14] Injuries to the trigeminal nerve result in increased signal in T2 sequences at the site of injury.

Furthermore, Zuniga's findings suggest that MRN can distinguish between different degrees of trigeminal neuropathy ranging from compression/entrapment in nontraumatic causations to compression/partial transection/transection and neuroma formation commonly found in traumatic injuries (**Fig. 6**). MRN can also demonstrate the normal IAN and LN anatomy, with a normal to intermediate signal thereby supporting the differential diagnosis of nonneural pain and sensory

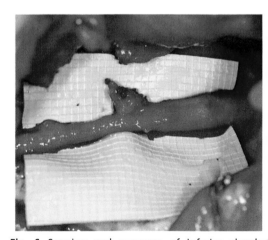

Fig. 6. Scarring and neuroma of inferior alveolar nerve.

disorder conditions. Based on Zuniga's findings it may be possible to correlate clinical findings, nerve injury classification, and surgical findings to a single imaging technique (**Table 3**).

PREVENTION OF INJURY

In some cases, an insult to the trigeminal nerve from surgery cannot be avoided, such as when resection of pathology involves branches of the nerve (see **Fig. 1**). For dentoalveolar procedures, localization of the IAN by panoramic radiologic imaging or cone-beam computed tomography is essential. For all surgeries, the plan formulated should involve the least amount of force, trauma, and development of postoperative edema to be placed on the neurovascular bundle.

Nguyen and colleagues[6] found that in the setting of an oral and maxillofacial surgery unit, with surgery performed by trainees and specialist surgeons, risk factors for permanent IAN injury were identifiable. These included increasing age (≥25 years old), surgery performed by trainees, surgery under general anesthesia, and mesioangular impaction.

Leung and Cheung[15] identified specific risk factors for IAN and LN injury in third molar surgery, as follows:

Inferior alveolar nerve injury
- Unerupted teeth (fully erupted 0.3%, partially erupted 0.7%, unerupted 3%)[15]
- Radiographic signs (Panorex assessment)
  - Diversion of IAN by root (30%)

Table 3
Correlation of MRN with trigeminal nerve injury classification, NST grading, and direct surgical findings

Sunderland Classification	Clinical NST Level and MRCS Level Grade Description	Surgical Findings by Direct Inspection	MRN Finding
I	Normal, S3+ or S4 by 3 mo	Intact with no internal of external fibrosis, normal mobility, and neuroarchitecture	Anatomic, homogenous, mild increased T2W nerve signal
II	Normal, S3+ or S4 by 6 mo	Intact with no internal of external fibrosis, restricted mobility, but neuroarchitecture intact	Anatomic homogenous, increased T2W signal and mild nerve thickening or constriction, perineural fibrosis
III	Mild or moderate injury, S2+, S3 by ≥6 mo	Intact with internal and external fibrosis, restricted mobility, and disturbance of neuroarchitecture (abnormal fascicle patterns and/or Fanconi bands not visible)	Anatomic, homogenous increased T2W signal of nerve and moderate thickening or constriction, perineural fibrosis
IV	Moderate or severe injury, S1, S2, S2+ by ≥6 mo	Partially transected nerve, but some amount of distal nerve present with or without neuroma in continuity	Anatomic, heterogenous T2W signal of nerve and neuroma in continuity, perineural and intraneural fibrosis
V	Severe or complete, S0, S1 by ≥6 mo	Completely transected nerve with or without amputation neuroma	Anatomic, discontinuous nerve with end bulb neuroma

Abbreviation: T2W, T2-weighted.

From Zuniga J, Mistry C, Tikhonov I, et al. Magnetic resonance neurography of traumatic and nontraumatic peripheral trigeminal neuropathies. J Oral Maxillofac Surg. 2018;76(4):727; with permission.

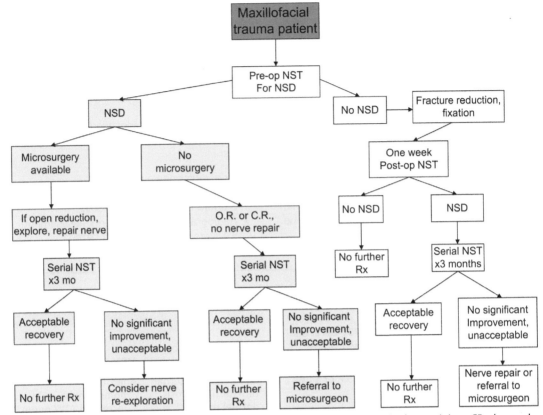

Fig. 7. Surgical decision-making algorithm for the patient with traumatic trigeminal nerve injury. CR, close reduction; NSD, neurosensory reduction; NST, neurosensory testing; OR, open reduction. (*Adapted from* Bagheri SC, Meyer RA, Khan HA, et al. Microsurgical repair of peripheral trigeminal nerve injuries from maxillofacial trauma. J Oral Maxillofac Surg. 2009;67(9):1797; with permission.)

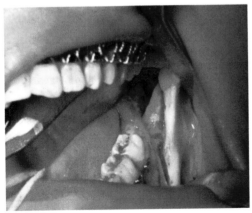

Fig. 8. Sagittal split osteotomy approach to inferior alveolar nerve.

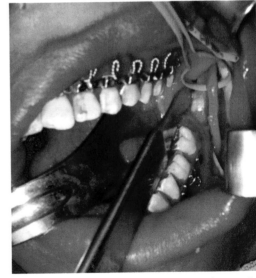

Fig. 9. Inferior alveolar nerve isolation after sagital split ramus osteotomy.

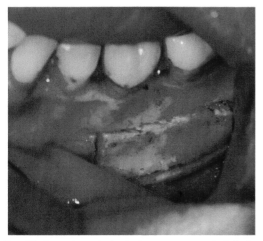

Fig. 10. Buccal cortical window to approach inferior alveolar nerve. Intraoral approach.

- ○ Darkening of the root (11.4%)
- ○ Deflected root (4.6%)
- IAN exposure in surgery (unexposed 1.1%, exposed 16.2%)
- Surgical approach (lingual split 5.7% > buccal approach 2.5% > coronectomy 0%)
- Surgeon experience (specialist 2.9% > trainee 1.3% > undergraduates 0.2%)
  - ○ Which may well represent operations of increasing risk being undertaken by more experienced clinicians

Lingual nerve injury
- Unerupted teeth[15]
- Distoangular impactions (distal impaction 4% > horizontal impaction 2.8% > mesial impaction 2.4% > vertical impaction 1.9%)
- Lingual flap retraction (3.1% vs no flap 3.1%)

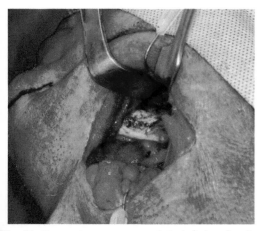

Fig. 11. Transcutaneous approach to inferior alveolar nerve.

- Lingual split approach (lingual split 9.3% > buccal approach 2.3% > coronectomy 0.7%)

Surgeons should be cognizant of the variability of the LN in relation to the area distal to the third molar with the nerve lying at or above the lingual alveolar crest in 10% of patients and in contact with the lingual plate in 25% of cases in the third molar region.[16] Where the IAN or LN is exposed, but not traumatized by the surgical procedure,[17] surgeons should consider protecting the nerve.[18]

MANAGEMENT OF INJURY
Medical Management

In the setting of an acute injury, there is evidence that some benefit is derived from anti-inflammatory medication. This is at present primarily based on experimental studies and the premise that ongoing neuroinflammatory processes can cause ongoing axonal damage.[19] Consideration should thus be given to administering steroids, nonsteroidal anti-inflammatory drugs, or both where there are no other contraindications.

The patient with trigeminal nerve injury may later experience dysesthesia resulting from either local or centrally driven mechanisms. Benoliel and co-workers'[20] review on this subject produced an evidence-based algorithm. Tricyclic antidepressants, serotonin norepinephrine receptor inhibitors (eg, duloxetine), and gabapentin or pregabalin all have a role. Their group found that amitriptyline was the medication of choice but may not be ideal in some patients because of poor tolerance of the side effects. However, these medications unfortunately only yielded benefits in 25% of patients, where 30% or greater symptom improvement was the goal.[21]

Zuniga and Labanc[22] suggested commencing therapy with the anticonvulsants gabapentin or pregabalin or combining these with tricyclic antidepressants/serotonin norepinephrine receptor inhibitors (amitriptyline, nortriptyline, duloxetine) where there is a failure of initial response. In their article, opioids are only considered when all other medical options have failed. We recommend that they only be used in the short term for acute injuries.

Surgical Management

When the nerve injury has occurred as a result of trauma or ablative oncologic surgery, the nerve is often visible and accessible in the surgical field. An immediate repair is ideal in this case where microsurgical expertise is available. Should the surgical necessary knowledge be lacking, or

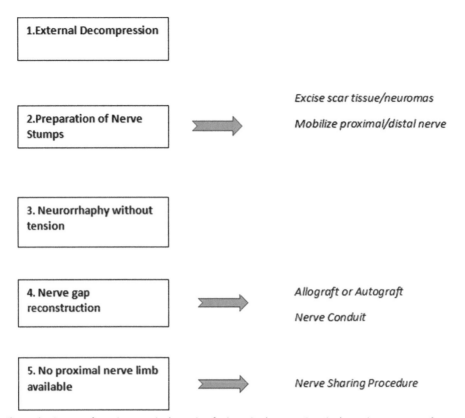

| 1.External Decompression |

| 2.Preparation of Nerve Stumps | → | *Excise scar tissue/neuromas*
Mobilize proximal/distal nerve |

| 3. Neurorrhaphy without tension |

| 4. Nerve gap reconstruction | → | *Allograft or Autograft*
Nerve Conduit |

| 5. No proximal nerve limb available | → | *Nerve Sharing Procedure* |

Fig. 12. Chronologic steps for microsurgical repair of trigeminal nerve. Surgical repair progresses from steps 1 to 3. Steps 4 and 5 are performed where tension-free coaptation is not possible or where there is no proximal nerve limb. (*Adapted from* Bagheri SC, Meyer R. Microsurgical reconstruction of the trigeminal nerve. Oral Maxillofacial Surg Clin N Am. 2013;25(2):292; with permission.)

conditions are unfavorable (a contaminated wound or patient who is medically unfit for further surgery), delayed primary repair within 1 week or secondary repair after granulation tissue has matured (1 month) are options (**Fig. 7**).

An unsuspected or unobserved nerve injury (the most common type in dentoalveolar mechanisms) benefits from surgical repair within 3 months of the insult. The reconstruction is best performed under general anesthetic with the use of an operating microscope.

The infraorbital nerve is approached transcutaneously or transorally. The LN and IAN are exposed transorally, through an sagital split ramus osteotomy for the IAN (**Figs. 8–10**) or through a submandibular skin incision (**Fig. 11**).

Surgical management in microneurosurgical operations is performed in a stepped manner (**Fig. 12**). The nerve's overlying bone, foreign bodies, and surrounding scar tissue are removed. The nerve is then carefully inspected, and neuromas are removed. Where indicated, a small segment of the nerve is removed and the discontinuous

fascicles are either apposed passively in good alignment and sutured within a conduit, or with an interpositional graft. Lack of tension is key for successful direct repair, with nerve stumps held together under tension tending to form scar tissue. In addition, the repair must be protected from the potentially hostile wound bed.

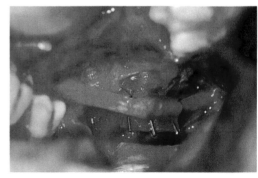

Fig. 13. Nerve protector around lingual nerve repair. Note the 1-mm gap between the proximal and distal segments.

Direct Repair with Suture

- Blood flow may be adversely affected by elongation of as little as 5%.
- Suture pull focuses tension at the coaptation site.
- Focuses localized inflammation from sutures in zone of regeneration.

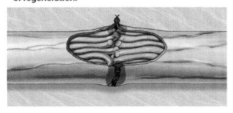

Direct suture repair concentrates suture irritation (shaded area) within critical zone of regeneration.[a]

Repair with AxoGuard Nerve Connector

- Allows some laxity in nerve stumps (up to 5mm gap).
- Alleviates tension at the coaptation site.
- Moves localized inflammation from sutures away from zone of regeneration.

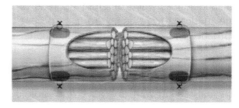

Use of AxoGuard Nerve Connector moves suture irritation (shaded area) away from critical zone of regeneration.[a]

Fig. 14. Comparison of direct repair with suture to repair with Axoguard implant. [a] Epineurium and connective tissue have been removed for illustration purposes. (Copyright© 2020 AxoGen. All rights reserved. Used with AxoGen's permission.)

The conduit and connector-assisted tensionless microsurgical nerve coaptation is associated with less sensory disturbances when compared with direct suture neurorrhaphy.[23] When tensionless repair is not possible the gap must be bridged with autograft, allograft, or conduit (Axoguard, AxoGen).[24] Safa and Buncke's[25] review found that in gaps of less than 6 mm, conduits consistently achieve functional sensory recovery. Processed nerve allograft (eg, Avance, AxoGen) consistently achieves functional sensory recovery in gaps up to 70 mm. These allograft results are similar to autograft, but without the additional donor site morbidity and surgical time.

The current practice is to use conduits for connector-assisted repair and as a nerve wrap around the coaptation site (**Fig. 13**).[23]

The benefits of conduits are as follows:

- Establishing a physical barrier between repaired nerve and physical environment.
- Preventing aberrant axonal growth and escape outside the nerve stumps.

Current research suggests that the conduit will contain the extracellular matrix proteins required for optimal healing at the site of repair, optimizing the microenvironment for healing (**Fig. 14**).

Once surgery has been decided on and the surgical approach decided (transcutaneous vs transoral), the chronologic steps in microsurgical repair of the peripheral nerve are as follows: external decompression (remove any tissue that may be exerting pressure on the nerve), then internal neurolysis (removal of scar tissue or adhesions). The surgeon should then prepare the nerve stumps for repair by mobilizing proximal and distal nerve tissue and excising any scar tissue or neuromas. The nerve is then repaired by coapting the segments without tension. Where there is gap of greater than 3 to 6 mm and/or tension in the closure then a graft should be considered for a nerve gap reconstruction. Finally, when there is proximal nerve limb available, consider a nerve-sharing procedure from a suitable local peripheral nerve (see **Fig. 14**). Postoperatively dexamethasone and vitamin B complex should be used to aid in healing.

SUMMARY

The branches of the trigeminal nerve are never far from the operating field of the oral and maxillofacial surgeon. The surgeon will increasingly be required to provide accurate diagnosis and grading of trigeminal nerve injury, and surgical management by oral and maxillofacial surgeons will increasingly become common.

Although trauma and ablative procedures for head and neck pathology can cause injuries, dentoalveolar surgical procedures remain an important cause of injury to the fifth cranial nerve, with the third division (V3) being the main branch affected. All oral and maxillofacial surgeons should be aware of strategies of avoiding iatrogenic injury, and know when referral and surgical management are appropriate. These injuries may cause significant functional deficits in patients, and litigation is becoming more common.

The advent of new imaging techniques, such as MRN, promises a new paradigm where surgeons can distinguish between different degrees of trigeminal neuropathy ranging from compression/entrapment in nontraumatic causations to compression/partial transection/transection and neuroma formation commonly found in traumatic injuries. The surgeon is increasingly able to correlate clinical testing with operative and radiologic findings.

Performing microneurosurgical repair in a stepped manner is key in producing a successful and predictable repair. The use of allogeneic nerve grafts, conduits, and nerve protectors eliminates the morbidity of autogenous harvest and is associated with less sensory disturbances post nerve repair.

Thanks to the efforts of numerous oral and maxillofacial surgeon and others in the health field, we are on the cusp of not only providing accurate diagnosis and management of these injuries, but providing effective rehabilitation and predictable outcomes.

DISCLOSURE

R. Tursun and A. Kaleem are compensated consultant for Axogen, Inc. P. Amailuk and H. Hatoum have nothing to disclose.

REFERENCES

1. Smith JG, Elias LA, Yilmaz Z, et al. The psychosocial and affective burden of posttraumatic neuropathy following injuries to the trigeminal nerve. J Orofac Pain 2013;27:293–303.

2. Libersa P, Savignat M, Tonnel A. Neurosensory disturbances of the inferior alveolar nerve: a retrospective study of complaints in a 10-year period. J Oral Maxillofac Surg 2007;65(8): 1486–9.

3. Tay AB, Zuniga JR. Clinical characteristics of trigeminal nerve injury referrals to a university centre. Int J Oral Maxillofac Surg 2007;36:922–7.

4. Renton T, Yilmaz Z. Profiling of patients presenting with posttraumatic neuropathy of the trigeminal nerve. J Orofac Pain 2011;25(4):333–44.

5. Ziccardi VB, Zuniga JR. Nerve injuries after third molar removal. Oral Maxillofacial Surg Clin N Am 2007;19(1):105–15, vii.

6. Nguyen E, Grubor D, Chandu A. Risk factors for permanent injury of inferior alveolar and lingual nerve during third molar surgery. J Oral Maxillofac Surg 2014;72:2394–401.

7. M.A. Pogrel nerve damage in dentistry. Current therapy in oral and maxillofacial surgery. Chapter 33,271-274.

8. Zuniga JR, Essick GK. A contemporary approach to the clinical evaluation of trigeminal nerve injuries. Oral Maxillofacial Surg Clin N Am 1992;4 353–67.

9. Zuniga JR, Meyer RA, Gregg JM, et al. The accuracy of clinical neurosensory testing for nerve injury diagnosis. J Oral Maxillofac Surg 1998 56(2).

10. Meyer R, Bagheri S. Microsurgical reconstruction of the trigeminal nerve. Oral Maxillofacial Surg Clin N Am 2013;25:287–302.

11. Seddon HJ. Three types of nerve injury. Brain 1943 6:237–88.

12. Sunderland S. A classification of peripheral nerve injuries producing loss of function. Brain 1951;74 491–516.

13. Jones RHB. Repair of the trigeminal nerve: a review. Aust Dent J 2010;55:112–9.

14. Zuniga J, Mistry C, Tikhonov I, et al. Magnetic resonance neurography of traumatic and nontraumatic peripheral trigeminal neuropathies. J Oral Maxillofac Surg 2018;76:725–36.

15. Leung YY, Cheung LK. Risk factors of neurosensory deficits in lower third molar surgery. A literature review of prospective studies. Int J Oral Maxillofac Surg 2011;40(1).

16. Behnia H, Kheradvar A, Sharokhi M. An anatomic study of the lingual nerve in the third molar region. J Oral Maxillofac Surg 2000;58(6):649–51 [discussion:652-3].

17. Susarla SM, Sidhu HK, Avery LL, et al. Does computed tomographic assessment of inferior alveolar canal cortical integrity predict nerve exposure during third molar surgery? J Oral Maxillofac Surg 2010;68(6):1296–303.

18. Selvi F, Dodson TB, Nattestad A, et al. Factors that are associated with injury to the inferior alveolar nerve in high risk patients after removal of third molars. Br J Oral Maxillofac Surg 2013;51(8) 868–73.

19. Shanti RM, Khan J, Eliav E, et al. Is there a role for a collagen conduit and anti-inflammatory agent in the management of partial peripheral nerve injuries? J Oral Maxillofac Surg 2013 71(6):1119–25.

20. Benoliel R, Kahn J, Eliav E. Peripheral painful traumatic trigeminal neuropathies. Oral Dis 2012;18(4) 317–32.

21. Haviv Y, Zadik Y, Sharav Y, et al. Painful traumatic trigeminal neuropathy: an open study of the

pharmacotherapeutic response to stepped treatment. J Oral Facial Pain H 2014;28(1):52–60.

22. Zuniga JR, Labanc JP. Advances in microsurgical nerve repair. J Oral Maxillofac Surg 1993;51(1 Suppl 1):62–8.

23. Ducic I, Safa B, DeVinney E. Refinements of nerve repair with connector-assisted coaptation. Microsurgery 2017;37:256–63.

24. Zuniga JR. Sensory outcomes after reconstruction of lingual and inferior alveolar nerve discontinuities using processed nerve allograft: a case series. J Oral Maxillofac Surg 2014;73: 734–44.

25. Safa B, Buncke G. Autograft substitutes: conduits and processed nerve allografts. Hand Clin 2016; 32:127–40.

UNITED STATES POSTAL SERVICE ®

Statement of Ownership, Management, and Circulation
(All Periodicals Publications Except Requester Publications)

1. Publication Title	2. Publication Number	3. Filing Date
ORAL & MAXILLOFACIAL SURGERY CLINICS OF NORTH AMERICA	006 – 362	9/18/2020

4. Issue Frequency	5. Number of Issues Published Annually	6. Annual Subscription Price
FEB, MAY, AUG, NOV	4	$401.00

7. Complete Mailing Address of Known Office of Publication (Not printer) (Street, city, county, state, and ZIP+4®)

ELSEVIER INC.
230 Park Avenue, Suite 800
New York, NY 10169

Contact Person
Malathi Samayan

Telephone (Include area code)
91-44-4299-4507

8. Complete Mailing Address of Headquarters or General Business Office of Publisher (Not printer)

ELSEVIER INC.
230 Park Avenue, Suite 800
New York, NY 10169

9. Full Names and Complete Mailing Addresses of Publisher, Editor, and Managing Editor (Do not leave blank)

Publisher (Name and complete mailing address)

DOLORES MELONI, ELSEVIER INC.
1600 JOHN F KENNEDY BLVD. SUITE 1800
PHILADELPHIA, PA 19103-2899

Editor (Name and complete mailing address)

JOHN VASSALLO, ELSEVIER INC.
1600 JOHN F KENNEDY BLVD. SUITE 1800
PHILADELPHIA, PA 19103-2899

Managing Editor (Name and complete mailing address)

PATRICK MANLEY, ELSEVIER INC.
1600 JOHN F KENNEDY BLVD. SUITE 1800
PHILADELPHIA, PA 19103-2899

10. Owner (Do not leave blank. If the publication is owned by a corporation, give the name and address of the corporation immediately followed by the names and addresses of all stockholders owning or holding 1 percent or more of the total amount of stock. If not owned by a corporation, give the names and addresses of the individual owners. If owned by a partnership or other unincorporated firm, give its name and address as well as those of each individual owner. If the publication is published by a nonprofit organization, give its name and address.)

Full Name	Complete Mailing Address
WHOLLY OWNED SUBSIDIARY OF REED/ELSEVIER, US HOLDINGS	1600 JOHN F KENNEDY BLVD. SUITE 1800 PHILADELPHIA, PA 19103-2899

11. Known Bondholders, Mortgagees, and Other Security Holders Owning or Holding 1 Percent or More of Total Amount of Bonds, Mortgages, or Other Securities. If none, check box ▶ ☐ None

Full Name	Complete Mailing Address
N/A	

12. Tax Status (For completion by nonprofit organizations authorized to mail at nonprofit rates) (Check one)
The purpose, function, and nonprofit status of this organization and the exempt status for federal income tax purposes:
☒ Has Not Changed During Preceding 12 Months
☐ Has Changed During Preceding 12 Months (Publisher must submit explanation of change with this statement)

PS Form **3526**, July 2014 *[Page 1 of 4 (see instructions page 4)]* PSN: 7530-01-000-9931 PRIVACY NOTICE: See our privacy policy on www.usps.com.

13. Publication Title	14. Issue Date for Circulation Data Below
ORAL & MAXILLOFACIAL SURGERY CLINICS OF NORTH AMERICA	MAY 2020

15. Extent and Nature of Circulation			Average No. Copies Each Issue During Preceding 12 Months	No. Copies of Single Issue Published Nearest to Filing Date
a. Total Number of Copies (Net press run)			620	546
b. Paid Circulation (By Mail and Outside the Mail)	(1)	Mailed Outside-County Paid Subscriptions Stated on PS Form 3541 (include paid distribution above nominal rate, advertiser's proof copies, and exchange copies)	487	449
	(2)	Mailed In-County Paid Subscriptions Stated on PS Form 3541 (include paid distribution above nominal rate, advertiser's proof copies, and exchange copies)	0	0
	(3)	Paid Distribution Outside the Mails Including Sales Through Dealers and Carriers, Street Vendors, Counter Sales, and Other Paid Distribution Outside USPS®	74	57
	(4)	Paid Distribution by Other Classes of Mail Through the USPS (e.g., First-Class Mail®)	0	0
c. Total Paid Distribution (Sum of 15b (1), (2), (3), and (4))			561	506
d. Free or Nominal Rate Distribution (By Mail and Outside the Mail)	(1)	Free or Nominal Rate Outside-County Copies included on PS Form 3541	43	25
	(2)	Free or Nominal Rate In-County Copies Included on PS Form 3541	0	0
	(3)	Free or Nominal Rate Copies Mailed at Other Classes Through the USPS (e.g., First-Class Mail)	0	0
	(4)	Free or Nominal Rate Distribution Outside the Mail (Carriers or other means)	0	0
e. Total Free or Nominal Rate Distribution (Sum of 15d (1), (2), (3) and (4))			43	25
f. Total Distribution (Sum of 15c and 15e)			604	531
g. Copies not Distributed (See Instructions to Publishers #4 (page #3))			16	15
h. Total (Sum of 15f and g)			620	546
i. Percent Paid (15c divided by 15f times 100)			92.88%	95.29%

* If you are claiming electronic copies, go to line 16 on page 3. If you are not claiming electronic copies, skip to line 17 on page 3.

16. Electronic Copy Circulation	Average No. Copies Each Issue During Preceding 12 Months	No. Copies of Single Issue Published Nearest to Filing Date
a. Paid Electronic Copies	▲	
b. Total Paid Print Copies (Line 15c) + Paid Electronic Copies (Line 16a)	▲	
c. Total Print Distribution (Line 15f) + Paid Electronic Copies (Line 16a)	▲	
d. Percent Paid (Both Print & Electronic Copies) (16b divided by 16c × 100)	▲	

☒ I certify that 50% of all my distributed copies (electronic and print) are paid above a nominal price.

17. Publication of Statement of Ownership

☒ If the publication is a general publication, publication of this statement is required. Will be printed
in the NOVEMBER 2020 issue of this publication. ☐ Publication not required.

18. Signature and Title of Editor, Publisher, Business Manager, or Owner

Malathi Samayan - Distribution Controller

Malathi Samayan

Date 9/18/2020

I certify that all information furnished on this form is true and complete. I understand that anyone who furnishes false or misleading information on this form or who omits material or information requested on the form may be subject to criminal sanctions (including fines and imprisonment) and/or civil sanctions (including civil penalties).

PS Form **3526**, July 2014 (Page 3 of 4) PRIVACY NOTICE: See our privacy policy on www.usps.com

Moving?

Make sure your subscription moves with you!

To notify us of your new address, find your **Clinics Account Number** (located on your mailing label above your name), and contact customer service at:

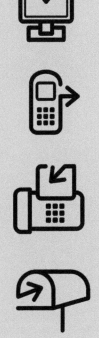

Email: journalscustomerservice-usa@elsevier.com

800-654-2452 (subscribers in the U.S. & Canada)
314-447-8871 (subscribers outside of the U.S. & Canada)

Fax number: 314-447-8029

Elsevier Health Sciences Division
Subscription Customer Service
3251 Riverport Lane
Maryland Heights, MO 63043

ELSEVIER

Printed and bound by CPI Group (UK) Ltd, Croydon, CR0 4YY

03/10/2024

01040306-0020